Nursing Care at the End of Life
Palliative Care for Patients and Families

Nursing Care at the End of Life
Palliative Care for Patients and Families

Joyce V. Zerwekh, RN, EdD
Professor and Director, Nursing Program
Concordia University
Portland, Oregon

 F. A. Davis Company • Philadelphia

F. A. Davis Company
1915 Arch Street
Philadelphia, PA 19103
www.fadavis.com

Printed in the United States of America

Last digit indicates print number: 10 9 8 7 6 5 4 3 2 1

Acquisitions Editor: Joanne DaCunha
Developmental Editor: Kristin L. Kern
Art and Design Manager: Carolyn O'Brien

As new scientific information becomes available through basic and clinical research, recommended treatments and drug therapies undergo changes. The author(s) and publisher have done everything possible to make this book accurate, up to date, and in accord with accepted standards at the time of publication. The author(s), editors, and publisher are not responsible for errors or omissions or for consequences from application of the book, and make no warranty, expressed or implied, in regard to the contents of the book. Any practice described in this book should be applied by the reader in accordance with professional standards of care used in regard to the unique circumstances that may apply in each situation. The reader is advised always to check product information (package inserts) for changes and new information regarding dose and contraindications before administering any drug. Caution is especially urged when using new or infrequently ordered drugs.

Library of Congress Cataloging-in-Publication Data

Zerwekh, Joyce V. (Joyce Valborg)
    Nursing care at the end of life : palliative care for patients and families
        / Joyce V. Zerwekh.
        p. ; cm.
    Includes bibliographical references and index.
    ISBN-13: 978-0-8036-1128-3 (pbk.)
    ISBN-10: 0-8036-1128-5 (pbk.)
    1. Palliative treatment. 2. Nursing. 3. Terminal care—Psychological aspects.
    4. Terminally ill—Family relationships. I. Title.
    [DNLM: 1. Hospice Care. 2. Nursing Care. 3. Palliative Care. 4. Terminally Ill.
    WY 152 Z58n 2006]
    RT87. T45Z47 2006
    616'.029—dc22

2005027123

Dionnetta Hudzinski, RN, MN
Nursing Consultant: Pain and Palliative Care
Instructor, Intercollegiate College of Nursing Yakima Campus
Washington State University
Yakima, Washington

Inge Klimkiewich, RN, MSN, CHPN
Fort Pierce Clinical Director
Hospice of the Treasure Coast
Fort Pierce, Florida

Elaine McIntosh, MBA
President and Chief Executive Officer
Kansas City Hospice
Kansas City, Missouri

Leslie H. Nicoll, RN, MBA, PhD
Editor, *Journal of Hospice and Palliative Nursing*
Hospice and Palliative Nurses Association
Pittsburgh, Pennsylvania

Theris Touhy, RN, ND
Assistant Dean for Undergraduate Program
College of Nursing
Florida Atlantic University
Boca Raton, Florida

Nancy Ann Cook, RN, MN
Professor of Nursing
Oklahoma City Community College
Oklahoma City, Oklahoma

Joan E. Dacher, PhD, RN, GNP
Graduate Program Director
The Sage Graduate School
Department of Nursing and Gerontology
Troy, New York

Linda M. Gorman, APRN, BC, MN, CHPN, OCN
Palliative Care Clinical Nurse Specialist
Cedars Sinai Medical Center
Los Angeles, California

Linda J. Keilman, MSN, APRN, BC
Assistant Professor
Gerontological Nurse Practitioner
Michigan State University
College of Nursing
East Lansing, Michigan

Carole A. Kenner, DNS, RNC, FAAN
Dean and Professor
University of Oklahoma
College of Nursing
Oklahoma City, Oklahoma

Jane Marie Kirschling, RN, DNS
Dean and Professor
University of Southern Maine
College of Nursing and Health Professions
Portland, Maine

Carol Meadows, MNSC, FNP, APN
Instructor
University of Arkansas
Eleanor Mann School of Nursing
Fayetteville, Arkansas

This book has taken shape over my 26 years in hospice nursing practice, leadership, education, and writing. I began teaching nursing in 1969. In 1997 I began practicing in home health and was privileged in 1979 to join three nurse colleagues, a social worker, and a chaplain, comprising the first paid team at Hospice of Seattle. We were one of the first hospice programs in the country and provided home care before the government or insurance companies became involved; that was when the only guidelines for practice were written in England. After that intense experience in developing bedside practice knowledge, writing about what we had learned, and speaking about it, I moved to inpatient hospice care to join a collaborative effort to plan and eventually open Seattle's first inpatient hospice, Hospice Northwest.

These early hospice experiences led me to co-author the 1984 *Hospice and Palliative Nursing Care* with Ann Blues (now Ann Widmer). In 1986, I joined the faculty at the University of Washington to teach in the last months of the Transition Services program, the end-of-life nursing graduate program that had been initiated by pioneering end-of-life nurse scholars Jeanne Benoliel and Ruth McCorkle. I have followed many paths since then, including completing my doctorate, teaching at several universities, and publishing a 1995 qualitative study of hospice nursing practice that proposed the hospice practice model, "The Hospice Family Caregiving Model," described in Chapter 1. This text integrates my many years of teaching nursing with my hospice expertise and deep appreciation for the clinical wisdom of nurses practicing at the bedside. I believe that nurses can make a profound difference in the quality of life at its end. *Nursing Care at the End of Life: Palliative Care for Patients and Families* systematically explores the knowledge base foundational for effective clinical practice.

With that in mind, I have chosen to organize the text into six distinct but integrated units:

- UNIT ONE, End-of-Life Care, examines the ground where the End-of-Life Caregiving Tree is planted. In other words, it looks at the context of caregiving in the United States, the environment in which end-of-life care can either grow or falter.
- UNIT TWO, Sustaining Yourself as a Nurse, explains that the tree must be deeply rooted in a foundation of self-care, in order to sustain caregiving.
- UNIT THREE, Reaching Out and Connecting, comprises the trunk of the tree, which connects the roots (self-care) to the branches that extend out to care for others. Unit Three explores core understanding

of the human experience of patients and develops the skills necessary to build relationships and provide emotional comfort.

- UNIT FOUR, Ethical and Spiritual Practices, examines these dimensions as a main branch of the Caregiving Tree, arising out of the connecting trunk.
- UNIT FIVE, Strengthening the Family, is likewise conceptualized as a main branch of the Caregiving Tree, arising out of the connecting trunk.
- UNIT SIX, Comforting, is symbolized by the leaves on the tree, which represent the extraordinary variety of interventions that provide physical comforting.

Each chapter begins with a Philosophical Reflection and Learning Objectives to focus learning. The chapters end with Concepts in Action, which is a clinical narrative and questions requiring thoughtful application of concepts discussed throughout the chapter. Throughout the text, the reader will find illustrative quotations from expert nurses who were interviewed by the author. Some can be found in my previous publications (Zerwekh, 1993, 1994, & 1995), but many are quotations from the original interviews that have never before been published. Planting the Seeds boxes offer practice-centered advice, and takeaway tips for nurses to use and integrate into their own work. Internet Reference Boxes call the reader's attention to strong information sources available on the Web.

UNIT ONE: End-of-Life Care: Chapters 1 and 2

This unit examines the ground where the Caregiving Tree is planted. Chapter 1 describes the context in which nurses practice at the end of life by identifying common characteristics of dying in America. Then it explores ten competencies of hospice nursing originally identified by the author.

Chapter 2, Hospice and Palliative Care, describes the end-of-life caregiving movements that continue to influence the quality of end-of-life care significantly. Modern-day hospices are programs to care for the dying that combine compassionate care with the finest pain and symptom management. The ideals of the hospice movement emphasize care of body, mind, and spirit, with judicious use of medical technology. Hospice emphasizes speaking the truth about dying and encourages patients to choose how they will spend their last days. Hospice care focuses on the needs of the entire family and fosters living fully until death. Palliative care also focuses on comforting at the end of life. Palliation involves reducing discomfort without curing. The contemporary palliative-care movement expands beyond the way hospice has been organized in the United States to incorporate palliative measures while still offering aggressive life-sustaining measures.

UNIT TWO: Sustaining Yourself as a Nurse: Chapters 3 and 4

Self-care and working with others comprise the roots of the End-of-Life Caregiving Model. The roots of the tree receive nourishment from the soil so that they can provide sustenance to the rest of the tree. Similarly, nurses receive nourishment from self-care and collaboration with other health-care practitioners so that they can nurture and care for patients and their families.

Chapter 3, Strategies to Stay Healthy, asserts that the effectiveness of work with the dying is determined by the nurse's self-awareness and effort to maintain personal well-being. The ability to care for dying individuals is sustained by tending to oneself. We bear up against difficulties because of our strong roots. We must deliberately nourish our body and spirit through healthy nutrition and exercise, as well as other strategies, such as developing a supportive community and finding meaning in transcendent spiritual reality. Only through deliberate self-care are we able to be strong enough, grounded enough, to confront the fear and suffering of patients and families.

Chapter 4, Collaborating with an Interdisciplinary Team, describes working relationships with many other caregivers. Nurses do not work alone. Consider the trees of the forest. On the surface, they appear to stand alone. Under the ground, their roots are intertwined. So it is that our roots are intertwined with those of other team members. The tree is rooted in and upheld by these collaborative relationships. The composition of each team is different. Hospice teams commonly include nurses, social workers, physicians, spiritual counselors, pharmacists, nursing assistants, therapists, and volunteers. Interdisciplinary teams work together to develop shared goals that consider the family and the patient as a whole entity. This requires mutual respect and careful listening to perspectives different from one's own.

UNIT THREE: Reaching Out and Connecting: Chapters 5, 6, 7, and 8

Firmly rooted in the ground, the crown is the neck of the root where it emerges above the ground and becomes the trunk of the tree. Nursing at the end of life involves reaching out to face fear and be in the presence of dying. The trunk of the tree connects the roots to the branches and is the ascending structure from which branches and leaves eventually develop. In the End-of-Life Caregiving Model, the trunk represents Reaching Out and Connecting. Connecting is defined as the process of joining in a relationship with the patient and loved ones. This unit explores the human experience of the dying person and the process of developing an authentic relationship with people who are dying. It also includes an examination of grief and cross-cultural differences because these components affect the human experience and the ability to make connections.

Chapter 5, Understanding the Dying Experience, considers how dying changes living. Connecting with the dying requires a fundamental understanding of the human experience at the end of life. This chapter explores the different types of death awareness. The experience of dying involves profound suffering that is unrelated to physical discomfort as the person faces disintegration of identity and threat to the continued existence of the self.

Nevertheless, many assert that dying can be considered to be a final stage of human development in which both families and patients can find meaningful growth and reconciliation.

Chapter 6, Connecting and Caring Presence, establishes a commitment to caring and compassion and provides concrete recommendations for establishing relationships with people nearing the end of their lives. Connecting involves active deep listening (often to difficult experiences of the dying), speaking the truth, and encouraging patient and family choice. Connecting requires the deliberate practice of caring presence, in which we deliberately focus attention on the other person, letting go of distractions, and being conscious of the other person as a human being.

Chapter 7, Grief and Mourning, explains current understanding of unhealthy and healthy grief. Elisabeth Kubler-Ross described five psychological reactions common to the grief process: denial, anger, depression, bargaining, and acceptance. Initially, these were understood as stages through which a person should proceed in a stepwise process in one direction toward healing. Now these reactions are understood as predictable dimensions of grief through which people move back and forth in a far more unpredictable way. Likewise, our understanding of how to help the grieving person has changed. Freud and other therapists once asserted that a grieving person must directly confront feelings through "grief work" in order to heal. Contemporary research demonstrates, however, that sharing feelings with others does not necessarily reduce the distress or foster readjustment of those grieving loss of a love. This means that nurses should offer active listening to the bereaved and those anticipating bereavement without forcing expression in any way. Grieving individuals should choose the extent to which they want to disclose feelings.

Chapter 8, Cross-Cultural Competency at the End of Life, asserts that we must go beyond the Golden Rule, which mandates that we should care for others as we ourselves would want. Instead, we should care for others as they would want. This requires opening our mind to ways of thinking and behaving that may be difficult to comprehend from our own perspective. Sometimes, cross-cultural competency requires bridging cultural gaps that challenge essential beliefs of the hospice and palliative-care movement. For instance, we believe that there comes a time when aggressive care is futile and causes purposeless suffering. At that point, it is time to focus entirely on comfort. However, African Americans and other minorities who have lived with discrimination in their lives sometimes believe that withdrawal of aggressive interventions is tantamount to neglect and abandonment.

UNIT FOUR: Ethical and Spiritual Practices: Chapters 9 and 10

Ethical and Spiritual Practices branches out from the connecting trunk in the End-of-Life Caregiving Model. One component of every relationship is attention to ethical and spiritual caring. Impending death causes us to confront ultimate moral and spiritual issues.

Chapter 9, Ethical Issues at the End of Life, presents major ethical issues that challenge us as nurses who provide care at the end of life. There may be conflicts around doing good and not doing harm. Individual decision-making is encouraged by the hospice movement, but when individuals lose their capacity for decisions, families can fall into extraordinary conflict over what is good and not harmful for their loved one.

Chapter 10, Spiritual Caring, differentiates between spirituality and religious faith and explains how spiritual understanding is essential to a holistic understanding of the person at the end of life. Spiritual needs at the end of life include hope, meaning, reconciliation, and transcendence. Nursing interventions can foster hope, meaning, and reconciliation in the dying patient, regardless of specific religious belief. The practice of being a healing or caring presence is a vital spiritual intervention that involves authentic listening, staying at the bedside, watching, and simply being there.

UNIT FIVE: Strengthening the Family: Chapters 11 and 12

Strengthening the Family branches outward from the connecting trunk. Caring relationships are integral to strengthening the family. Patients cannot be considered in isolation. They are members of families and have circles of friends. Their dying profoundly affects family functioning, and often the family provides extensive caregiving at the end of life. Families need special help when children are involved, either as survivors or as patients.

Chapter 11, Understanding and Strengthening Families, describes working with American families when a family member is dying to provide emotional support and to strengthen their caregiving ability. The family goes through a major transition that involves redefining the entire family life and struggling with the paradox that the patient is both living and dying. The burden of caregiving is highly stressful as caregivers learn to manage the illness and respond to the suffering of their loved one. Nurses guide families by assisting with the transition and redefinition of family life, and developing the families' capacity to provide physical and emotional care.

Chapter 12, Children Facing Death, describes normal behavior of grieving children at each developmental stage and presents caring strategies for each age group. The chapter also describes essential features of palliative physical and emotional care when the child is the one who is dying. Children often suffer needlessly because of the contemporary compulsion to save life at all costs. Both clinicians and parents have difficulty accepting it when life prolongation no longer makes sense. Likewise, both clinicians and parents may fail to acknowledge the child's suffering; children's pain is notoriously undertreated.

UNIT SIX: Comforting: Chapters 13, 14, 15, 16, and 17

Five chapters comprise this unit on comforting. Providing physical comfort is illustrated as foliage on the End-of-Life Caregiving Tree. The extensive number of leaves illustrates the multiplicity of ways to relieve a person's discomfort.

Chapter 13, Understanding and Anticipating the Course of Terminal Disease, examines the process of end-of-life prognostication and explains the pathophysiology and predictable set of symptoms for the top causes of death. Predicting the course of end-stage disease enables the nurse to antici-pate patient needs, provide anticipatory guidance for patient and family, and prevent crisis instead of waiting for crisis to occur. One important nursing role is to encourage patients to ask questions and speak truthfully about con-cerns. Permission to speak openly about difficult subjects, like pain and fear, is a hallmark of effective nursing at the end of life.

Chapter 14, Comforting and the Essentials of Pain Relief at the End of Life, presents foundational concepts for pain control. The subjectivity of the pain experience leads many clinicians to doubt patients when they report pain. This leads to a significant problem with undertreatment. Nurses must not accept pain as a normal experience that patients must endure as a conse-quence of their illness or surgery. Unfortunately, we risk being in the pres-ence of pain without seeing, hearing, or comforting. Unrelieved pain is known to shorten life, cause hopelessness, and consume the energy of the dying so that they are unable to have any quality of life in their final days.

Chapter 15, Medicating for Pain at the End of Life, provides a founda-tion for understanding analgesic drugs. Selected essential concepts include around-the-clock scheduling of drugs to maintain a stable blood level; use of long-acting preparations to sustain the blood level; oral administration as the first choice of route; careful adjustment and readjustment of drug, dose, and interval; and use of opioids, nonopioids, and adjuvant medication. Fear of opioids remains a major barrier to comforting the dying. When carefully titrated to terminal pain, opioids cause neither addiction nor death from res-piratory depression.

Chapter 16, Management of Physical Nonpain Symptoms, provides detailed guidance to understand medical and nursing interventions to relieve common end-of-life symptoms. As with pain, the foundation of symptom assessment is carefully questioning patients about their symp-toms. End-of-life nurses should continually refocus family and professional caregivers on maintaining comfort for the dying person. The nurse needs to assume a courageous role as patient advocate when physical suffering is ignored.

Chapter 17, Caring in Different Settings When Death Is Imminent, pre-sents the signs and symptoms that are indicators of imminent death and explains their management. At the very end of life, nurses support patients letting go and provide spiritual caring. This chapter describes the challenges of creating a caring environment for life to end in the intensive care unit, nursing home, and home. Death at home requires a trained family that is clear about whether it will call paramedics when breathing and heartbeat slow and stop. Medications must be on hand to manage the common, pre-dictable symptoms that may arise.

I hope you will find *Nursing Care at the End of Life: Palliative Care for the Patient and Family* to be informative and provocative. The intent is to delve below the surface of the most common end-of-life issues. Consider how you may apply the ideas to practice wherever you nurse. As you read, ask yourself the following questions:

What is the quality of nursing at the end of life in your current practice or in clinical practicum settings where you are a student?

What would you like to change in your individual actions? How could you provide greater physical, emotional, and spiritual comfort for your dying patients and their families? What do you need to know and do? Who can help you?

What kinds of organizational changes are necessary for system-wide change to improve nursing at the end of life where you work or where you are a student? What are the barriers, and who can come together to facilitate change?

Remember the famous quotation by Margaret Mead, "Never doubt that a small group of thoughtful, committed citizens can change the world. Indeed, it is the only thing that ever has." That is the way the hospice movement began and so it will be with every program and policy that humanizes end-of-life care.

References

Zerwekh, J. (1993). Transcending life: The practice wisdom of hospice nursing experts. *The American Journal of Hospice and Palliative Care, 10*(5), 26–31.

Zerwekh, J. (1994). The truth-tellers: What you can learn from hospice nurse experts. *American Journal of Nursing, 97*(3), 30–34.

Zerwekh, J. (1995). A hospice family caregiving model for hospice nursing. *The Hospice Journal, 10*(1), 27–44.

CONTENTS

UNIT FOUR

ETHICAL AND SPIRITUAL PRACTICES

UNIT FIVE

STRENGTHENING THE FAMILY

UNIT SIX

COMFORTING

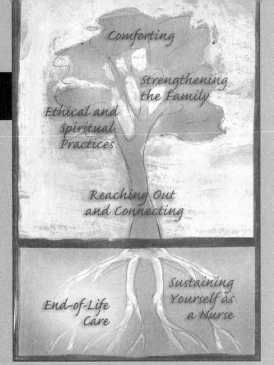

Comforting

Strengthening
the Family

Ethical and
Spiritual
Practices

Reaching Out
and Connecting

End-of-Life
Care

Sustaining
Yourself as
a Nurse

END-OF-LIFE CARE

CHAPTER 1

The End of Life and End-of-Life Caregiving

Philosophical Reflections

"Ivan Ilyich suffered most of all from the lie, the lie, which, for some reason, everyone accepted: that he was not dying but was simply ill, and that if he stayed calm and underwent treatment he could expect good results."

LEO TOLSTOY, *THE DEATH OF IVAN ILYICH*

Learning Objectives

1. Explain how the contemporary circumstances of death in America can result in a dehumanizing experience.
2. Describe how the original Hospice Family Caregiving Model was developed.
3. Describe the 10 original hospice caregiving competencies and give examples of how to implement them in nursing practice.

Nursing practice at the end of life intimately influences the quality of life in patients' final days. When a dying patient requires care, many factors present in American health-care settings come into play—from finances to technology. Nurses can make the difference between a dehumanizing experience for a dying patient and his family, and enable last days that are peaceful and person-centered. And when all is said and done, it is the nurse who is present for the patient and family to ensure comfort and guide them toward closure. This chapter introduces readers to both the realities of dying in America and the ideals of dying in America. It explains the Hospice Family Caregiving Model, which was developed 20 years after the American hospice movement started improving the circumstances of American death. This initial model for hospice nursing was the predecessor to the End-of-Life Caregiving Model used to organize this entire text. Both models visualize end-of-life nursing as a tree. Importantly, this chapter sets the scene for the nursing interventions and ideas that follow in the remainder of the text.

END OF LIFE IN CONTEMPORARY AMERICA

To highlight the unmet needs of dying people, it is important to grasp the context of death and dying in America today. After all, it is within this context that nurses must advocate, comfort, and care for dying patients and their families. This is the ground in which the End-of-Life Caregiving Tree is rooted. Death in contemporary America is characterized by institutionalization, uncertainty, the battle against disease, social isolation, and professional detachment.

Institutionalization

Before the mid 20th century, throughout the developed world, death occurred at home. But since then and currently, most people die in institutions and in the care of strangers. Approximately 75% of deaths occur in hospitals or nursing homes (Hooyman & Kiyak, 2005). There is significant variation between the states, however. Utah and Oregon have the highest number of deaths in the home (Oregon Hospice Organization, 2005). For instance, the 2004 statistics for Oregon reveal that 30% of deaths were in hospitals, 29% in long-term care centers, 34% at home, and 7% in other locations (O'Neill, 2005). Contemporary American hospitals provide acute care only for people with rapidly changing conditions. The hospital focus is on avoiding death at all cost. Dying in the hospital is permitted only if it happens incidental to managing acute pathophysiology. Reflecting this way of thinking, under Medicare, there is no Diagnosis Related Group (DRG) for imminent death or palliative care.

Despite the statistics, most people say they would prefer to die at home (Oregon Hospice Association, 2005); but there are a number of limiting factors:

- Absence of family or friends who can provide care
- Lack of social and economic support for available caregivers
- Preoccupation with medical treatments to sustain life

- Absence of medical and nursing resources and expertise to provide end-of-life care in the home

As dependency needs increase, many dying people simply have no one available in the home who is able to provide their physical care. Many children, spouses, siblings, and friends are unable to give up their jobs to become full-time caregivers. In the case of the very old, potential caregivers may be too frail themselves to become caregivers. Even if potential caregivers exist, their capacity is limited if there is no extended network among friends, family, and the community to support them. Since most life-threatening diseases today are considered to be chronic and treatable, many people end up cared for in hospitals and nursing homes, which are considered to be the only environments capable of providing complex treatments. Whereas in the past, many conditions were considered to be rapidly terminal, today disease courses are longer and prognoses more uncertain, leading to extended stays in institutions.

Uncertainty

Uncertainty and denial pervade end-of-life care. Most Americans do linger and experience a prolonged end of life, living with an uncertain future. Two-thirds of dying people have been chronically ill; diseases are detected early and medical regimens keep them alive for months and years (Moller, 2000). Therefore, prognoses are uncertain. The time to say good-bye is never clear. Physicians, patients, and families have difficulty speaking openly about death. They seek to deny its possibility and focus on potential for life. Uncertainty makes it difficult, if not impossible, for individuals to avail themselves of the hospice benefit, which requires that a physician certify that a patient has 6 months or less to live. Even when the patient is weeks or days from death, contemporary medicine always offers one more intervention. It is hard for fearful patients and families to say, "Enough!"

Fighting Disease

In the beginning of the 21st century, the battle against "evil" death seems to be the primary focus of health care. Physicians are preoccupied with solving the riddle of disease (Nuland, 1994) and conquering death. The more specialized the physician, the greater his or her primary drive and unspoken professional code requiring intervention after intervention to battle disease. Dr. Ira Byock (1997), trained in the battle against death, describes the "jolt" he experienced with his own father's dying. He asserts that the emphasis at the end of life needs to be on the human being and those who love that person, not on a set of medical problems needing to be solved. As a physician, he had been socialized to fight death down to the finish line. Everything possible had to be done to save the patient at all costs:

> Every patient with a pneumonia or fever from bacteria in their blood received intravenous antibiotics. Those who died only did

so after an emergency code was called over the loudspeaker and a team was summoned to perform CPR, invading the body with tubes, compressing the chest hard enough to pump blood manually (and sometimes crack ribs), and applying electrical jolts to try shocking the heart back into a rhythm. I wondered what it was permissible to die from (p. 27).

Contemporary medicine has been accused of suffering under the delusion that we can actually win the battle against disease and death (Callahan, 1999). The costs of such hopes can be seen in the escalating prices of drugs and technological interventions that are stressing the economies of nations around the world. To be sure, many of these drugs and technological advances help to save lives and preserve quality of life for individuals. But on the other side, turning fatal conditions into expensive chronic illnesses strains societal ability to afford care and creates a growing population of sick people. Technological interventions are perceived as the instruments for winning the battle against death. Americans believe that technology can restore our polluted planet, conquer our enemies, and conquer death. Human problems are transformed into technical problems with technical solutions (Moller, 2000).

66 | *Turning fatal conditions into expensive chronic illnesses strains societal ability to afford care and creates a growing population of sick people.*

As a result, maintaining the function of physiological systems becomes a primary function of the nurse, while the patient is in danger of becoming an object in a dehumanized and routine-focused health-care system. The contemporary work of the nurse is to keep all body systems functioning. In the hospital, we give highly toxic drugs to maintain circulation, respiration, and elimination. We expertly monitor gases and pressures and rhythms and rates; we measure the input and output of bodily fluids. We maintain machines and machine connections to the person. In the skilled nursing facility, we must have technological expertise but are also expected to keep up weights and food and fluid intake and to promote mobility and skin integrity until the end of life. When people die, nurses pound on their chests and breathe for them. Death is perceived as defeat. When the perceived battle is lost, patients are often alone.

Social Isolation

Social death involves no longer being acknowledged or seen by other persons (Kastenbaum, 1995). Social death occurs as the seriously ill are progressively isolated from the living. In our action-oriented, beauty-preoccupied society, people who are chronically ill with life-threatening illnesses often experience social death before their actual physical death. These individuals experience little eye contact, minimal communication, and minimal caring. They may be discussed as if they are not there. Such discussion is an unfortunate and difficult-to-extinguish practice that takes place during medical rounds and when several nursing staff work together at the bedside of a patient.

Until very recently in human history, death was an everyday reality that was impossible to deny. It did not occur in isolation. From early childhood, children witnessed the passing of siblings and parents, aunts and uncles, cousins and neighbors. Frequently, grandparents died before grandchildren ever knew them. Usually death came quickly; there were few measures to treat acute infection and injury, and little to prolong life with chronic illness. Caregiving was a family responsibility and the rituals before and after death offered comfort and meaning. Religious and social expectations surrounding death were a common and public part of community life.

Today, most death occurs behind closed doors in institutional settings with professional caregivers. Many people are isolated from supportive communities and estranged from religious and/or spiritual practices. After the ill person enters the health-care system, he or she can expect social isolation. The spiritual and emotional realms are commonly ignored by caregivers whose focus is on solving the puzzles of disease and battling against death. Hospitalization involves removal of clothes and possessions, a work-up, confinement in a narrow uncomfortable bed in a room without privacy, tests, punctures, intubations, and absolute obedience to strangers who often do not identify themselves. There often is no room to speak of anguish in a bureaucratic system that is moving faster and faster to process and discharge patients. The individual feels lost and abandoned when activities focus on the body and disregard spirit and emotion.

In contrast, the hospice and palliative-care movements, described in the next chapter, seek to draw the patient and family into a supportive community that affirms humanity and quality of living at the end of life. Nursing at the end of life must challenge social isolation and reject professional detachment.

Professional Detachment

Exacerbating social isolation and in preparation to fight the war against death, physicians and nurses are socialized by colleagues and mentors to become detached from the humanity of those suffering. Medical students learn to redefine human problems as depersonalized biomedical puzzles. Likewise, the nurses who are role models for nursing students sometimes demonstrate ways to withdraw from patient involvement in order to maintain professional composure. Often the focus is on maintaining routines and completing ordered regimens.

This book invites all nurses to resist these dehumanizing tendencies when caring for the dying. Nurses should practice with appropriate technical expertise, but be aware of the tensions in society and within health care that tend to reduce the dying person to an object for technological intervention rather than a fellow human being. See Box 1-1, Humanization Goals, to identify nursing goals that humanize the dying person and deliberately counter the dehumanizing forces described in this chapter. "The mechanistic view of human beings is the single greatest threat to professional nursing and to practices that seek to uphold human dignity, freedom, and quality of life"

> ## Box 1-1 ■ HUMANIZATION GOALS
>
> - Learn who the dying person is. Listen to his or her story.
> - Honor the dying person's wishes.
> - Question preoccupation with complicated medical interventions that ignores the reality of death approaching.
> - Question inappropriate technology that is burdensome and futile.
> - Create a comforting person-centered environment for caring.
> - Insist on physical, emotional, and spiritual comfort.
> - Refuse to participate in the conspiracy of silence about dying.
> - Prevent isolation and abandonment of the dying. Encourage providers and loved ones to draw near.

(Mitchell, 2001). In the United States, the hospice movement has directly challenged the dehumanizing forces at the end of life. Described in detail in the next chapter, hospice was established in the United States in the 1970s to humanize care of the dying.

THE HOSPICE FAMILY CAREGIVING MODEL

In the mid 1990s, 20 years after the first American hospices opened, the author interviewed 32 home visiting hospice nurse experts who had been recommended by their supervisors as nurses to whom others turned for hospice clinical advice (Zerwekh, 1995). The goal of the study was to capture the essence of hospice nursing practice by clearly describing the competencies of expert hospice nurses. The informants were asked to describe home visits during which they believed they were practicing hospice nursing at its best. Their 95 anecdotes of home visits were analyzed qualitatively to name nursing competencies that were repeated in the stories. The names of the categories were refined by a focus group comprising 10 of the nurses originally interviewed. Ten nursing competencies were identified at that time:

- Sustaining oneself
- Reaching out to meet fear
- Connecting
- Encouraging choice
- Speaking truth
- Strengthening the family
- Caring spiritually
- Guiding letting go
- Comforting
- Collaborating (Zerwekh, 1995)

The tree drawing also emerged from this focus group. The group envisioned an organizing framework that symbolized the relationship among the hospice nursing competencies. An outline did not work to explain the inter-relationships. Geometric diagrams were also rejected. The group sought an organic model to explain their practice, and so a tree began to grow. The tree made the most sense as a metaphor for practice. Nursing at the end of life requires ongoing self-care for the nurse, and likewise the tree needs to be deeply rooted or it will fall over. Caregiving grows through connecting relationships and branches out with various competencies. See Figure 1-1, The Hospice Family Caregiving Model.

Figure 1-1 The Hospice Family Caregiving Model.

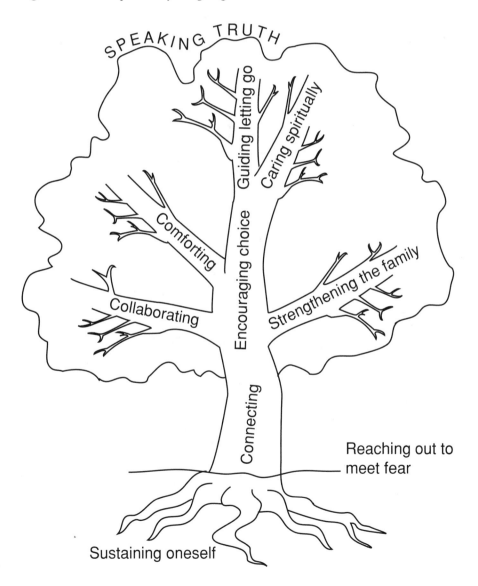

The original hospice nursing competencies are running themes throughout this text. The reader will find them expanded and used to illustrate major points in many chapters. They are described below, beginning with the roots of the tree. Each is illustrated by selections from the nurses' stories. Some of these anecdotal accounts will reappear elsewhere in the text as they vividly illustrate practice concepts.

Sustaining Oneself

The root stabilizes the tree and draws in nourishment. The individual nurse must be strongly rooted in order to provide nursing at the end of life. See Figure 1-2, The Root of Hospice Caregiving. The stories of the interviewed nurses clearly revealed five rootlets involved in sustaining oneself:

- Giving and receiving
- Staying healthy and open
- Grieving
- Letting go of personal agenda
- Replenishing oneself

Giving and receiving is illustrated by nurses who describe learning about living from those who are dying, feeling enriched and energized by the experience of knowing people who are living in their last days. One nurse explained:

Figure 1-2 The Root of Hospice Caregiving.

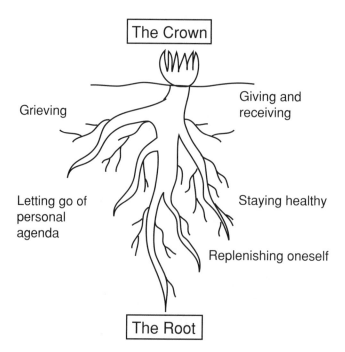

> I feel so honored to be part of these peoples' lives. I feel like they have given me such a gift. They are open to me in a time of their life that is so tender and so painful. It teaches me about being a nurse, being a human being, being respectful.

Staying healthy and open involves the willingness to be involved and sincerely concerned with the welfare of patients and families. Dying people are sensitive to whether someone actually cares about them. Sincere concern requires maintaining one's own emotional health:

> I think we have to be pretty together inside. We have to be emotionally secure. That means we're vulnerable and we have to be willing to risk.

Grieving is an essential dimension of continuing to care for those who are suffering and dying. An expert nurse laments the lack of grieving in her current work environment:

> There has to be a place to express the enormous amount of grief. In my hospice job we could just go into the office and break down and cry together. Now I'm in a highly reserved culture. Everything is nice, nice, nice. God forbid you should be anything but nice. I don't see feeling expressed by the team. I miss crying and soul.

Not everyone needs to cry and talk, but everyone needs to grieve in their own way. One nurse explains her own unique process:

> You have to learn to grieve or you will be eaten up, burned out. For me, I watch sad dog movies.

Letting go of personal agenda is learned through experience in nursing at the end of life. The realities of what can be accomplished realistically lead to the necessity of putting aside one's own goals and aspirations. A nurse explained when she first understood this:

> I will forever be grateful to the night nurse on an oncology unit. I was caring for an AIDS patient and I thought he should accept that he was dying so he could finish his end-of-life business. She educated me that he had to do it in his own way. So I didn't go in with my do-goody intentions. It would have been a bad mistake. That wasn't what he wanted.

Replenishing oneself involves deliberate efforts to renew oneself. This may include sleeping, exercising, praying, music, and being with friends and loved ones. After a particularly difficult encounter with a dying woman just her age, a hospice nurse describes going home:

> I filled the bathtub. I added bubbles and it smelled like roses. I poured a glass of wine. I put on the Beatles and slipped into the warm water. For a while, I lost track of time.

Reaching Out to Meet Fear

The crown is the neck of the root of the tree. The crown is the place where the tree reaches above ground. The hospice nurses spoke about their practice requiring courage to reach out to meet fear. The nurse must confront her or his own fears of death and suffering while calming the patient's fears. There are so many fears that need to be put at rest. For example, one nurse describes calming a terrified patient:

> She was dreadfully afraid of dying gasping for breath, having horrendous air hunger as her last vision on this earth. She even felt that if there were too many people in the room, too much talk, there would be a drop in oxygen level in the room. I was the essence of calm and slow emotions. I let her tell me what she needed. I didn't label her fears as rational or irrational. I wasn't in her body breathing.

Connecting

The trunk of the tree reaches upward and connects the roots to the branches and leaves. In the Caregiving Tree, the process of connecting involves nurses developing a relationship with patient and loved ones before they can truly care for them. An authentic relationship is possible when the nurse is deeply rooted. Connecting includes three dimensions: Being there, hearing and asking, and deliberately building trust. Being there involves the practice of caring presence. As one nurse explained, "The essence of me is sharing with the essence of them beyond the words we're talking about." Hearing and asking involves deep listening to the stories of patient and loved ones. For example, a nurse explains, "I go in and they just need to tell their stories. I try to give them space to tell me where they're coming from." Expert nurses also ask difficult questions such as, "Tell me what exactly is hardest for you right now." These are the kinds of questions that many are afraid to bring up, because the answers are painful to hear.

The third dimension of Connecting is deliberately building trust. A nurse describes building trust in an extremely challenging environment:

> She lived without furniture in her roach infested apartment and she wouldn't talk to me. We just spent a long time together. I knew that she was basically waiting to find out what I would say. Sometimes Black people see White people and are just waiting for the insults, the indirect racism, whatever. God knows we do it! Finally, I told her, 'you know, I might make some mistakes. I want you to be patient with me. I'm here to listen, and to make sure you don't have pain, and I'll do everything I can to keep you at home and to hold your children next to you.' And she started crying and said that's all she wanted.

The nurses deliberately used strategies to ensure that patients saw them as trustworthy. Those included taking time, respecting privacy, making concrete interventions requested by patients, encouraging patients to stay in control, and consistently speaking the truth.

Encouraging Choice

The Family Caregiving Model envisions this competency as a branch growing upward out of the practice of Connecting. In the United States, promoting self-determination is so essential to hospice care that all other competencies extend as limbs from Encouraging Choice in the center. Hospice nurses firmly believe that people should die as they choose. This competency involves believing that people should choose, explaining options, assessing their choices, accepting those choices, and facilitating the patient decision process. One nurse summarized, "We empower them to live and die the way they want to." Sometimes the nurses advocated for choice when the medical or social system resisted. In the process of facilitating patient and family choices, the nurse must sometimes completely let go of her own agenda and respect theirs:

> I had to go along with a lot of compromises about cleanliness and asepsis in the way they did all his bandages and bags and IVs in order to give them control. There was a tremendous amount of technical care in the last couple of weeks. Then he started bleeding, and actually he wanted to be in the tub, she helped him in. There was blood everywhere. The water turned bright red.

Speaking Truth

Truth telling is visualized in the model as encircling the entire top of the tree, illustrating that speaking truth encompasses the entire practice. Choice is made possible only when patients understand the truth about their condition. Hospice nurses are willing to speak openly about terminal illness, the meaning of symptoms, end-of-life processes, and realistic goals that can be achieved with curative and palliative therapies. The hospice nurse is sometimes "the first person they can talk to about the issues that happen." Dimensions of speaking truth include asking difficult questions and saying difficult words, speaking truthfully when the truth is in transition and often uncertain, and facing the normal human tendency to avoid and deny the truth. One nurse describes truth telling at a family conference:

> I began, 'Well you know your mother's got this illness and is not curable and she will die from this. And that's what we're all here about, to try and figure out what your Mom would want.' Then there was silence and a sense of relief. Then one of the daughters started to cry and then they started to ask questions. What does this symptom mean? How can we help her? What about eating? And I explained that their mom could only eat so much. There really isn't anything we can do about that. Let her eat what she wants and if she wants to eat, great, and if not, let her alone. Then I went into the discussion of codes. They decided they didn't want

to resuscitate her. So, it's just the ability to be where people are at, and to just use the words that need to be said.

Strengthening the Family

Hospice care in the home requires caregiving by family, defined as people who are related by blood, marital ties, or personal commitment. Strengthening the family is a branch of the tree that develops out of encouraging choice. The nurses shared extensive anecdotes about their work to strengthen families. Under the Hospice Medicare Benefit, a person cannot receive hospice care unless they have a competent family caregiver. Strengthening the family involved assessment, developing family ability, going between family members to discuss issues they could not face in direct conversation, and recognizing family caregiving limitations. One nurse described family caregiving at the end of life as "shepherding them through confusion." The complexity of this task is illustrated in one nurse's story:

> With this particular family, they were trying to do good, but they didn't even know where to begin. The decline of this lady was very rapid. They were real proud of themselves because they had gotten her home with hospital bed and commode. Very rapidly she had become bedbound. They needed to figure out how to provide her physical care and still continue life as a family. When you go into a house, you not only have to watch the main caregiver and that person's support, but you have to watch the rest of the family and how they are dealing with it. They had a teenager and a 9-year-old, both acting out, and grandma was dying.

Caring Spiritually

Caring spiritually involves recognizing spiritual issues, dialogue about spiritual issues, fostering reconciliation, and sharing near-death experiences. Caring spiritually is a branch on the Caregiving Tree. Recognizing spiritual issues involves acknowledging matters of religious belief as well as struggles with issues such as the meaning and purpose of life, forgiveness of past hurts, and transcendence. Hospice team members believe that unresolved spiritual issues, "unrest in the soul," sometimes cause pain and agitation that is very difficult to relieve. Dialogue about spiritual issues involves deep listening and shared reflection. Nurses ask questions like, "What has life really meant for you?" Fostering reconciliation involves resolving relationships with others and with God. Nurses encourage this period as "a window of opportunity" to heal past estrangements. They also "need to integrate their life with their beliefs and somehow find congruence." A nurse described a dramatic experience with a suicidal patient:

> As he began to process all these things that were coming up from his past, he became extremely upset. He decided that he was

going to kill himself because he was not worthy of living because of some of the things in the past. I got a phone call one Sunday, and instead of going to church, I talked to him for a good hour and a half about why he was so desperate and considering using a gun in front of his wife. The challenge is to be nonjudgmental and allow people to know that they were doing the very best job with the skills they had at that time in their life. If we can be non-judgmental, then they can be less judgmental. After that day, he started work with our chaplain.

Guiding Letting Go

Illustrated as another branch at the top of the Caregiving Tree, the process of helping people let go of the life they have known is unique to end-of-life nursing and was vividly described in the hospice nurse anecdotes. This involves letting go of former activities and hopes, letting go of life, predicting imminent dying, and being present at the moment of death. Guiding a dying person to let go involves listening to emotions and helping the person find resolution as he or she must give up activities, relationships, and life itself. The losses involved are extraordinary and occur over and over again until the moment of death. When patients linger close to death, hospice nurses often look for unresolved issues that prevent patients from relaxing and dying. What business is unfinished? What words remain unspoken? Experience nursing at the end of life often results in nurses being able to predict imminent death. Being present at the time of death elicits memorable nursing experiences. Nurses alert the family that death is imminent, explain the meaning of signs and symptoms, attempt to gather the family, and encourage final good-byes and traditional rituals as chosen. Here is an example from the author's experience with an extended Filipino family:

> The dominating sound, overcoming gunfire coming from the T.V., is the 40-in-a-minute rasping, gurgling breaths from the emaciated shrunken occupant of the bed. I touched this family patriarch tentatively, as family members ranging from toddlers to young adults gathered around the bed. They had placed a Crucifix in his hands. His pupils were fixed, one midpoint and one constricted. His lips were cracked and his tongue covered with brown-red debris. With and without a stethoscope, his lungs were overcome with wheezing and crackles. His heart was regular at 124, but failing to move the blood all the way into the periphery. His feet and legs were icy purple without pulses. Maybe 100 cc of thick dark brown urine sat stagnant in the bag hanging from the side of the bed. Until today, they had been giving him liquids like orange juice, which it sounded like he was unable to swallow, so that it went right into his lungs and led to fits of coughing. He was without any signs of suffering. I reviewed basic care measures with the oldest son, particularly care of his mouth and lips, turning, and how to use morphine under the

tongue if he had any signs of distress with breathing. I talked about hearing being the last sense to be lost before dying. Death appeared imminent, so I urged them to say their good-byes and pray together. Hearing my prediction, the family decided to call the priest.

Comforting

Comforting branches out of Connecting and Encouraging Choice. The interviewed nurses described an extraordinary range of comforting strategies. Comforting at the end of life requires close collaboration with the physician and strengthening the family, the primary caregivers for hospice home care. The nurses interviewed in the early 1990s practiced with a high level of autonomy and flexibility to provide comforting interventions. Their stories identified eight overlapping comforting approaches:

- Providing hands on care
- Anticipating comfort needs
- Trying multiple options
- Balancing pharmacological effects
- Organizing and reorganizing regimens
- Making major changes in regimens
- Initiating nontraditional therapies
- Facing limits

Assertive comforting strategies and a high level of collaboration with physicians are vividly described in the nurses' narratives. Following are two that illustrate the high level of nurse expertise in pain and symptom management to markedly improve end-of-life quality:

She needed to be on TPN because they still hoped she would be getting better and that her fistula would heal. She had a lot of shortness of breath and rales. She had edema from head to toe. Her legs were like planks. They were doing periodic paracentesis for the ascites. It was obvious to me that she was getting too much fluid. So, I called the doctor and we reduced the dextrose and lipids and the total volume she received. She lost 15 pounds in a week and a half, and her lungs cleared.

This man had been on increasing doses of MS Contin and was on sublingual morphine for breakthrough pain and finding no relief from an intractable left shoulder pain that appeared to me to be likely due to bony mets. He also had a nerve component with sharp, shooting pain that went down his fingertips, and at times left him without function of his left side. It incapacitated him completely, left him grumpy and distanced from his family. We started him on Trilisate 750 mg every 12 hours. We use Trilisate as our NSAID for pain because it doesn't affect platelet aggregation. Twenty-four hours after starting the Trilisate, he was having side effects from the morphine: somnolence, constricted pupils, respiratory depression. So we backed off on the morphine and let the Trilisate work. He remained comfortable for several weeks until he started having sharp, shooting pains. We put him on Tegretol, and he started getting out of bed. This man had been in bed for months.

Collaborating

All hospice nursing practice requires collaboration, illustrated as an essential branch on the Caregiving Tree. Hospice teams confer around the table and are constantly conferring with each other in one-to-one conversation in person and by telephone. Collaborative practice with physicians and other providers with prescribing privileges is essential to providing comfort. The nurses had many stories of mutually respectful and cooperative relationships. Most physicians were described as listening and honoring their experience and recommendations. Physicians who were resistant to hearing and honoring nurse expertise presented special challenges. Nurses struggled to approach them in a way that they would listen. One nurse described this challenge:

> Some feel like you're trying to tell them what their business is. You have to be tenacious even when a physician may feel that you're being a pain. You know that there are things that can be tried.

The nurse is usually the first visitor to assess needs in the home, and then she or he brings in other team members that might include social workers, spiritual counselors, nursing assistants, therapists of various kinds, and volunteers. The nurse experts believed that patient and family were better understood and served through an interdisciplinary approach. Frequently, the nurse is challenged to pull in help when there is family or patient resistance. Such resistance is caused by shame at needing any help; denial of progressive dependency needs; and families with boundaries to outside interference, feelings of need to control, and desires for privacy. A nurse describes victory over resistance:

> It took me 3 to 4 months to get her to accept anyone beside me to come in. Finally, the daughter agreed to relinquish her need to be sole caregiver for her mother. We finally were able to bring in a home health aide they trusted. We placed a volunteer who works quite a bit with children to give them all kinds of attention. It was a real victory for me. Not just to get them more help, but because I really like working as a team. Having team input makes you see other aspects of somebody and do a better job of caring for them as whole people.

Transformation of the Hospice Family Caregiving Model

The Hospice Family Caregiving Model was published 10 years before completion of this text. *Nursing at the End of Life* introduces a new drawing and reorganized framework that is more current and tailored to a comprehensive textbook and that more accurately represents end-of-life care today.

CONCEPTS IN ACTION

Jeanne M., age 44, was a divorced single mother of two teenage sons. Over the previous 3 years, Jeanne had lived with advanced ovarian cancer for which she received aggressive chemotherapy. She continued to work as a teacher's aide, using up all her sick leave, until her final hospitalization. Although Jeanne and her mother, a retired registered nurse, both feared that Jeanne was not improving, all conversation with her health professionals had been about therapies and the function of her various body organs. They wanted to stay positive, so there had been no conversations about code stats or a living will. She expressed no wishes about the future of her sons and had not spoken to them about her possible death. Although a practicing Catholic, she had not requested the Sacrament of the Sick (last rites) and no one had suggested it.

Then she became acutely ill and was admitted to the medical intensive care unit with renal failure and acute respiratory distress. In the ICU, she was immediately placed on a ventilator and dialyzed. Her blood pressure dropped and blood appeared in her Foley catheter. Sepsis with disseminated intravascular clotting was likely. Throughout her final evening, Jeanne was agitated and confused, complaining of severe pain throughout her tumor-distended abdomen and extending into her right hip. She had received meperidine (Demerol) 50 mg IM twice in the previous 24 hours. Her mother and sister had been allowed to visit for no more than 10 minutes at a time, until encouraged to "go home and get some rest." They were assured that her lab values were improving. Jeanne arrested. A full code failed at 10:03 PM, 23 hours after admission.

1. How would you characterize Jeanne's last day of life?
2. How did prognostic uncertainty affect how she died?
3. How did social isolation and professional detachment affect the way her care was managed both before her acute episode and during it?
4. What more might have been done to care for Jeanne and her family during her treatment for aggressive ovarian cancer? Consider the Humanization Goals in Box 1-1.
5. In Jeanne's case, technological interventions were appropriate with significant probability of reversing her condition. Nevertheless, explain how her care could have been humanized in the ICU.
6. Imagine an alternative ending with Jeanne discharged home, stable but close to death. Following a hospice referral, apply the 10 competencies to propose hospice nursing interventions for Jeanne and her family.

References

Byock, I. (1997). *Dying well: peace and possibilities at the end of life.* New York: Riverhead Books.

Callahan, D. (1999). *False hopes: overcoming the obstacles to a sustainable, affordable medicine.* New Brunswick, NJ: Rutgers University Press.

Hooyman, N., & Kiyak, H. (2005). *Social gerontology* (7th ed.). Boston: Pearson.

Kastenbaum, R. J. (1995). *Death, society, and human experience.* Boston: Allyn & Bacon.

Mitchell, G. (2001). Pictures of paradox: Technology, nursing, and human science. In R. Locsin (Ed.), *Advancing technology, caring, and nursing.* Westport, CT: Auburn House.

Moller, D. W. (2000). *Life's end: Technocratic dying in an age of spiritual yearning.* Amityville, NY: Baywood Publishing.

Nuland, S. B. (1994). *How we die: Reflections on life's final chapter.* New York: Alfred A. Knopf.

O'Neill, P. (10 April, 2005). Same fate, different ways. *The Oregonian,* pp. B1–B2.

Oregon Hospice Association. (2005). Hospice FAQ. Retrieved from www.oregonhospice.org.

Zerwekh, J. (1995). A hospice family caregiving model. *The Hospice Journal, 10,* 27–44.

CHAPTER 2

Hospice and Palliative Care

ELAINE MCINTOSH AND JOYCE ZERWEKH

Philosophical Reflections

"She was calm, she seemed ready. Her affairs were in order. She was respected and loved. In short, Mrs. Davis was having an excellent death. A week later, when she had actually died, I felt this all the more because she had left, in me, the indelible knowledge that such a death is possible. For myself, for all of us, I want a death like Mrs. Davis'. When we will ripen and ripen further, richly as fruit, and then fall slowly into the caring arms of our friends and other people we know."

ALICE WALKER

Learning Objectives

1. Identify the social forces that led to the hospice movement.
2. Contrast the ideals of the hospice movement with the philosophy of patient care that continues to dominate American health care.
3. Explain the uniqueness of St. Christopher's Hospice and the contributions of Cicely Saunders.
4. Describe key features of American hospices and requirements of the Hospice Medicare Benefit.
5. Explain the effects of hospice on individual patient experiences.
6. Explain the reasons for the palliative-care movement.
7. Explain the advantages of a hospital developing a palliative care program.
8. Articulate values and practices within contemporary health care that are contrary to palliative goals.
9. Be able to explain hospice services to dying patients and their families.

This chapter provides a foundation for understanding hospice and palliative care, which are organized to provide quality end-of-life care. The hospice and palliative-care movements have provided the groundwork that sustains practice illustrated by the End-of-Life Caregiving Model. *Hospices* are programs that comfort and care for the dying. *Palliative care* is defined as comforting and person-centered measures for those with advanced, life-threatening illness. *Palliative-care programs* are expanding the number of people who can receive palliative care beyond those receiving care in hospices, which have narrow eligibility requirements for patients to be admitted. This chapter examines the hospice movement, including its development in England and in the United States. The Medicare hospice requirements are presented and contemporary trends and limitations explored. The chapter continues with a description of the palliative-care movement in the United States and reasons for resistance to the integration of palliative goals into mainstream medicine.

THE HOSPICE MOVEMENT

Into the last quarter of the 20th century, as pharmacological and technological treatment of the diseased body became more and more successful, attention to the mind and spirit was sidelined. When treatment failed to extend life, the humanity of the dying person was often forgotten in the maze of aggressive treatment regimens. The end result was often a helpless dehumanized person, penetrated by many tubes and lines. Families were restrained, allowed only limited visiting, lest they interfere with increasingly futile interventions. Death was not discussed; the subject was forbidden. Death meant failure. Medical decisions were paternalistic, based on the physician's desire to offer the most aggressive life-prolonging care available. The voices of the patient and family were seldom heard.

But with consumerism on the rise in health care, patients began to take more of a role in steering the course of their care. Patients and their loved ones began to question whether yet another round of chemotherapy was worth the suffering it would cause. Medical ethics began to strongly emphasize patients' autonomy and rights to make their own health-care decisions. Some outspoken physicians began to recognize that just because a medical technology or treatment exists, does not necessarily mean that it should be used. Some outspoken nurses began to recognize that death is a natural part of life, and that there comes a time when the most appropriate goals for the patient are:

- Comfort
- Quality of life
- Reconciliation of conflicts with loved ones
- Making a time of final illness also a time of peace

It was in this environment that the hospice movement developed. It grew out of four societal mandates for change that became prominent in the 1970s. The mandates asserted that:

1. Terminally ill persons should have access to appropriate care that attended to body, mind, and spirit.
2. Death should not be a taboo subject.
3. Medical technology needed to be applied more judiciously.
4. Patients had the right to be more involved in their own treatment decisions.

In addressing these public concerns, hospice took a more holistic view of health and health care, recognizing the need to care for the entire person: body, mind, and spirit. The overriding principle behind hospice was the notion that patients needed and deserved an alternative to an aggressive, cure-oriented, hospital-based system of care that generally failed to address the real issues of concern to the dying.

> *The overriding principle behind hospice was the notion that patients needed and deserved an alternative to an aggressive, cure-oriented, hospital-based system of care that generally failed to address the real issues of concern to the dying.*

The early developers of hospice, often nurses, were highly idealistic and passionate in their drive to create a better way to care for the dying. Reacting to the "cure at any cost" syndrome, which characterized most of medicine, health-care professionals and lay people alike began to realize that people with terminal illnesses were often denied the truth of their situations and given aggressive treatments well beyond when there was hope of cure or remission. Sometimes they were forced to endure pain and suffering as pain-relieving medications were withheld due to the lack of knowledge of physicians, fears of addiction, and a general lack of priority on keeping the patient comfortable. When all possible treatments aimed at curing the disease had been exhausted, often it was said, "There is nothing more that can be done." Hospice challenged that idea with another way of talking. For example, a hospice representative might say to the patient, "Although we may not be able to cure your disease, there is a great deal we can do for you. We can keep you comfortable, help you achieve quality of life for however much time remains, help your family, pray with you, and stay with you until the end."

The hospice movement has been compared with the childbirth education movement, which emerged in the 1960s. Until that time, fathers were barred from delivery rooms, mothers were often heavily anesthetized, and patients received little education about what to expect. Now, most women have the opportunity to attend childbirth education classes and have the "coach" of their choosing with them in the delivery room. Women have choices about what type and amount of pain-relieving efforts they want during labor and delivery, unlike the days when the physician made every decision. Hospice parallels the values expressed in the childbirth movement: inclusion of family, encouraging the patient to be in control of decisions, appropriate comfort measures, compassion and support during an important and difficult time.

> 〝 *Hospice parallels the values expressed in the childbirth movement: inclusion of family, encouraging the patient to be in control of decisions, appropriate comfort measures, compassion and support during an important and difficult time.*

England to North America

Hospice is derived from the Latin words *hospes,* meaning both host and guest, and *hospitium,* referring to an inn or a place of refuge for travelers. Hospices began in medieval Europe as refuges for the sick and dying. The founders of the early hospices in America first looked to England where a new model of care for the dying had already been developed. In 1967, a British physician, Cicely Saunders, founded St. Christopher's Hospice. Dr. Saunders expanded her professional credentials from nurse to social worker to physician (Stoddard, 1978). As a social worker, she was moved by witnessing a young man named David struggle with terminal cancer. Having talked openly about his dying, they discussed the need for a place better suited to caring for terminal patients than a hospital ward. At his death, he left her a gift of 500 English pounds. He had told her, "I will be a window in your home." Although it took her 19 years, she opened St. Christopher's Hospice in Sydenham, England, and credits this young man, David Tasma, as her source of inspiration (Saunders, 1976). As Americans began to study the needs of the dying, many made the pilgrimage to study with Dr. Saunders in England. The early hospice literature is filled with moving accounts of what they found at St. Christopher's.

Thelma Ingles, former chair of the graduate program at Duke University School of Nursing, traveled to St. Christopher's to work as a staff nurse and study the care. She told the story of a man who worked there. "I remember the gentle kindness of the man who delivered the morning paper to the patients. He knew each patient by name, always had a few pleasant words to say, and was ready to make an extra effort to fulfill any unexpected request. One morning I said to him, 'Do you know how much the patients love you?' He looked at me quietly for a moment and then said, 'St. Christopher's does this to you, you know. Here there is always room for love' " (Hamilton & Reid, 1980, p. 48). Cicely Saunders' affirmation of the dignity of each dying person is expressed in her famous quote, "You matter because you are you. You matter to the last moment of life, and we will do all we can, not only to help you die peacefully, but also to live until you die" (Stoddard, 1978, p. 91).

> 〝 *You matter because you are you. You matter to the last moment of life, and we will do all we can, not only to help you die peacefully, but also to live until you die. (Saunders in Stoddard, 1978, p. 91)*

In addition to the patient-oriented, loving kindness found at St. Christopher's, sophisticated medical care aimed at ensuring patient comfort was given the highest priority. A striking feature of St. Christopher's was the demonstration that oral opioids administered around the clock were highly effective to control pain. Previously, it had been assumed that only injections would control pain, and that they had to be administered sparingly, only when the patient's complaint became severe.

English hospice was within the walls of inpatient facilities, designed and built specifically to service the hospice population. When the Americans began to seriously develop hospices, home care emerged as the primary setting in which to deliver hospice care.

In North America, two individuals pioneered the development of specialized programs to care for the dying (Stoddard, 1978). Dr. Balfour Mount founded the Palliative-Care Program at the Royal Victoria Hospital in Montreal, Canada. Dr. Mount inspired many American physicians who sought a philosophy of medicine that recognized that death is natural and dying needs excellent medical management. Florence Wald was Dean of the Yale School of Nursing and the founder of the first American hospice in Branford, Connecticut.

The American Translation—Focus on Home Care

In the United States, concerns about escalating health-care costs were already well established at the beginnings of the hospice movement in the 1970s. Growing emphasis was being placed on saving money by shortening hospital stays and keeping patients at home. This meant that finding funds to build more inpatient beds in order to provide hospice care was unlikely. Therefore, the American hospice developers focused on providing hospice care in the patient's home.

The American version of hospice emerged with certain characteristics: emphasis on home care, control of symptoms, emotional and spiritual counseling for patient and family, bereavement support, volunteers providing important services, and programs to support team members. See Box 2-1, Common Characteristics of American Hospices.

An interdisciplinary team delivers the care. The hospice team consists of nurses, social workers, chaplains, a medical director, home health aides, and volunteers. Other services often include dietary counseling, physical therapy, and occupational therapy. Art or music therapy, massage, therapeutic touch, or other complementary therapies have sometimes been added. Some hospice programs have developed as separate health-care organizations, but most are now services provided by hospitals or home health-care agencies.

The Medicare Model

In the early days of the American hospice movement, there was a philosophy and program of care, but there was no consistent funding. It came to pass

---

Box 2-1 ■   COMMON CHARACTERISTICS OF AMERICAN HOSPICES

- Coordinated home care, with inpatient care being provided if needed under the direction of the hospice
- Emphasis on control of pain and other symptoms
- Provision of emotional support and counseling
- Availability of spiritual care
- Recognition that the entire family constitutes the unit of care
- Bereavement support after the patient's death
- Active role for volunteers
- Programs to support staff and address burnout

---

that hospice care could not be made available to broad numbers of people without Medicare and private insurance coverage. Because hospice held the promise of saving money by keeping people at home rather than in hospitals, in 1982, Congress created a hospice benefit in the Medicare program (Public Law 97-248, 1982). (See Box 2-2.)

Congress feared that the hospice program might cost far more than originally envisioned. In turn, certain provisions were built into the program to restrain its costs and to ensure that the emphasis in hospice continued to be on home care. These requirements include the following (Marrelli, 1999):

- The patient has a prognosis of 6 months or less.
- Hospice care is to be "palliative" or comfort-oriented, rather than curative.

Box 2-2 ■   SERVICES COVERED UNDER THE MEDICARE HOSPICE BENEFIT CARE BY NURSE AND PHYSICIAN

- Home health aide and homemaker
- Occupational, physical, and speech therapy
- Counseling and social work
- Chaplain
- Volunteer help to visit, shop, transport, do chores
- Medical equipment and supplies
- Medication to relieve symptoms
- Inpatient respite care to relieve caregivers

Source: From Scala-Foley, Caruso, Archer, and Reinhard (2004).

- The payment is a flat rate paid to hospice for each day the patient is in the program, regardless of the cost of care. This is a departure from the previous method of payment, which was based on actual cost.
- The patient "elects" or signs up for the hospice benefit and in so doing waives regular Medicare benefits. That is, the patient exchanges the benefits received from the normal Medicare program in order to receive the benefits from the hospice Medicare program.
- Care across all settings is coordinated and arranged by the hospice. This makes the hospice team both the clinical case manager and the financial case manager.
- Four levels of care have been created: 1. Routine home care; 2. Continuous home care when the patient's condition is acute and death is imminent; 3. Inpatient care (usually in a hospital) for acute symptom relief; 4. Respite care (usually in a nursing home) to relieve family caregivers.
- No more than 20% of the days of care can be in either of the two institutional levels of care.
- There must be 24-hour/7-day-a-week availability of hospice staff for consultation or emergency visits. Previous to hospice, it was rare that anyone other than the attending physician "took call." When hospice came along, nurses began to respond to the patient's emergency needs in the middle of the night.

Congress also recognized that in order for hospice to work, patients had to have access to medications, supplies, and services that would allow them to remain at home. Therefore, for the first time, coverage for prescription drugs for routine ongoing use at home was included in the Medicare payment for hospice.

Internet Reference Box

See the Web site for the National Hospice and Palliative Care Organization at *www.nhpco.org*. Hospice Net at *www.hospicenet.org* is designed to be a resource for patients and families. The Medicare Hospice Benefit is clearly outlined at this site.

The Role of the Nurse in Hospice

Although the interdisciplinary group comprises the care team, the nurse's role on the team is central. The nurse is the case manager and usually visits the patient more frequently than other team members, often two to three times a week, whereas the other team members might visit once every week or every other week. Patients come to know and depend on their nurse as their guide, teacher, comforter, communicator, and liaison to the physician.

Nurses guide the symptom management and work closely with the patient's personal physician to ensure the patient's comfort. One nurse explains her role in controlling symptoms for patients at home:

> My understanding of pathophysiology and pharmaceuticals makes me more confident during home visits. You always have to consider options in keeping ahead of symptoms. If one combination of medications doesn't work, try organizing pills in a different way or time. Maybe we need a different drug or a different dose. Maybe we should try complementary therapies. I feel like I'm making a little custom-made suit every time I go on a visit. I tailor the plan to where they're at with physical and psychological comfort. The doctors trust my recommendations.

❝ | *I'm making a little custom-made suit every time I go on a visit.*

Hospice practice presents remarkable opportunity for nurses. It is perhaps the most independent practice role available, short of a nurse practitioner, and offers the opportunity—actually the requirement—that the nurse treat the patient as a complex being, with physical, spiritual, and emotional dimensions. The expert hospice nurse makes comprehensive assessments and is deeply knowledgeable about pain and symptom management, including the pharmacology, side effects, and efficacy of sophisticated medications and treatments. She is also very strong in psychosocial nursing skills. The course of care for the patient is largely determined by the nurses' intervention. The well-managed hospice case is uneventful and proceeds without trips to the hospital or emergency room, largely because each crisis or change has been anticipated. It is the nurse who makes this smooth final course of illness possible. See Box 2-3, Speechless in Seattle, to consider the author's story of easing the final course of illness during an initial home visit.

❝ | *The well-managed hospice case is uneventful and proceeds without trips to the hospital or emergency room, largely because each crisis or change has been anticipated. It is the nurse who makes this smooth course of illness possible.*

Planting the Seeds

WHAT TO LOOK FOR WHEN REFERRING TO HOSPICE

- Is the medical director certified in hospice and palliative medicine?
- Medical oversight should be undertaken by physicians with symptom management expertise.
- Is there leadership by a nurse who is certified in hospice and palliative nursing?

Box 2-3 ■	**SPEECHLESS IN SEATTLE: FIRST HOME HOSPICE VISIT**

The hospice nurse secured her bag over her shoulder and inched along the ramp that sloped down to the tiny weathered houseboat. A stoop-shouldered man with red eyes and a red nose greeted her and pulled her into a smoky bedroom. He was Earl, the patient's husband. His wife was a new referral to hospice for an expanding brain tumor. His words tumbled out of his mouth, "Yesterday she was fine. Today she's choking on water. She won't talk to me. She can't stand up. What can I do? What does it mean? It's a nightmare." The nurse investigated further to learn that Marge had eaten Swiss steak and peas the evening beforehand and was able to walk to the kitchen table. She had been able to speak in brief sentences and could follow instructions. The nurse examined her head-to-toe to identify a flat expression, moon face, no ability to follow instructions, evidence of urinary incontinence, cyanosis, mottling in her lower legs, BP 76/30, and periods of 30 second apnea.

Nursing interventions included calling the physician to report her terminal status and ask him to consider prescribing an increased dose of dexamethasone that might reduce the swelling around the tumor. He had a long-standing collaborative relationship with the nurse, and agreed to increase the dose in hopes of achieving temporary improvement. The nurse sat down at the kitchen table with Marge's sister, her son, and Earl to discuss the disease course, possible reasons for Marge's deterioration, and what to expect. They concocted a thick frozen yogurt shake that she was able to swallow. This meant that the dexamethasone, analgesics, anti-convulsants, and laxatives could be administered by this route until she stopped swallowing. The family returned to the bedroom to learn how to care for an incontinent bedridden patient. The nurse ordered a hospital bed and diapers from a medical supply house. The signs of imminent death were reviewed with Earl, and the nurse gave him the hospice on-call nurse number. Before she could leave, the nurse facilitated an emotional 20-minute family discussion of whether or not they would call 911 if she stopped breathing. They all agreed that they would call the hospice instead of the paramedics. They agreed to a visit from the hospice chaplain and considered beginning 24-hour continuous care because death was imminent.

- Does the hospice have a staff person whose job is to evaluate and ensure quality of care?
- What kind of bereavement program is offered? Is the service provided by qualified staff who are not volunteers?
- What is the staffing ratio of nurses to patients? One home visiting RN to every 10 patients indicates quality.

• Is the hospice for-profit or not-for-profit? The not-for-profit health-care organization focuses on its mission. The for-profit hospice must make money to compensate owners or shareholders. Both can provide good care.

Growth and Changes in Hospice over Time

Who receives hospice, for how long, and from what type of organization has changed considerably since hospice's inception. Initially, nearly all hospice patients had cancer because its terminal phase was predictable. Eventually, patients with other diagnoses began to be admitted, including those with end-stage cardiac and respiratory illness; neurological diseases, especially ALS; kidney or liver disease; Alzheimer's dementia; and general debility of the frail elderly who are dying of multiple causes. Originally, nearly all patients were cared for in their private homes. In the mid 1980s, Medicare allowed hospice to admit patients who were residents of nursing homes. After initially limiting payment for hospice care to a maximum of 210 days, in 1990, Congress authorized payment for care for an unlimited length of time, as long as the patient meets certain clinical criteria (Omnibus Budget Reconciliation, 1990). The average length of stay in hospice has shortened. With uncertainty surrounding the lifespan of individuals with diseases that were once rapid death sentences, referrals are made very late in the disease process. For instance, AIDS used to be a rapid death sentence and now it is a chronic life-limiting disease.

As time has passed and hospices have become more a part of the mainstream of health care, they have been subject to some of the same challenges other types of health-care providers experience, as well as some that are unique to hospice. These obstacles include abuse by some unscrupulous organizations, financial pressures, competition, and labor shortages. Death denial in American culture continues to plague the hospice movement so that patients and their providers limit discussion about end-of-life issues, patients are referred too late or not at all, and their symptoms too often are not relieved until hospice admission. The median length of hospice stay before death is 15 days (Later Referrals, 2004) with many patients receiving hospice care for only 2 or 3 days before death. Short hospice stays limit the possibility of making a difference at the end of life.

From Charity to Business

Hospices began as highly idealistic, not-for-profit organizations, largely supported by grants and donations. For the first 15 years of their development, hospices were almost exclusively nonprofit. However, once reimbursement from Medicare and other insurers was firmly established and the patient population expanded to include residents of nursing homes, profit-driven organizations have been eager to establish themselves as hospices. Medicare payment for hospice is highly reliable, so that profits can be abundant. In many communities today, there is incendiary competition for the hospice "market share." Unless restricted by state law, almost anyone can open a hospice with very little investment or necessarily any expertise. The proliferation of hospice organizations has resulted in uneven quality, and, in some communities, considerable confusion about what the consumer can expect from a hospice. To understand the impact of quality hospice care, let's turn to the experience of one patient.

Mrs. Albert was 78 years old. After 35 years of marriage, she went through a very painful divorce and returned to the city of her birth to live alone, but close to her two adult children. About 1 year after her move, she was found to have metastatic lung cancer with seizures caused by brain metastases. She received radiation and chemotherapy, which achieved a period of stability. After a few months, seizure activity resumed, pain became a problem, and she chose not to undergo a new course of chemotherapy because of her rapid decline.

During a brief hospitalization brought on by a respiratory crisis, her oncologist talked with her and her children, told them that further treatment was unlikely to help, and said that it was a good time to start hospice care. The family agreed, so the physician made a referral to the community hospice. During the initial visit, the hospice nurse identified the history and general physical needs of the patient and the practical aspects of her living situation. She observed the son had some distress and anger directed at the physicians and hospital, and that the daughter was not confident in her ability to provide the needed care, given her job and responsibility for her own teenage children. The nurse also observed Mrs. Albert's pattern of appeasing her son and trying to go along with his wishes, and that communication between the son and daughter was limited and somewhat stilted. This initial assessment provided information upon which to begin the plan of care. The nurse ordered medications, oxygen, a hospital bed, and wheelchair, all to be in the home at the time of the patient's arrival.

The plan of care for this family included the following elements:

- Teaching regarding the disease course and comforting care
- Maintaining the patient's comfort and independence as long as possible
- Providing support and opportunity for the son to address his emotional distress
- Developing emotional and practical support for the daughter to permit her to meet family and job obligations
- Developing a caregiving system to allow Mrs. Albert to remain at home if at all possible, or, if not, to ensure a smooth transfer elsewhere
- Assisting with family communications through the course of care

Over the subsequent 4 weeks, hospice nurses, aides, social workers, and a pastoral counselor all became involved with the family. The patient's primary symptoms were pain and shortness of breath. After a period of adjusting drug dosages, she felt comfortable with a long-acting opioid and doses of short-acting medication for events when the pain broke through. She also needed medications for sleeping and anxiety, which the hospice nurse suggested to the attending physician who was familiar with hospice and with ordering whatever was needed for symptom management. In her last 2 weeks, she became almost entirely bed-bound, and the family chose to supplement their own caregiving with privately hired nurses' aides. The nurse instructed the family in turning, positioning, bathing, and managing bowel and bladder needs. In her last week of life, she had severe difficulty breathing, which the hospice nurse had anticipated with emergency medications ready in the kitchen cupboard and family instructed in their use. To control seizures, the medications and routes were changed several times by the hospice nurse working closely with the prescribing physician.

The psychosocial and spiritual issues that surfaced during the care provided opportunity for everyone to review their family's biography and speak of memories, both good and bad. As the social worker and chaplain made their visits, their gentle inquiries revealed the family's pivotal events: the parents' divorce and the loss of another daughter who was killed in a drunk-driving accident. Although both of these events occurred many years ago, everyone still felt great pain; these subjects were never discussed. Neither of the adult children was in contact with their father, who had remarried. He was very well off financially and the rest of the family did not enjoy great financial success. The son felt abandoned and resented his father's success.

Ultimately, the social worker and nurse facilitated several important conversations. The siblings spoke together of their parents' divorce and its impact on them. The patient spoke of the loss of her daughter and, in a visit with the chaplain, sobbed over this and her subsequent loss of faith. Conversations about family finances, the funeral, and other practical matters were made possible because of the neutral and therapeutic presence of the hospice team members. The hospice team encouraged the involvement of the grandchildren, 10 and 15 years old. Small tasks were given to the children. They were informed about what was happening, and encouraged to visit their grandmother as much as possible. A special bond had always existed between the patient and her 15-year-old granddaughter, who ultimately read a poem at her funeral.

Mrs. Albert died one night about 3 AM. Her death came less than a month after admission to hospice. The hospice intervention allowed the family to honor the patient's wish to be at home, and helped the family address long-neglected emotional turmoil. A major issue was whether they would call their father to let him know of their mother's death. Finally, they decided he would be informed, in a brief letter, which would include a copy of the obituary and funeral program, plus an offer to call if he'd like to talk. The bereavement staff from hospice continued to offer support to the family, which was welcomed by the daughter and her family. The patient's son was less interested in continuing the counseling offered by hospice.

This story illustrates the possibilities for growth that hospice involvement can bring to a family. If hospice had not been involved, this patient's course of final illness might well have been chaotic, with a series of emergencies, and probably two or three hospitalizations, and a possible nursing home admission for her last 2 weeks of life. Hospice provided the opportunity for her to remain in her own surroundings, for her family to emerge from the experience feeling satisfied that they had done well in their care for her, and for emotional hurts of long ago to begin healing.

Barriers to Accessing Hospice

For all the beauty of hospice, an almost insurmountable barrier exists for many people to access this care. Medicare hospice admission requires that a patient have 6 months or less to live. This poses a tremendous barrier because prognostication is an imperfect science and physicians tend toward optimistic prognostication. Another obstacle to hospice access is the Medicare requirement that the patient must acknowledge that he or she is dying by choosing hospice care at the expense of other life-extending treatment. Continuing certain treatments, chemotherapies, medication regimens, and interventional procedures may not be financially possible with the current system of hospice reimbursement, but may foster quality of life at the end of life. This decision has been called "the terrible choice." Forcing that terrible decision is a deterrent to hospice referral for both physicians and patients. As a result of the obstacles built into the hospice model, a new form of care is emerging. Palliative-care programs attempt to do all the things hospice does, yet they do so earlier in the course of life-threatening illness and without the requirement that the patient must give up any treatment or care options.

THE PALLIATIVE-CARE MOVEMENT

Palliative care focuses on easing suffering as the patient chooses. It is not necessary to give up more aggressive life-sustaining care in order to receive palliation. *Palliation* means lessening pain and symptoms without curing. Therefore, an intervention that is *palliative* is intended to relieve pain and other symptoms without curing underlying disease. Palliative care actively seeks to relieve discomfort and promote quality of life for patients and loved ones. The aim of the contemporary palliative-care movement is to expand beyond the limitations of the hospice movement to relieve suffering at the end of life, and to incorporate palliative measures even as aggressive life-sustaining care is still being offered. To do this, palliative services are offered through hospitals, clinics, hospices, and home-care agencies. Box 2-4 describes the goals of such palliative services.

> 66 | *Palliation can be defined as lessening pain and symptoms without*
> *curing.*

Currently, most people living with life-threatening illness have months to years to live. Two-thirds of them will die in institutions, some receiving aggressive resuscitative care in hospitals, and some receiving only superficial

| Box 2-4 ■ | **PALLIATIVE GOALS** |

- Sustain relationships and refuse to abandon the patient.
- Promote independence and physical function as long as possible and as chosen by the patient.
- Aggressively seek to relieve symptoms and promote comfort as chosen.
- Provide physical, psychosocial, and spiritual support.
- Consider the patient within the context of family and community.
- Define who is a family member and involve them as the patient chooses.
- Pay careful attention to spiritual and cultural viewpoints.
- Determine goals based on the values and choices of patient and family.
- Meet needs through an interdisciplinary team approach.
- Acknowledge and seek to relieve the burdens of family caregivers.
- Build a system of support within the home and community.

Source: Adapted from Scanlon (2001).

custodial care in nursing homes until the moment of death. Prognoses are notoriously difficult to determine for those with chronic organ failure: cardiac, pulmonary, hepatic, or renal. Their courses of illness are up and down and difficult to predict. Individuals living with progressive neurological disability, particularly stroke or dementia, may endure long, stretched-out periods at a low level of functioning. Cancer and AIDS, once rapidly fatal, have uncertain prognoses because of advanced therapies. All of these people need palliative care coupled with continued active treatment if it is effective. As mentioned earlier, hospices require that patients relinquish active treatment.

Even in hospitals with well-developed hospice programs, hospice usually becomes involved in only a small percentage of deaths (Santa Emma, Roach, Gill, Spayde, and Taylor, 2003). In many circumstances, it is simply not reasonable to relinquish all efforts at life saving and to certify that patients are within 6 months of death. Patients often continue to focus on whatever more can be done to treat their disease and prolong their life.

As symptoms and quality-of-life issues become growing concerns for people at the end of life, existing hospital, home care, and nursing home structures are often not in place to assist with parallel needs for active treatment, open communication, patient choice, comforting care, and end-of-life management. This is why palliative consulting teams, inpatient units, and transitional home-care teams are being developed. Box 2-5 identifies Mainstream Medical Focus Contrasted with Palliative Focus. Palliative care should be offered throughout the course of disease and should incorporate

Box 2-5 ■	MAINSTREAM MEDICAL FOCUS CONTRASTED WITH PALLIATIVE FOCUS
MAINSTREAM FOCUS ON MEDICAL PROCESS	PALLIATIVE FOCUS ON HUMAN PROCESS
Therapies to maintain physiological systems	Therapies to comfort and meet individual goals
Death as defeat	Dying as opportunity for growth
Silence without discussion of dying	Open discussion if patient chooses
Withdrawal from dying people	Gathering around dying people
Avoidance of opioids and sedatives	Careful adjustment of opioids and sedatives to comfort and permit optimal function

Source: From Zerwekh (2002b).

the best of curative medicine in a process that has been called "simultaneous care" (Myers & Linder, 2003).

Consider the case of 64-year-old Lyle. During routine health screening, he was found to have advanced prostate cancer. His uncertain prognosis was discussed with him from the beginning. Three years after surgery, his prostate-specific antigen (PSA) rose, and he was effectively treated with radiotherapy. Two years after that, his PSA increased again and he was treated with hormones to eliminate androgen production. Three years later, he developed bone lesions in his pelvis, right shoulder, and right upper arm. His pain was effectively managed with extended release morphine and nonsteroidal anti-inflammatories. As a pathological fracture was treated with internal fixation, Lyle realized through dialogue with the palliative-care providers that the disease was gaining the upper hand. He and his wife chose to travel while he still could; he also deepened his long-standing spiritual practice. Lyle enrolled in a succession of two clinical trials, but the tumors did not respond. His pain escalated and required adjuvant medication, as well as high doses of the morphine, continually adjusted. At that point, he chose hospice care.

 As symptoms and quality-of-life issues become growing concerns for the people at the end of life, existing hospital, home-care, and nursing home structures are often not in place to assist with parallel needs for active treatment, open communication, patient choice, comforting care, and end-of-life management.

Planting the Seeds

Palliative care should be a goal in all health-care settings. In childbirth, we should focus on patient choice and comfort measures to promote a person-centered birthing experience. When young children are ill, the focus should be on parent choice and comfort measures to promote the child's well-being, not just treat a disease process. When people are living with chronic illness, we should focus on their own choices and definitions of quality, and provide comfort measures to enhance well-being. When people are aging and living with multiple illnesses, the focus should not be on disease management, but on their own choices and desire to be comfortable and live as well as possible. All our patients deserve palliation.

Palliative-Care Structure

A leader in the palliative-care movement, Dr. Joanne Lynn, has asserted that a good palliative system would continue active medical treatment with proven effectiveness while offering an individually customized plan to provide comfort, ensure continuity of care, emphasize end-of-life planning, use resources thoughtfully, and assist the person to make the best of every day (2001). It has been difficult to mobilize palliative home-care programs because little reimbursement is available. Nevertheless, hospitals are finding great advantages to developing inpatient palliative teams.

Consulting Teams

When patients with life-threatening illnesses are admitted acutely ill to the hospital, they often expect their disease to be managed and their condition stabilized once again. Often, even when it becomes apparent that these goals may not be achievable, health-care providers fail to acknowledge the futility and perform aggressive measures until death occurs after the last resuscitation fails. Alternatively, such patients often are discharged to a nursing home without palliative goals in mind. Comfort and choice are neglected; routine medical practice commonly does not consider these to be priorities. But palliative teams are able to implement palliative goals for patients in these settings.

Consider the circumstances of Johnnie, a 3-year-old head-injured child with no reflexes who has been in the intensive care unit on a ventilator for 14 days, surviving several cardiac arrests. Physicians and family had been hopeful about aggressive measures, but now the measures are failing.

Among family members, grief, anger, and denial prevail. Fortunately, the hospital has a palliative-care team. Following the neurologist's referral, the team social worker sits down with the family and asks them "What do you see happening?" The family members reveal their fears that the hospital staff wants to let Johnnie die "because we have no money." The social worker explains that this is not true and asks the palliative team physician to sit down with the family. After introductions he begins, "Let's go over what medical treatment can and cannot do to help Johnnie." In time and after repeated explanation, they ask to have their minister's counsel. Over the next 2 days, amidst many conversations, the family makes arrangements for Johnnie to be weaned from the ventilator while at the same time being medicated to avoid agonal respirations. All of this is performed in the presence of family and clergy, praying together.

Consider also the experience of Barbara, a middle-aged woman with extensive pulmonary cancer and liver metastases, admitted to the hospital for dehydration and pain management. She wants to continue to fight her disease, but her quality of life is poor due to the side effects of therapies. Not only does she not want "to give up," but her oncologist believes that she may well have longer than 6 months to live. Again, the palliative-care team goes to her bedside to initiate a plan focused on comfort and a safe plan for living at home after discharge. Barbara does not want to stop aggressive treatment, but she does want to have her pain, nausea, and dyspnea controlled. She also wants the emotional support from the palliative team social worker, who has demonstrated his compassion and sensitivity to her wishes. The palliative team has helped her with end-of-life decisions, including a living will and health-care proxy. The palliative team coordinates care throughout her hospital admissions, home care, and eventual nursing home admission.

As yet, there is no special reimbursement for palliative home care through insurance or government programs. Nevertheless, palliative-care consulting teams and inpatient palliative units are spreading rapidly across the country. They are saving money for hospitals by reducing the cost of care of seriously ill patients (wwww.capc.org). Remember that Medicare reimburses hospitals at a fixed rate for diagnosis-related groups, for a predetermined number of days. When length of hospitalization exceeds the days allowed by Medicare for that diagnosis, reimbursement drops dramatically and the hospital begins to lose money. Palliative programs can cut costs of care at the end of life by reducing the use of expensive but futile technologies and moving the patient from high-cost intensive-care beds to less expensive beds and then to appropriate care in skilled nursing facilities or at home. In addition, palliative programs save time for the entire productivity-focused health-care team by assuming responsibility for communication and coordination with these patients and families who have such compelling needs. The regular staff members are freed from these responsibilities.

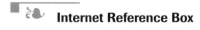

Internet Reference Box

The Center to Advance Palliative Care is located at *www.capc.org.*
Note their description of how palliative-care programs ease burdens on
staff and improve patient satisfaction and outcomes, as well as the hospital
bottom line financially.

Resistance to Addressing Suffering and Dying

The palliative-care movement continues to face resistance from the mainstream health-care community. There are two primary barriers: (1) preoccupation with aggressive life-saving interventions, and (2) fear of acknowledging suffering and using drugs to palliate. Before the 20th century, palliation was essentially all physicians and nurses could offer. In the beginning of the 21st century, however, palliation gets lost in the biomedical preoccupation with aggressive measures to investigate disease and prolong life as long as possible. Nuland has described the greatest challenge of contemporary medicine to be "not primarily the welfare of the individual human being but, rather, the solution of The Riddle of his disease" (1994, p. 249). Death is forbidden and we, as nurse technicians, often become the instruments of technology that insists on life at any cost. Box 2-5 contrasts this mainstream medical focus with palliative focus.

Another primary reason that palliation is resisted has to do with fear and avoidance of suffering and the means to relieve it. Physicians and nurses fear their own vulnerability if they pay attention to the suffering:

> Many of us have spent our entire nursing career learning how not
> to react to suffering: a neutral face, a steady hand, no eye contact.
> We regard patient's complaints with suspicion. We admire those
> who silently endure; they allow us to avoid confronting their suffering (Zerwekh, 2002a, p. 89).

Opioids and sedatives also provoke fears of suppressing respiration, reducing consciousness, causing addiction, and being deceived by patients who we suspect are exaggerating their pain. Physicians may fear being investigated for over-prescribing opioids. Fear of comforting and becoming comfortable as a nurse using these medications safely is discussed extensively in Chapters 14, 15, and 16.

OPPORTUNITIES FOR CHANGE

Participation in the palliative-care movement permits us to practice our own deepest values, to live caring and extend comforting to the entire population of people who are suffering emotionally, spiritually, and physically at the end of their lives. Palliative understanding and action must be extended into all health-care settings where people are living their last days.

CONCEPTS IN ACTION

Hannah Smith is a 43-year-old woman with terminal ovarian cancer, against which she has struggled for 10 years. She has received multiple aggressive interventions, including debulking surgeries, chemotherapy, and radiation therapies. She now suffers from an inoperable large bowel obstruction, massive ascites, pleural effusion, and kidney failure. Her mother and grandmother are able to provide care in her home, which she is now choosing. She asks not to return to the hospital and refuses all aggressive measures. Her physician has signed a Do Not Resuscitate order. Imagine you are the hospice nurse explaining hospice services to Ms. Smith, her husband, and her adolescent son. How would you tell them what hospice can do? What words would you use? How would her family care-givers benefit? How might the different members of the hospice team be helpful?

References

Byock, I. (1997). *Dying well: Peace and possibilities at the end of life.* New York: Riverhead Books.

Center to Advance Palliative Care (www.capc.org)

Hamilton, M., & Reid, H. (1980). *A hospice handbook: A new way to care for the dying.* Grand Rapids, MI: William B. Erdsman.

Later Referrals Do Not Allow Time. (2004). *Quality of Life Matters, 5*(4), 2–3.

Lynn, J. (2001). Serving patients who may die soon and their families: The role of hospice and other services. *Journal of the American Medical Association, 285*(7), 925–932.

Marrelli, T. (1999). *Hospice and palliative care handbook.* St. Louis: Mosby.

Meyers, F., & Linder, J. (2003). Simultaneous care: Disease treatment and palliative care throughout illness. *Journal of Clinical Oncology, 21*(7), 1412–1415.

Nuland, S. B. (1994). *How we die: Reflections on life's final chapter.* New York: Alfred Knopf.

Omnibus Budget Reconciliation Act (OBRA) of 1990. 42 Code of Federal Regulation 418.21.

Public Law 97-248, Tax Equity and Fiscal Responsibility Act (TEFRA) of 1982, Section 122.

Santa-Emma, P., Roach, R., Gill, M. A., Spayde, P., & Taylor, R. (2002) Development and implementation of an inpatient acute palliative care service. *Journal of Palliative Medicine, 5*(1), 93–100.

Saunders, C. (1976). *Care of the dying* (2nd ed.). London: Nursing Times.

Scala-Foley, M., Caruso, J., Archer, D., & Reinhard, S. (2004). Medicare's hospice benefits. *American Journal of Nursing, 104*(9), 66–67.

Scanlon, C. (2001). Public policy and end-of-life care: The nurse's role. In B. Ferrell & N. Coyle (Eds.), *Textbook of palliative nursing* (pp. 682–689). New York: Oxford University Press.

Stoddard, S. (1978) *The hospice movement.* New York: Stein and Day.

Zerwekh, J. (2002a). Fearing to comfort: A grounded theory of constraints to opioid use in hospice care. *Journal of Hospice and Palliative Nursing, 4*(2), 83–90.

Zerwekh, J. (2002b). Home care of the dying. In I. Martinson, A. Widmer & C. Portillo (Eds.), *Home health care nursing* (2nd ed., pp. 274–295). Philadelphia: WB Saunders.

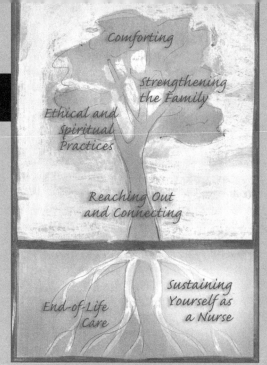

Comforting

Strengthening
the Family

Ethical and
Spiritual
Practices

Reaching Out
and Connecting

End-of-Life
Care

Sustaining
Yourself as
a Nurse

SUSTAINING YOURSELF AS A NURSE

CHAPTER 3

Strategies to Stay Healthy

Philosophical Reflections

"Even when you yourself are in need—and you are—you can help others and, in so doing, help yourself. He who calls forth the helping word in himself, experiences the word. He who offers support strengthens the support in himself. He who bestows comfort deepens the comfort in himself."

BUBER, 1957, P. 110

Learning Objectives

1. Explain the importance of knowing yourself in order to practice healthy caring.
2. Reflect about your own feelings and experiences related to death and dying.
3. Identify sources of stress as a result of working with dying patients and their families.
4. Identify sources of stress due to problems within the work environment.
5. Apply strategies of fostering a healthy work environment.
6. Apply Maslow's Hierarchy to sustaining personal well-being.
7. Apply to your own nursing practice the five dimensions of staying healthy as described by expert hospice nurses.

The End-of-Life Caregiving Model is rooted in strategies to stay healthy. To care for others and sustain compassion, nurses need to stay healthy. There are many ways nurses can sustain their own health, some of which this chapter explores in detail. This chapter also offers advice from expert hospice nurses about how to stay healthy and be able to reach out courageously to patients and families in the midst of their fear.

STAYING HEALTHY

If you imagine caregiving as a tree, then the root is the part of the tree below ground that holds the tree in position and draws sustenance from the soil. Effective nurses understand that in order to care for others, they must tend to the roots of the tree—themselves—first. After all, without strong, healthy roots, the tree will not grow. A study of 32 expert hospice nurses revealed five fundamental ways that nurses tend to themselves and stay healthy so that they can effectively care for their patients (Zerwekh, 1995). Expert nurses were defined as being those having at least 5 years of experience and those to whom other nurses turned for clinical advice. They sustained themselves by:

- Giving and receiving
- Letting go of agendas
- Grieving
- Being open and clear
- Replenishing themselves

Giving and Receiving

The expert nurses describe receiving emotional and spiritual gifts from caregiving that are in balance with their own continual giving:

"I am a consultant and a learner."
"I have been taught about living in the present and enjoying the moments of our lives."
"I feel so honored to be part of these people's lives. They have given me such a gift."

When a nurse feels that she or he is only giving and no longer receiving, stress and dissatisfaction are tipping the balance. Sometimes nurses are able to renew themselves by deliberately becoming mindful of the gifts they receive through their work. Sometimes it is necessary to change the circumstances of work in order to renew the experience of receiving.

Letting Go of Agenda

Effective work alongside the dying requires letting go of predetermined care plans and idealistic hopes. This is a developmental process that takes time because it is not instinctual to many nurses who keep trying to fix things in ways they think are best. When nurses stop trying to dictate how patients should behave at the end of life, it frees patients to live and die as they want for themselves. Nurses new to this work want control over end of life and need time to realize what is and is not possible. The nurse experts explain how they give up their desire to control:

> "I put aside my own wants, subordinate them or figure out how to modify them."
>
> "You have to have aspirations and not put yourself down when you don't reach them."
>
> "When there are complicated psychosocial problems, I'm not going to change them. I don't worry about them. I help people where they are emotionally."
>
> "When I see that patients are doing things in ways that are not healthy, I'm able to point it out to them, but it doesn't drive me crazy."

There are so many challenges to our preferred care plans. You may walk into a home that is dirty and vermin-infested. You will need to let go of your goal to improve the housekeeping. You may work with a patient who believes he must suffer for his sins and therefore is noncompliant with your recommendations for controlling his symptoms. You may have a goal that a broken family is reconciled, but family members themselves reject any proposal for forgiveness and closure. We need to respect patient and family autonomy, and recognize circumstances that we can and cannot influence. Thus, developing realistic goals and letting go of our own agendas are essential skills to sustain us in this work.

Grieving

Beyond attending funerals and memorials, the expert hospice nurses describe their insights into how to cope with enormous grief:

> "If staff doesn't have a safe place to deal with the emotional burden of facing that level of suffering, you are going to have burnout."
>
> "You have to learn how to grieve or you will be eaten up, burned out, unable to meet your client's needs, much less your own. For me, I watch sad dog movies."

Nurses who are effective at the end of life must find ways to grieve, and agencies must find ways to assist them in this persistent need. Lamendola (1996) explains that all intense feelings, including sadness and grief, need to be acknowledged regularly and expressed. Emptying ourselves of these feelings is essential or he warns that we will become "too full" to give or receive. One poetic nurse proclaimed, "We need to fall apart, then come together again. Out of the ashes we become powerhouses."

Being Open and Clear

Expert nurses insist that emotional openness and clarity are vital to sustaining themselves. At the end of life, patients are quickly aware of insincerity and false words:

"It's not what you do, it's who you are and your openness to inte
grate that into what you do."

"Your sincerity will show. If you're not sincere, there's very little
true contact that you are going to make. Dying people are really
sensitive to whether you care."

"Having decided that it was better to be emotionally honest in
regular life just transferred over to my nursing."

At the end of life, patients want to speak to someone who is truly listening and comprehending their circumstances, not someone who is pretending
to listen and care. We must choose to be present emotionally with the person,
not simply to nod and paraphrase their words while our mind is otherwise
disengaged. When we are open and clear, we have the gift of truly coming to
know another human being.

Replenishing Yourself

Expert nurses find ways to replenish themselves. Identify those things in
your life that give you pleasure and make room for them. Balancing your life
will make you a better nurse. After work, find ways to restore your energy in
activities that fit your personality. Perhaps you will seek renewal through
silence. Perhaps you will be renewed with joyful music. Perhaps you are at
peace when you go to the forest, prairie, river, or ocean. Become involved or
strengthen your involvement in church, synagogue, mosque, temple, or
other organizations that meet your needs. Let yourself be nurtured through
your community. Rest and exercise. Surround yourself with good people.
Seek out beauty. Avoid commitments beyond your capacity. Laugh. In order
to stay healthy and replenish yourself, it is first necessary to understand
through self-reflection what works with you and what does not.

WWW.   **Internet Reference Box**

Learn some ways to replenish yourself using these resources:

www.howmuchjoy.com/links.html

www.inspiredathome.com/v.1/18.htm.

KNOWING YOURSELF

Replenishing yourself first involves knowing what works for you and what
does not, understanding your own perspectives and your own emotions. In
other words, before caring for patients who are dying, you must first know
yourself.

Emotional Clarity

Self-awareness is a life-long challenge. Your ability to understand your own
emotions and reactions will help you provide quality end-of-life nursing

care. Nurses are constantly experiencing a variety of emotions and reacting in ways that may or may not be caring. For instance, one patient may have a tone of voice that you associate with someone you dislike. Because of that association, you might have trouble listening to his problems; you should be aware of your inclination to avoid him. Another patient may have a condition from which your beloved relative died and you noticed that you develop headaches whenever you care for him. Self-awareness would help you make the connection. Another example might involve a nurse's distress at home. For instance, you might have had a morning argument with your teenager about going to school; you may find yourself still too angry and distressed to listen to a patient's distress. It is important to reflect inwardly and to be aware of how our feelings influence our ability to care.

> *Your ability to understand your own emotions and reactions will help you provide quality end-of-life nursing care.*

We are all products of our own histories. Many of us are recovering from childhood emotional injuries that led to unhealthy patterns like guilt, severe self-criticism, overwork, attention-seeking, or angry behavior. For instance, some of us had mothers whose criticism was constant. Now we play a never-ending message in our heads that we are not good enough. Such a past might lead to a tendency to try to prove oneself by working extra shifts, taking on extra projects, and otherwise interfering with relationships with those we love. Many have experienced adult traumas, betrayals, or losses, such as divorce or the premature death of a loved one. We may still be angry and project that anger on patients and coworkers. In short, we have all developed ways of coping with our own suffering that determine how we care for suffering in others. Some of these patterns may not be healthy for us or helpful to others. A nurse who may have always suppressed criticism from her mother may also be ineffective in handling a patient who is expressing distress over criticism from his mother. Emotional clarity requires us to come to terms with unhealthy coping mechanisms so that we can provide effective care.

Planting the Seeds

Coming to terms with your own issues involves:

- Being curious about yourself
- Resolving to grow in self-awareness
- Looking at how your family history and life experiences have influenced your emotions
- Identifying how you usually feel in a typical day
- Identifying your most important needs
- Noticing what situations and relationships make you uneasy and distressed

- Recognizing personal judgments, fears, and anger intruding upon relationships with patients
- Choosing to put aside these automatic feelings and reactions in order to be more effective in all relationships

FACING DEATH

We are a death-denying culture and most of us have had few encounters with death before becoming nurses. In the hospital, home, and nursing home, we focus on keeping physiological systems functioning and technological interventions running smoothly. We sometimes overlook the fact that caring for people who are dying requires paying attention to their human experiences. We must stop, listen, and look into the faces of those close to death. To do this, we must develop some comfort in facing death ourselves and exploring our own personal beliefs and fears.

66 | *We must stop, listen, and look into the faces of those close to death.*

Reflecting on death is a great challenge in our culture because social prohibitions keep us from talking about and thinking about death. Other cultures perceive death differently. For example, death and suffering are subjects of common reflection and acceptance in Hindu culture (Kemp & Bhungalia, 2002). Traditional Hindus actively anticipate the next life. The elderly and terminally ill do not deny their dying. By contrast, among the elderly and terminally ill in America, there are often strong social prohibitions against saying anything about death. Recently, a hospice nursing supervisor reported that her 90-year-old mother refused to watch a highly recommended television program about death because her friends considered the subject "morbid."

Not only is discussion of death considered to be inappropriate in our society, but the mention of death also brings up strong feelings of fear, anger, and sadness. We are afraid of the unknown, angry that death unfairly intrudes upon life, and sad about our own losses. If we have been caregivers for a while, we often have feelings of chronic sorrow about all of our patients who have died. "Feelings that we don't acknowledge remain hidden in the shadow" (Larsen, 2002, p. 88).

66 | *Feelings that we don't acknowledge remain hidden in the shadow*
    | *(Larsen, 2002, p. 88).*

Acknowledging repressed feelings allows us to understand ourselves better. It allows us to let our defenses down so that we can come to know people who are dying instead of maintaining boundaries against them because of our own fear. Take time for reflection by examining the questions

Box 3-1 ■   FEELINGS ABOUT DEATH

1. Reflect about whether your family talked about death and how it was discussed or avoided when you were a child. Can your family discuss this topic today?
2. Consider your first encounters with death. What do you remember?
3. What do you currently believe about what happens after death?
4. What feelings do you have about your own death? What would be your greatest fears?
5. What feelings do you have about the death of those you love? What would be your greatest fears?
6. What would be your own last wishes? What business would you want to complete? With whom would you want to reconcile? What rituals would you choose at the end of your life?
7. What are your greatest fears in talking to a dying person?
8. Would your family and friends be able to talk to you about your dying? Would you be able to talk to them about their dying?
9. What feelings do you have about encountering end-of-life symptoms?
10. What feelings do you have about dead bodies and doing post-mortem care?

in Box 3-1, Feelings about Death. It is not until we can reflect upon our own feelings about death that we can care for others encountering death.

Our feelings about death have an impact on the care we can provide. For example, if all talk of death has been avoided in our family, we need to learn to talk about it deliberately. If we do not believe in an afterlife, we may be deeply troubled to work with patients who we believe face a final termination. If we have experienced bereavement ourselves, we may have unresolved feelings that lead us to a desire to avoid future encounters with death. If we associate death with dark forces and evil spirits, we may be terrified to be in the presence of death. For example, one student was assisting with post-mortem care, when suddenly, she froze in position and would neither move nor speak. The traditional belief system of her childhood culture had taught her that nonrelatives risked their souls by touching dead bodies. She had to be half-carried out of the room and referred for counseling. In order for her to provide effective end-of-life care, she needed guidance to work through her thoughts and feelings about death.

HEALTHY CARING

Knowing yourself and recognizing your feelings about death is the basis of a strong foundation for healthy caring. Healthy caring requires self-awareness to be able to purposefully enter into the world of a suffering person to understand his or her experience, while maintaining enough detachment to be of practical usefulness and to retain our own emotional health. We seek to "feel without being overwhelmed, to care without being overcome, to participate without losing identity" (Blues & Zerwekh, 1984, p. 333). This is a career-long challenge for all nurses. Martin Buber, the famed Jewish philosopher, believes that when we are compassionate toward others, our own lives are enhanced and we are comforted in our own suffering (1957). In other words, Buber assures us that we will actually become stronger, not weak and overwhelmed, as we develop this practice of compassion. The prequisites of compassion include a strengthened sense of self and greater comfort for our own hurts.

The practice of compassion brings great rewards, including the joy of being able to relieve suffering and the opportunity to know the sufferer as a fellow human being. Despite these rewards, the ability to sustain such compassion ebbs and flows throughout our lives and careers. Lamendola (1996) calls this phenomenon "burning brightly and burning dimly." Sometimes we are energized and feeling well so that we can fully engage in caring; other times we suffer from "compassion fatigue" and can barely listen to calls for caring. Nurses suffering from compassion fatigue are aware of their diminishing empathy as they suffer growing emotional distress over their continual encounters with suffering. Alternating burning dimly and burning brightly is a normal human pattern for all of us, and to avoid compassion fatigue, we need to stop and consider ways to be self-aware and care for ourselves.

STRESSORS IN END-OF-LIFE CARE

Nurses have personal stressors, patient and family stressors, and work environment stressors, all coming into play at the same time. Understanding the sources and impact of the stressors, and learning ways to combat them, can go a long way toward making you a better nurse and a happier person.

WWW.   Internet Reference Box

For more reading on the stressors associated with end of life nursing, refer to *www.hospiceresources.net/hospicearticleabstracts/*.

Sources of Stress

Nurses working at the end of life encounter two kinds of stress: (1) stress arising directly from their work with patients and families, and (2) stress arising from within the work environment.

Patients and Families

Vachon (2001) has extensively studied the causes of stress for nurses working with dying patients and their families. Patient and family stressors include experiencing patient decline and death, lack of control, and being in the middle of family conflict. When patients with whom they have long-standing relationships gradually deteriorate, nurses become stressed. We witness suffering of patients and families and may at times feel overwhelmed with feelings of sorrow. In addition, conflict between stressed family members often erupts right in front of our eyes. For example, one family member might want to give adequate morphine to relieve pain of the suffering patient, while another fears addiction and withholds pain relief. The nurse is in the middle, seeking to mediate conflict so that the dying person can be comforted.

In addition to having limited control over dying, nurses also cannot control how other people feel about and act when dying. Patients or family members may seek more aggressive therapies than are appropriate or give up too soon. Nurses may question the wisdom or morality of decisions that are not theirs to make. We are caught between idealistic expectations of fostering a "good death" and the realities of how people choose to live and die. For example, some people carry hatred to their deathbed. Some choose to accept physical and emotional abuse from loved ones, as they have done through life. Others may choose to live alone and refuse help. We witness people making troubling choices at the end of life. Caring for the dying requires coping with lack of control and deliberately letting go of one's own agenda, which many find stressful.

Organizational Sources

Despite the obvious difficulties of being immersed in end-of-life patient and family suffering, Vachon (2001) proclaims that organizational conflicts actually cause more stress than witnessing the suffering. Nurses often experience great responsibility and high expectations to relieve suffering without the power and resources to meet those expectations, which can impose great emotional burdens. We strain to narrow the gap between idealistic goals and real possibilities. Contemporary work environments, which emphasize productivity and finances, can threaten quality practice that nurses have previously been able to provide. We desire to provide holistic care for every patient and family, yet the organization might expect us to make more visits every day. Our visits end up being too short to spend the needed time listening. We seek to offer spiritual care, yet the hospice chaplain might have a caseload so large that he cannot respond effectively to our referral for spiritual counseling. We want to serve the poor, yet the hospice cannot survive by making visits to patients without a funding source. In the early days of the hospice and palliative-care programs, nurses had generous time to respond to complex patient and family challenges. However, we are now often stretched to our limits with a growing workload.

Lack of control may be a critical stressor at work. In some agencies, the nurse's freedom to provide comforting care may be constrained by other professionals. For instance, in one agency, social work leaders insisted that they were the only profession who could intervene in psychosocial issues and that nurses could not document regarding patient or family emotional issues. As nurses, we are prepared to care for the whole person: body, mind, and spirit. Denying nurses' psychosocial role reduces us to focusing on the body alone and prevents us from practicing an essential dimension of our profession. In another agency, physicians refused to write standing orders so that every change in medication dosage or route required the extended and stressful process of contacting the physician and getting a response. The nurses were unable to modify regimens readily to ensure stable control of symptoms, and patients suffered as a result.

Manifestations of Stress

Stress imposes tension and strains our coping mechanisms. Moderate stress mobilizes our personal resources. It stimulates us to activity and accomplishment. However, excessive stress causes so much distress that it can produce symptoms affecting our body, spiritual well-being, emotional state, and professional behavior. Physical symptoms include headache, appetite change, weight change, substance abuse, gastrointestinal disturbances, fatigue, sleep disturbances, shortness of breath, and palpitations. Spiritual effects include apathy, cynicism, and hopelessness. Emotional effects include anxiety, anger, sadness, depression, guilt, frustration, inadequacy, and powerlessness. We may withdraw from significant relationships or create conflict with our loved ones or colleagues. Refer to Box 3-2, Symptoms of Stress, to familiarize yourself with additional symptoms of stress.

When nurses lack power, whether it be from a personal or organizational source, anger commonly results (Droppleman & Thomas, 1996). Too often, nurses direct anger inward and develop depression or risky health behaviors such as overeating. In addition, nurses sometimes become more and more hostile toward coworkers in a process called "horizontal violence." This dynamic, first observed among oppressed people in third world countries, involves attacking peers and family members rather than confronting policies and practices that keep us powerless. See Box 3-3, Defensive Organizational Behaviors.

Management of Stress

Work environments can be created to minimize stress and maximize nurse satisfaction and healthy coping (Vachon, 2001). Fast-paced agencies may be focused on survival or expansion to meet organizational goals or respond to community health needs. Leaders must nonetheless make it a priority to develop a caring culture in which nurses can thrive. Otherwise, they will function poorly or leave. Nurses must be involved in problem-solving to

---

Box 3-2 ■   SYMPTOMS OF STRESS

PHYSICAL

Headaches	Major weight changes
GI disturbances	Sleep problems, fatigue
Shortness of breath	Palpitations
Unhealthy eating	Alcohol or drug abuse

SPIRITUAL

Apathy	Hopelessness
Cynicism	Emptiness
Withdrawal from faith community	Inability to forgive

EMOTIONAL/SOCIAL

Anxiety	Powerlessness
Anger	Withdrawal from others
Depression	Hostility toward others
Guilt	Persistent frustration

---

improve work conditions and participate in major organizational decisions that affect patient care. Likewise, we need to be able to control our professional practice decisions and not have them seriously limited by agency policy. Nurses so empowered can work constructively with agencies and see themselves as participating in shaping their own destinies. For example, a

---

Box 3-3 ■   DEFENSIVE ORGANIZATIONAL BEHAVIORS

In times of fear and uncertainty, horizontal violence manifests itself in angry, defensive organizational behaviors (Ryan & Oestreich, 1991). Cynicism deepens and organizational staff and leaders withdraw from each other, resist problem-solving, deny responsibility, backbite, blame, scapegoat, and go after those who try to make changes. The moral environment declines when people lie because they believe it is necessary to protect themselves. In contrast, consider Kritek's (2002, pp. 355–356) proposed personal epitaph as she seeks to address nurses developing moral courage in the face of conflicts, "She was invited to cynicism daily, and she said no. . . . She cherished her personal integrity." Consider how to word a resolution for yourself.

hospice or home-health agency aiming to reduce RNs and increase a new RN/LPN partnership model must provide for active input at the staff nurse level to develop strategies that will work. There must be meetings with small groups of staff in which active listening by supervisors eventually results in observable change. Staff ideas must be taken seriously. Without staff-level participation in change, withdrawal and sabotage are predictable defensive behaviors.

Nurses must also be involved in discovering and developing ways to make the health-care organization emotionally friendly. Respect and appreciation from leaders and coworkers are essential. An affirming work environment may involve strengthening social and professional support with regular group sessions or professional "buddies." This may appear expensive in the short run because professional nurse time is expensive. However, in the long run, the agency benefits because nurses who feel supported by others are more likely to stay than those who feel isolated and alone in providing for their patients. In addition, meaningful, collaborative relationships predict organizational effectiveness. We solve problems together instead of alone.

Nurses must have ways to tell their stories, but they often cannot do that at home. They cannot always count on loved ones to respond to such intense experiences. Any agency strategy that fosters healthy grieving will foster staff health. Nurses should be encouraged to attend wakes and funerals and to participate in agency memorials, such as monthly rituals that name every patient who died during the month. They need to share their joys and sorrows in simple ways, like recognizing birthdays and graduations and tragedy among loved ones, in ways that fit the group culture.

When there is cause for anger and fear, healthy responses include speaking openly about it to those we trust and emphasizing that everyone in the agency is in today's challenging health-care environment together; the "us" versus "them" mentality must be defeated at every turn. It is important to identify outside forces that are affecting the agency's ability to care. The group should be encouraged to develop common goals and group strategies with everyone at the table. As an individual staff nurse, you can reject anger to promote a healthy work environment by the following:

- Offering to help others on your team
- Refusing to participate in gossip
- Offering positive solutions to unit or agency problems
- Rejecting a role as angry martyr
- Being aware of your own health as well as the health of coworkers
- Refusing to accept abuse and making an honest effort to help others in the face of such treatment

For example, Ruth is a new nurse on an oncology unit that offers palliative chemotherapy and radiation therapy to many patients with terminal prognoses. Ruth has observed that several of the nurses on her shift spend a significant amount of time complaining about their workload, about the nursing assistants, and about one physician in particular, who is rumored to be at fault in a malpractice suit she is facing. It has become clear to Ruth that her own mood and physical well-being will be affected if she becomes part of that subgroup. She decides not to contribute to the negativity and to be helpful and positive with the aides and physicians. Whenever coworkers are rude, she quietly asks them to treat her with respect before the conversation can continue. When one of the aides is publicly humiliated by loudly spoken criticism in the middle of the nurse's station, Ruth is able to bring both the aide and the nurse into an office where the door can be closed. She offers to mediate to discover the point of view of each member of the team and resolve the conflict.

Howard is another example of a nurse who has chosen to manage organizational stress in a healthy, productive way. Howard has become aware of his own health and realizes the adverse effects of stress on his blood pressure and eating habits. He has organized a Saturday morning yoga practice for fellow employees. He deliberately avoids nonproductive group complaining about overwork and instead has chosen to work on a staff governance committee that is looking at ways to limit overtime demands on staff nurses.

Planting the Seeds

When you find yourself in a situation where you feel violated, take a deep breath and perhaps even a time out, then assess and take constructive action. Accept responsibility for mistakes, but look beyond to improving the system. Seek to channel your anger into patient advocacy, problem-solving at the unit level, or productive agency-wide changes. Asserting this level of constructive activity in the organization should be grounded in deliberate efforts to take care of yourself.

MASLOW'S HIERARCHY APPLIED TO SUSTAINING OURSELVES

You can develop life-long habits of managing stress and self-renewal through listening to your mind and body, and practicing compassion for yourself. Imagine applying Maslow's Hierarchy (see Fig. 3-1) to your own self-care. At the base of the triangle you will find breathing, followed by nutrition, physical exercise, exercise for the mind, human community, and exercise for the spirit at the top of the triangle. Each level of the triangle will be discussed in turn.

Breathing

Breathing is necessary for life itself. Stress and worry have an impact on the way we breathe; our state of mind has a direct impact on our breathing pattern (Kahn & Saulo, 1994). When under stress, we tend to breathe rapidly and

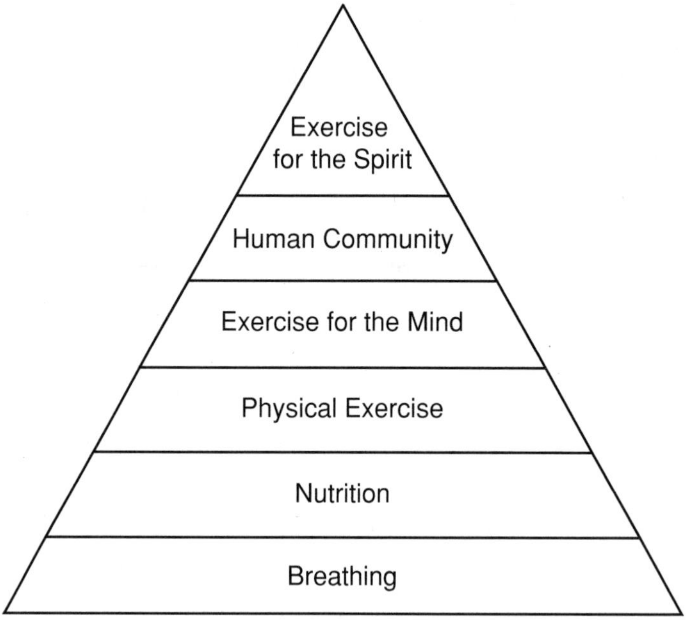

Figure 3-1 Maslow's Hierarchy Applied to Sustaining Yourself. (Adapted from Maslow, 1970.)

shallowly, reducing oxygen levels in our blood. In contrast, slow, deep abdominal breathing increases oxygenation of cells. Deep breathing is helpful for calming and for increasing energy and mental clarity. Try practicing deep relaxation breathing by following the steps in Box 3-4. Imagine that a frightened patient in severe pain has just yelled at you for not responding immediately to her call light. First, you should breathe deeply, then respond with compassion.

Nutrition

It is said that we are what we eat. Are you eating healing foods or harmful foods? Do you follow the same healthy nutritional guidelines that you teach your patients? Healthy means lots of fruits and vegetables and not a lot of fatty meat, simple carbohydrates, and salt. Do you skip meals and then double up on fast food? Do you eat slowly and mindfully or do you inhale your meal rapidly while multitasking? Does your stomach hurt? Be mindful of the food you ingest and it will enhance your physical, emotional, and intellectual well-being. Too often we survive through a nursing shift by eating high-salt, high-fat, and refined-sugar snacks, and drinking caffeinated beverages. Examine Box 3-5, Nutrition Self Appraisal, and be aware of how you can best sustain yourself. With just a little bit of extra forethought and effort, we can make a positive impact on the care we provide by practicing the healthy eating habits we preach to patients.

Box 3-4 ■   DEEP RELAXATION BREATHING

Sit in a comfortable position with your back straight and your eyes closed. While you are learning this technique, rest your right hand on your abdomen and your left on your chest . . . Exhale completely through your nose, and then inhale deeply. Feel your abdomen filling with air and your right hand rising. Continue to inhale as you fill your chest with air, and note how your left hand rises as your chest expands. Inhale even more, filling your lungs and feeling your collarbone rise.

Hold your breath for as long as is comfortable. Exhale in the reverse order from the way you inhaled. Release the air slowly, first from your lungs, then from your chest as you feel the contraction in this area. Lastly, allow the air to be released from your abdomen, contracting your abdominal muscles to expel as much air as possible.

Source: From Kahn & Saulo (1994), p. 92.

Physical Exercise

Exercise maintains physical fitness and has wide-ranging positive physiological effects, including heart and bone health. Exercise increases energy and relieves anxiety and depression. Exercise allows us to relax. So, why don't we do it more? Each of us has our own personal set of reasons. Nevertheless, practicing compassion for yourself includes creating an exercise plan

---

Box 3-5 ■   NUTRITION SELF APPRAISAL

Evaluate the following elements in and factors related to your diet:

Fresh fruit and vegetables _____

Whole grains _____

Fatty meat _____

Saturated fat _____

Simple sugars _____

Salt _____

Fast food _____

Daily calories _____

Eating slowly _____

Skipping meals _____

that fits your life. Don't aim too high. Make a plan that is achievable; plan for small successes. In addition to aerobic exercise, a growing number of people are adopting practices such as yoga, which focus on breathing and concentration with movement (Kahn & Saulo, 1994).

Exercise for the Mind

Moving up Maslow's triangle, we reach exercise for the mind. Thoughts, including words and images, have power. Cognitive restructuring is a field of psychotherapy that focuses on the power of the messages that we repeat to ourselves (Beck, 1976). It emphasizes becoming aware of negative messages, controlling the thoughts, and then planning to challenge the negative thoughts systematically with healthy affirmations. To practice cognitive restructuring, examine the words you speak to others and to yourself. During the course of a day, write down the thoughts that cycle through your mind. Examine how you persistently think about yourself and others. Some of us engage in constant self-criticism. By catching the thought and replacing it with a healthy one, you can choose to challenge an inner voice that is telling you, for example, "Nothing you ever do is good enough." You can deliberately change that inner voice by silently repeating more positive messages such as, "You are doing enough good. Take time for yourself."

Just as words have power, so do mental images. Athletes are using visualization to create a new reality (Kahn & Saulo, 1994). This involves carefully developing mental images of what you would like to achieve. A usually quiet nurse, for example, can repeatedly visualize herself speaking out about a change that she perceives as necessary in the work environment. One day, she finds herself speaking out during a meeting. Now imagine yourself approaching a physician who believes that high morphine doses will kill her dying patient. Get a clear picture of her and her expected words and nonverbal behaviors. Then imagine yourself walking up to her with confidence. Your breathing is slow and deep. Imagine your posture and your other nonverbal behavior as positive and strong. Your back is straight. Your smile is welcoming. Imagine yourself speaking assertively. Systematically develop your evidence-based argument. See yourself presenting the evidence on behalf of your client, and picture the physician who then agrees to collaborate with you on a pain-management solution.

Human Community

The extreme individualism of contemporary American society instructs us that self-reliance is the highest good. Throughout the history of humanity, however, we have needed each other to meet our basic survival needs. Even in these times of e-mail and labor-saving devices, online shopping, and reproduction without intercourse, humans cannot survive in isolation. Especially if we are caring for others, we need to develop and nurture a caring community to hold us up in good times and bad. Research demonstrates that emotional and physical health is enhanced wherever the bonds between people are strong (Aday, 1993). People who have strong extended families are healthier than people who live alone without a social network. People who live in communities where neighbors are actively involved in local schools, faith communities, and political groups are healthier than are those who live in isolation.

Exercise for the Spirit

Finally, consider the top of the Maslow triangle. In spiritual practice, we seek a transcendent reality beyond ourselves. We find meaning beyond self satisfaction and beyond human relationships. We may find renewal through the grandeur of nature or that of glorious art or music. We may worship and pray according to our tradition.

Meditation is practiced by many religious traditions, and also by people outside of faith communities. Meditation seeks a connection with a transcendent reality, which may be Spirit, God, the universe, nature, or a collective human consciousness. People practicing regular meditation tend to be calmer, more focused, and at peace with life (Kahn & Saulo, 1994). They have learned to quiet themselves even when surrounded by agitating circumstances. Meditation may focus on breath, a word, a sound, or an affirming thought. See Box 3-6 for a simple meditation exercise that focuses on breathing and a single word. Meditation can be extended beyond a meditative session to the practice of mindfulness in daily life (Hanh, 1976). Mindfulness includes slowing down and focusing on breath and awareness during activities such as eating, walking, and housework. A few moments of meditation before a challenging work situation permit a nurse to respond constructively and calmly.

Box 3-6 ■   A SIMPLE MEDITATION

- Sit comfortably with your spine straight
- Breathe through your nose deeply and slowly
- Exhale slowly
- Continue with your attention focused entirely on the breath, in and out
- Watch your thoughts and consciously let them go whenever they bubble up
- Refocus back on your breathing
- You might choose to focus on a word or phrase with each inhalation. For example, on inhalation think "peace" and on exhalation "like a river." Choose words that have the greatest meaning for you.

CONCEPTS IN ACTION

A hospice nursing supervisor describes Sandy, one of her nurses, as "burned out." This is the supervisor's story:

Yesterday I came in at 8:00 A.M., after Sandy had been on for an hour, and there were actually two patients sitting in wheelchairs at the nurse's station who grabbed me and said they were desperate for pain medication. Two hospice patients in pain! One was crying. I checked with Sandy who told me, "They are always complaining. They shouldn't be having that much pain!" I medicated them both for breakthrough pain. Sandy is a very hard worker with 9 years of nursing experience. She arrives on the unit and never takes a break all day. She expects everyone to work hard and to do what she tells them to do. Patients and families are actually afraid to question her. She drinks coffee and consumes donuts while charting. Sandy is recently divorced; her husband continues to attend their community church, but Sandy has stopped going because she sees him there and all her friends from church seem to be comforting him with many invitations to meals and outings. Sandy tells everyone, "The only thing I have left is this darn job."

- Why is Sandy unable to practice compassion?
- What symptoms of stress is Sandy experiencing?
- Examine Sandy's experience in terms of Maslow's Hierarchy Applied to Sustaining Ourselves.
- If the supervisor has had a long-term, good relationship with Sandy, what recommendations might she make to improve Sandy's health?
- Explain the relationship between Sandy's health and her ability to provide effective end-of-life care.

Only by caring for ourselves are we able to confront the level of fear experienced by patients and families. Only through practicing compassion for ourselves are we able to witness and respond to needs that one expert nurse described as "cavernous." Rooted in self-care, we are able to reach out with courage to the broken and terrified at the end of their lives. Gifted by knowing them and relieving their suffering, we become "powerhouses." Such power is not practiced in isolation, however, but through working with a team. The next chapter describes how collaboration with an interdisciplinary team strengthens our ability to care.

References

Aday, L. (1993). *At risk in America.* San Francisco: Jossey-Bass.

Beck, A. (1976). *Cognitive therapy and the emotional disorders.* New York: New American Library.

Blues, A., & Zerwekh, J. (1984). *Hospice and palliative nursing care.* Orlando, FL: Grune & Stratton.

Buber, M. (1957) *Pointing the way.* New York: Harper & Row.

Droppleman, P. G., & Thomas, S. P. (1996). Anger in nurses: Don't lose it,

use it. *American Journal of Nursing,*
96(4), 26–31.

Hanh, T. N. (1976). *The miracle of mind-*
fulness: A manual on meditation.
Boston: Beacon Press.

Kahn, S., & Saulo, M. (1994). *Healing*
yourself: A nurses' guide to self care and
renewal. Clifton Park, NY: Delmar.

Kemp, C., & Bhungalia, S. (2002). Culture and end of life: A review of major
world religions. *Journal of Hospice and*
Palliative Nursing, 4(4), 235–242.

Kritek, P. (2002). *Negotiating at an*
uneven table: Developing moral courage
in resolving our conflicts (2nd ed.).
San Francisco: Jossey-Bass.

Lamendola, F. (1996). Keeping your
compassion alive. *American Journal of*
Nursing, 96(11), 16R–16T.

Larsen, L. (2002). *Facing the final mys-*
tery. First Books. (self-published).

Maslow, A. H. (1970). *Motivation and*
personality (2nd ed.). New York:
Harper & Row.

Nouwen, H. (1972). *The wounded healer.*
Garden City, NY: Doubleday.

Ryan, K., & Oestreich, D. (1991). *Dri-*
ving fear out of the workplace. San
Francisco: Jossey-Bass.

Vachon, M. L. S. (2001). The nurse's
role: The world of palliative care
nursing. In B. R. Ferrell & N. Coyle
(Eds.), *Textbook of palliative nursing.*
New York: Oxford University
Press.

Zerwekh, J. (1995). A family caregiving
model for hospice nursing. *The Hos-*
pice Journal, 10(1), 27–44.

CHAPTER 4

Collaborating with an Interdisciplinary Team

LESLIE H. NICOLL

Editor-in-Chief, *The Journal of Hospice and Palliative Nursing*

Philosophical Reflections

"Far and away, the best prize that life has to offer is the chance to work hard at work worth doing."

THEODORE ROOSEVELT

Learning Objectives

1. Compare and contrast four models of teamwork, including multidisciplinary, interdisciplinary, cross-functional, and transdisciplinary.
2. Identify benefits to patients and families that accrue from delivery of care by an interdisciplinary team.
3. Describe the differences between primary, secondary, and tertiary palliative care.
4. Identify the key members of the hospice interdisciplinary team and list at least three core competencies for each member.
5. Discuss external and work stressors that may influence functioning of the interdisciplinary team.
6. Explain the importance of individual and organizational support to enhance the functioning of the team.
7. Discuss strategies that can be used to provide support to the interdisciplinary team.

End-of-life care is provided to terminally ill and dying patients by an interdisciplinary team. Interdisciplinary caregiving is at the roots of the End-of-Life Caregiving Model. This chapter will describe the nature of teams in health care, with an emphasis on end-of-life care, and will describe team members and their roles. It will also cover strategies for helping team members to collaborate effectively and to manage team-related stress.

MODELS OF TEAMWORK

Teams are an integral component of end-of-life care and have been described as "the glue that holds together the hospice approach" (Beresford, 1993). The purpose of the team is to build a caring community, with the patient and family at the center. Care providers, including nurses, physicians, pharmacists, social workers, chaplains, and volunteers, come together as an integrated whole to respond to each patient's needs, 24 hours a day, 7 days a week. Figure 4-1 illustrates the interdisciplinary team. The team is responsible for addressing the diverse needs of the patient and family, including pain and symptom management, psychosocial concerns, spiritual distress, and bereavement counseling for the family after the patient's death.

In hospice and palliative care, the team is usually defined as "interdisciplinary" but there are other models of teams, including multidisciplinary, cross-functional, and transdisciplinary, that need to be understood for a full appreciation of the importance of the team approach.

Figure 4-1 Interdisciplinary Team Focused on Patient and Family.

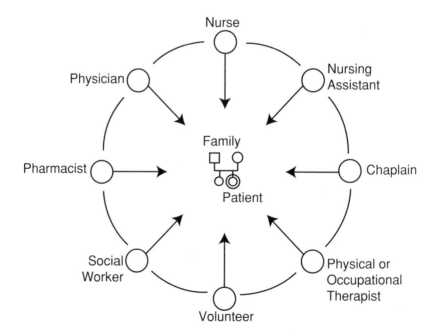

Multidisciplinary Teams

In many health-care settings, multidisciplinary teams serve as the norm for care delivery. A multidisciplinary team entails a variety of health professionals all working together on behalf of the patient. On a multidisciplinary team, individuals are known first by their professional identity and second as a member of the team. Leadership is often hierarchical and in many cases the physician is the "captain of the ship." Information is shared not in meetings but through the medical record and as a result, team members often work in relative isolation (Ajemian, 1994). Each member has a clearly defined place in the overall care of the patient, contributing to the care through his or her expertise. Goals for the patient are formulated individually by each practitioner and reflect the expertise of the practitioner. The focus is not necessarily on an integrated understanding of the patient, but instead, on the separate expertise each discipline has in relation to the patient (Egan & Labyak, 2001). A pie analogy is useful to describe the multidisciplinary team. Each practitioner represents a separate piece (Crawford & Price, 2003); while each contributes to the whole pie, the quality of the whole is *not* necessarily greater than the sum of its parts.

The lack of collaborative care-planning and goal-setting can be detrimental to the patient. The different approaches can be inconsistent and haphazard, resulting in discontinuity of care. This, in turn, is frustrating for the patient and family, and may result in poorer outcomes and diminished quality of life.

Interdisciplinary Teams

The interdisciplinary team, by contrast, has members who share information and work interdependently. The team provides expert medical and nursing care, pain management, and emotional and spiritual support expressly tailored to the patient and family's wishes and needs (Lipman, 2002). Team membership and the identity of the team supersede individual professional affiliations and roles. Leadership is task dependent and tasks are defined by the patient's changing situation. Again, Crawford and Price (2003) use an analogy, this time of a hand, to describe team functioning. The individual digits alone have differing abilities, functions, and dexterity but when they work together they can "achieve more than the sum of the individual fingers" (p. S33).

Care management by an interdisciplinary team is a process, not an event (Egan & Labyak, 2001). To be effective, the team must have an ongoing, collaborative practice that incorporates shared goals, care-planning, role-blending, and shared leadership. Frequent dialogue between different team members with differing expertise and perspectives fosters continuing development and evaluation of therapeutic approaches. For instance, the chaplain shares his concern about the patient's uncontrolled vomiting; the nurse speaks of the patient's worries about divine judgment; the social worker notes that the primary caregiver is uncomfortable with bathing the patient. The plan of care evolves as they interact with each other. A high level of trust and effective interactional process is vital to the success of the team.

Cross-Functional Teams

A team concept developed in business, but not used widely in health care, is the notion of a cross-functional team. In this model, a team is assembled with an eye to creating a skill set specific to the purpose at hand. Team members are recognized as experts who are ready to move quickly and be flexible to meet changing demands. The synergy created by the team is beneficial to all involved (Parker, 1994). In end-of-life care, this synergy would provide support to the team as well as translate into improved processes for care for the patient and family. "Successful teams may possess combinations of skills that no single individual demonstrates alone" (Crawford & Price, 2003).

> 66   *Successful teams may possess combinations of skills that no single individual demonstrates alone (Crawford & Price, 2003).*

In a sense, a cross-functional team may be seen as an extension of the traditional interdisciplinary team. Although an interdisciplinary team does have some role-blending, in a cross-functional team this is taken one step further. Members learn how to cover for each other—perhaps not in the areas of highest specialization—but in areas of patient support and caring. They minimize each other's weaknesses and maximize their strengths. A cross-functional team provides a powerful forum for creative problem-solving, as every member's contribution is genuinely solicited and respected (Crawford & Price, 2003).

Transdisciplinary Teams

At the farthest end of the continuum is the transdisciplinary team. In this model, "role release" occurs. Roles and responsibilities are shared and there are few seams between the members' functions (Parker, 1994). To the patient, it does not matter if the practitioner is a nurse, social worker, or physician. Again, this model is not predominant in health care, but it is present in hospice. For example, Mazanec and colleagues (2002) described a transdisciplinary model of pain management. In this model, every member of the team was empowered to assess and manage a patient's pain. Whether a nurse, physician, or nursing assistant, everyone was expected to screen and intervene, at a level appropriate to their expertise, to minimize a patient's pain. During the implementation of the project, it was found that nursing assistants, who had frequent patient contact, often identified subtle changes in patients' behaviors that were indicative of discomfort. In a traditional process for documentation, their notes would not be included with the notes of the other team members. This process was changed and their assessments and interventions became part of the transdisciplinary patient-care record.

The "Zero Acceptance of Pain" (ZAP) cancer pain-assessment protocol is another example of a transdisciplinary approach to pain management (Fortner et al., 2003). This protocol was developed by cancer pain specialists, with funding for its implementation and testing provided by the Anesta Corporation. The protocol was designed for oncology practices and physicians' offices. Once again, every member of the practice, from receptionist to physician, was empowered to screen and assess a patient's pain. They were given tools to assess and document pain, and protocols to intervene appropriately. Patients were taught that they could call and say, "I am experiencing pain" and it would be treated. The roles and identities of team members truly were transparent to the patient who made the call and needed help.

Benefits of Team Processes

Although interdisciplinary teams have been the traditional name given to teams in end-of-life care, many teams may read these descriptions and realize they are functioning at a higher level—perhaps cross-functional or even transdisciplinary. Whatever the name, there are many benefits of a comprehensive, collaborative team approach to end-of-life care, including:

- Working for common goals
- Pooling of expertise
- Having a forum for problem-solving
- Having opportunities for personal growth and development
- Being able to share burdens and offer personal support, particularly for professional self-care (von Gunten, Ferris, Portenoy, and Glajchen, 2001)

The skills of multiple disciplines are required in providing thorough end-of-life care. Patients are whole persons with many dimensions. Patients need a social worker, for example, to focus on emotional and social health. They need a physician to focus on treating disease. They require a nurse to focus on treating the human response to pathology. They may want a chaplain to focus on spiritual health. Patients and families have different needs and vulnerabilities, and may express these needs to different providers. Team members bring not only their expertise, but their personalities and life experience to their patient encounters. Moreover, caring for patients at the end of life can be physically demanding and emotionally draining. Having a team with which to share these feelings is an important component of personal self-care.

LEVELS OF INTERDISCIPLINARY CARE DELIVERY

The interdisciplinary team is the vehicle for providing end-of-life care. Care provided by the team can be delivered at three levels. Von Gunten and colleagues (2001) describe *Primary, Secondary, and Tertiary Model of Palliative Care Delivery*.

Primary Palliative Care

By definition, primary palliative care is provided by all health-care professionals, no matter what their setting or practice. Primary palliative care is offered by the interdisciplinary team in doctors' offices, clinics, hospitals, nursing homes, and home-health agencies. All individual practitioners are expected to have a basic competency in primary palliative or end-of-life care. The initiative of the Joint Commission on Accreditation of Healthcare Organizations (JCAHO) to ensure that all patients are assessed for pain would be an example of primary palliative care (von Gunten et al., 2001). Ensuring that patients have been given information to make informed decisions regarding advance directives would be another example. In general, primary palliative care is provided by and is an expectation of all health-care practitioners. At this level, they are not providing care as part of an interdisciplinary team per se, although, of course, they are part of the health-care team.

Secondary Palliative Care

Specialized services, provided by an interdisciplinary team, constitute secondary palliative care. In secondary palliative care, the members of the health-care team have advanced knowledge and expertise that exceeds that of providers of primary palliative care. Practitioners provide services to patients in settings such as inpatient or outpatient hospice, or are members of palliative-care teams.

Nurses who choose to become certified in hospice and palliative nursing have developed a level of expertise and knowledge that demonstrates their competency in secondary palliative care. Certification is offered through the National Board for Certification of Hospice and Palliative Nurses (NBCHPN). The credential for those who successfully meet the requirements and pass the examination is "CHPN." Physicians can also be certified as palliative medicine specialists by the American Academy of Hospice and Palliative Medicine (AAHPM).

WWW.   Internet Reference Box

For more information on certification in hospice nursing, visit the NBCHPN Web site at *http://www.nbchpn.org/*.

For more information on physician certification, visit the AAHPM Web site at *http://www.aahpm.org/*.

Tertiary Palliative Care

Tertiary care exceeds the ability of secondary care. Practitioners work at referral centers and have expertise in difficult problems. Tertiary palliative care is generally provided in academic medical centers where specialist knowledge for the most complex cases is practiced, researched, and taught (von Gunten, 2002). The types of problems these patients may experience include severe pain syndromes, terminal agitation, and terminal restlessness. It should be noted that a patient may move between requiring secondary and tertiary care. For example, a patient may require a brief in-hospital stay on a tertiary-care unit because of severe pain that is not being well controlled by the current regimen. Once a new pain-treatment plan has been developed, implemented, and evaluated for its success, the patient may very well return home with care again being provided by the members of the secondary-level team.

MEMBERS OF THE HOSPICE INTERDISCIPLINARY TEAM

By regulation in the United States, the hospice interdisciplinary team must include, at a minimum, a doctor of medicine or osteopathy, a registered nurse, a social worker, and a chaplain or spiritual counselor. In addition, the hospice must employ, or have a formal agreement with, a licensed pharmacist to provide advice on ordering, storing, administering, disposing, and record-keeping of medications (Lipman, 2002). With the comprehensiveness of this role, the pharmacist is typically a full member of the interdisciplinary team (Arter & Berry, 1993; Berry, Pulliam, Caiola, and Eckel, 1981). A variety of other professionals may also be team members, including:

- Ethicists
- Specialists, such as psychiatrists, psychologists, or practitioners with expertise in pain management
- Therapists (occupational, physical, art, and music)
- Dieticians or nutritionists
- Bereavement counselors

Important nonprofessional members of the care team include licensed practical nurses, nursing assistants, and volunteers. Their roles will be discussed more fully in a subsequent section.

Physician

The physician member of the team is responsible for the medical component of the patient's care. The physician serves as a liaison between the patient's primary care physicians and the hospice program staff (Lipman, 2002). Physicians working in hospice tend to come from a wide variety of backgrounds, including surgery, anesthesia, family medicine, oncology, psychiatry, and internal medicine, to name a few (Ajemian, 1994). To be effective in end-of-life care, the physician must have a broad base of clinical expertise, plus a commitment to a philosophy of care that sees the patient as a total person. "Physicians are called to be healers with their whole person, and in addition to their professional competence will need the personal qualities of compassion, patience, maturity, and confidence that enable this to happen"

Box 4-1 ■	CORE PHYSICIAN COMPETENCIES FOR THE INTERDISCIPLINARY TEAM

- Understands human health and disease, especially end-of-life disease processes
- Possesses expertise in end-of-life diagnosis and symptom control
- Communicates effectively
- Leads palliative treatment planning
- Helps to clarify the goals of care by affirming and listening to other team professionals
- Facilitates decision-making

(Swanson, 1990). The core competencies of the physician member of the interdisciplinary team are listed in Box 4-1. The physician is responsible for diagnosis of disease progression and prescription of palliative treatment. He or she maintains current palliative knowledge and enjoys ongoing communication with the rest of the team to provide care for the whole person.

> *Physicians are called to be healers with their whole person, and in addition to their professional competence will need the personal qualities of compassion, patience, maturity, and confidence that enable this to happen (Swanson, 1990).*

Registered Nurse

Many of the qualities that draw people into nursing—intimacy, equality, nurturing, and conscience—are the same qualities that draw nurses into end-of-life care (Fagin & Diers, 1983). The registered nurse is the team member who will spend the most time with the patient and family, at home or in an inpatient setting. This gives the registered nurse the unique opportunity to know the patient intimately, even when there may be only days left in the patient's life.

The registered nurse has responsibility for the patient's physical and psychosocial comfort, as well as for care coordination. It is important for the nurse to have excellent skills in end-stage physical assessment, disease progression, and pain and symptom management. The nurse has an important role in teaching the patient and family about their role in caregiving, including medication administration, equipment use, skin care, and management of daily living. Like the physician, the nurse must have a commitment to listening and counseling the whole person and family. The registered nurse will have responsibility for supervising the other nursing-related personnel on the team, including licensed practical nurses, certified nursing assistants, and home-health aides (Egan & Labyak, 2001). Day-to-day coordination of

> ### Box 4-2 ■ CORE PROFESSIONAL NURSE COMPETENCIES FOR THE INTERDISCIPLINARY TEAM
>
> - Performs skilled psychosocial and physiological assessments
> - Communicates patient needs and status to the team
> - Supports patient and family participation in decision-making
> - Advocates for the patient and family
> - Organizes the patient's environment to minimize loss of control
> - Plans and implements palliative nursing interventions in concert with other disciplines
> - Educates patient and family regarding course of disease and interventions
> - Provides psychosocial support

care and maintaining communication among the team members are important responsibilities. The nurse must also oversee the plan of care and evaluate its effectiveness in meeting patient goals. Core competencies for the registered nurse are listed in Box 4-2.

Social Worker

A social worker with expertise in end-of-life care is a central member of the team, but as von Gunten and colleagues (2001) note, the discipline of social work is often poorly understood. Social workers have extensive knowledge and expertise in psychology and family systems. Their goal is to help the patient and family deal with the personal and social problems of illness, disability, and impending death.

Social work interventions typically involve one of two types: instrumental services, such as referral to needed community services; or emotional support, including individual counseling, family counseling, and after death bereavement counseling. Many professionals are familiar with the social worker's instrumental interventions but are less knowledgeable about their expertise in counseling. Unfortunately, for social workers, counseling is often the work that they often find more compelling and important, especially in end-of-life care. Thus, it is particularly important for social workers to clarify their role on the interdisciplinary team (Ajemian, 1994). Core competencies for social workers are listed in Box 4-3.

Spiritual Counselor

The spiritual component of care is significant in end-of-life care. The spiritual care professional may have a variety of titles, among them chaplain, clergy person, spiritual counselor, pastoral counselor, or pastoral care worker. The

Box 4-3 ■	CORE SOCIAL WORKER COMPETENCIES FOR THE INTERDISCIPLINARY TEAM

- Assesses the patient and family reaction to the illness and the implication of the illness for their lives
- Determines physical and social resources
- Provides needed psychosocial information
- Mobilizes needed health and community resources
- Promotes effective communication with the patient/family unit
- Fosters insight and adjustment to social consequences of illness and loss
- Assists in practical planning
- Helps with financial challenges and insurance benefits
- Offers counseling and emotional support
- Provides bereavement services for complicated grief after the patient's death

Source: Adapted from von Gunten, Ferris, Portenoy, and Glajchen (2001).

spiritual care professional on the hospice interdisciplinary team may be grounded in a strong religious tradition, but does not evangelize and comes to the dying person in an open way that is nondenominational, nonsectarian, and all-inclusive (Lipman, 2002). Care may be provided by the spiritual care professional in coordination with the patient's own clergy, if such a person is a part of the patient's life.

The goal of hospice spiritual care is to support the patient and the family. The approach is nonjudgmental and focuses on healing, forgiveness, and acceptance. Spiritual interventions are many and varied, and can include prayer, rites, rituals, singing, and assistance in planning and performing funerals. The core competencies for the spiritual care professional are listed in Box 4-4.

Box 4-4 ■	CORE CHAPLAIN COMPETENCIES FOR THE INTERDISCIPLINARY TEAM

- Assesses spiritual distress and opportunities for spiritual growth
- Provides support and counseling to the patient/family
- Leads or promotes supporting rituals, as appropriate
- Promotes linkages to the faith community

Source: Adapted from von Gunten, Ferris, Portenoy, and Glajchen (2001).

Pharmacist

The pharmacist plays a key function on the interdisciplinary team, with activities that are a blend of both traditional and expanded roles. Responsibilities fall in the areas of clinical practice, administration, and support to other team members. Larger hospices may have their own pharmacist; smaller hospices will have contracts with consulting pharmacists.

Pain and symptom management are always key goals of pharmacist care. The pharmacist maintains medication profiles and monitors all medication use, both prescription and nonprescription, for safety and effectiveness. He or she provides medications to patients within a time frame that ensures continuous symptom control and avoids the need for emergency medical services (Lipman, 2002). Pharmacists also work to provide medications in nonstandard forms and dosages to meet specialized patient needs.

Pharmacists have a role in educating other team members about medication therapy, including dosage forms, routes of admission, costs, and availability. They can provide advice to the team about the potential for toxicity from and interactions with dietary supplements and alternative and complementary therapies.

The scope of practice for pharmacists recognizes their authority and responsibility. They must meet the same standards as other providers for quality and continuity of patient care. They must demonstrate requisite knowledge and skills and must maintain their knowledge through ongoing education and specialty residencies. Core competencies for hospice pharmacists are listed in Box 4-5.

Box 4-5 ■ CORE PHARMACIST COMPETENCIES FOR THE INTERDISCIPLINARY TEAM

- Assesses the appropriateness of medication orders
- Ensures the timely provision of effective medications for symptom control
- Counsels and educates the hospice team about medication therapy
- Ensures that patients and caregivers understand and follow the directions provided with the medications
- Provides efficient mechanisms for extemporaneous compounding of nonstandard dosage forms
- Addresses financial concerns
- Ensures safe and legal disposal of all medications after death
- Establishes and maintains effective communication with regulatory and licensing agencies

Source: Adapted from von Gunten, Ferris, Portenoy, and Glajchen (2001).

Other Team Members

As previously noted, there are many other workers who may be called to action as part of the interdisciplinary team, depending on the patient's and family's needs and situation.

Certified Nursing Assistant/Home-Health Aide

These team members provide basic physical and functional care where there is a need, and they also offer family support. They can provide assistance with activities of daily living, such as bathing, grooming, skin care, mouth care, and positioning. They are usually selected from those with extensive training and experience in home health, skilled nursing facilities, and hospitals.

Homemaker/Companion

In contrast to the certified nursing assistant, these team members do not provide direct hands-on care. The homemaker can assist with light housekeeping, meal planning and preparation, laundry, shopping, and companionship. For many elderly patients who live alone, a homemaker is the member of the team that allows them to remain independent in their home until their death.

Ethicist

End of life is a difficult time, fraught with discussions and decisions that must be made in the context of a terminal illness. We would all like to believe in a "good death" and family units that are functional, articulate, cohesive, and able to adapt to changing situations (Fisher, 2003). Unfortunately, that is not always the case and there are times when professional intervention is required to help family members have a meaningful discussion and make difficult decisions. Ethics consultation may be the required forum for resolving these differences (Dalinis, 2004; Hayes, 2004). Larger hospices contract with ethicists to consult about ethical dilemmas at the end of life. Often, an ethics committee meeting is convened to explore ethical decision-making.

Therapists

A variety of therapists, including physical, occupational, art, and music, may be called on to share their expertise. A physical therapist can help a patient maintain a realistic level of activity in light of diminishing muscle strength. Interventions such as massage and range-of-motion exercises can improve circulation and help prevent contractures. An occupational therapist can also assist the patient to maintain an independent level of function through adaptive equipment selection and use. Finding a balance between the "medical milieu" and play/leisure is also an important role of the occupational therapist (Ajemian, 1994). Therapists in music and art can provide expressive languages that may be necessary alternatives for the patient at a time of need.

WWW.   Internet Reference Box

"The Journey Home: Stories from Hospice" was a production by KUED-TV in Salt Lake City, Utah. This Web site features commentary from different members of the hospice interdisciplinary team. Read, in their own words, what it means to be a member of the team: *http://www.kued.org/productions/journey/team/.*

Volunteers

Volunteers fill a very important position in end-of-life care. Since the beginnings of "modern" hospice in the United States, volunteers have played a crucial role in providing a wide variety of services, from direct care to companionship, to "behind-the-scenes" administrative work in hospice program offices. Almost 90% of California hospices surveyed provide bereavement support at no charge to the bereaved; much of this support is offered by volunteers (Foliart, Clausen, and Siljestrom, 2001).

In many communities, the delivery of end-of-life care has changed over time. Many of the hospice programs that exist today began as all-volunteer programs. They have evolved to become professional organizations with a strong volunteer component (Steinhauser, Maddox, Person, and Tulsky, 2000). Within this context, the role of the volunteer becomes even more important. As Ajemian (1994) notes, "There is often a major gulf between the professional world of the institution or healthcare program and the community it serves. Volunteers bridge this gulf, bringing a special dimension of community support to the program and reminding healthcare professionals of the particular needs of that community" (p. 20). Ideally, volunteers come from the neighborhoods and communities they serve. Thus, a Latino volunteer may be able to relate to a patient from the same community and interpret her needs to the interdisciplinary team. Likewise, a senior volunteer who has lived all her life on a farm is able to make special connections and explain the values and needs of her neighbors.

66 | *There is often a major gulf between the professional world of the institution or healthcare program and the community it serves. Volunteers bridge this gulf, bringing a special dimension of community support to the program and reminding healthcare professionals of the particular needs of that community (Ajemian, 1994, p. 20).*

Who serves as a volunteer? Volunteers come from all areas of the community and have diverse backgrounds. Many nurses begin their work in end-of-life care as volunteers and many volunteers come to hospice through personal experience with bereavement (Gaydos, 2004; Payne, 2001). Volunteers are men and women of all ages and walks of life, even teens can be trained as junior hospice volunteers (Letizia, Zerby, Hammer, and Tinnon, 2000).

Some of the most compelling stories of hospice volunteers come from prisons. There is a growing movement in this country to develop hospice programs within prisons (Craig & Craig, 1999) to serve the needs of prisoners who die while serving their sentence. For instance, in the Louisiana State Penitentiary in Angola, 85% of the 5108 inmates are expected to die at the prison (Evans, Herzog, and Tillman, 2002). Because of statistics like this, the California Medical Facility in Vacaville has an active inmate hospice volunteer program with more than 50 trained participants (Linder, Knauf, Enders, and Meyers, 2002). The volunteers perform many duties, including sitting vigil with actively dying inmates and providing bereavement services to other inmates, staff, and members of the free community.

■
WWW.   **Internet Reference Box**

Learn more about the prison hospice program at the National Prison Hospice Association Web site: *http://www.npha.org/index.html.*

All hospice volunteers undergo some form of training. Typically, a volunteer orientation session lasts 24 to 36 hours and is held over several weeks. The curriculum covers topics such as the physical, psychological, emotional, financial, spiritual, and social concerns of the patient and family. Training is provided by professionals and by experienced hospice personnel.

Once the training program is complete, the volunteer is assigned to a role according to personal interest and hospice need. Most opt to work directly with the dying patients and families, but many take on other responsibilities, including providing administrative support, participating in fundraising, or serving as consultants on public relations and community education.

■ ह▲ **Planting the Seeds**

Consider contacting a local hospice to learn more about its volunteer program. This is often an ideal introduction to the world of hospice and palliative care. You will learn about both physical and emotional support for dying people and their families. Whether you ever choose to practice as a hospice or palliative-care nurse, you will find that your new skills will be relevant to most areas of nursing practice. You will deepen your ability to care for the whole family and individuals who are experiencing loss and physical, as well as emotional, suffering.

TEAM WORK AND TEAM SUPPORT: PUTTING THE PIECES TOGETHER

Successful teams require a high level of commitment from the members, development of trust, and openness to communication and problem-solving. Twelve characteristics of effective teams are presented in Box 4-6. For instance, consider the impact of an interdependent team that works as an organic whole. The team's problem has been that Frank Chen will not take his oral morphine around-the-clock as ordered. He waits until the pain is really extreme. The total picture that explains his nonadherence gradually emerges as the volunteer comes to understand his Chinese family background, the chaplain learns about his religious beliefs, and the social worker uncovers his stoical values through expert interviewing. Then, the nurse proposes incorporating traditional Chinese healing methods and the physician changes the

---

Box 4-6 ■   CHARACTERISTICS OF EFFECTIVE TEAMS

1. A team is organic, a whole that is greater than the sum of the individual component players.
2. A team is interdependent, all members succeeding together or failing together.
3. A team is stimulating, and spurs individual members to greater achievement.
4. A team is fun, with members enjoying a sense of belonging and camaraderie.
5. A team is civilized, structured, with members submerging their individual aspirations in a larger objective, as they learn to share and interact.
6. Teams demand a certain conformity, but not uniformity.
7. Team members must share their vulnerabilities as well as their strengths.
8. Difficult conversations are best conducted face-to-face.
9. Confident teams allow flexible professional roles.
10. Difficult decisions need to be shared.
11. Personal exchange can lead to professional growth.
12. Formal review improves future performance.

Source: Adapted from Ajemian (1994).

prescriptions to an opioid that is long-acting and need be taken only once daily. The wisdom of the whole is greater than the sum of its parts.

Many people have described caring for those at the end of their life as a privilege. But at the same time, the work can be emotionally draining and extract a toll from the individual. This is also true for the interdisciplinary team, which may face losses on an almost daily basis. Therefore, it is essential that the team have a process in place to provide for support of its members. Without this, the team is doomed to functional problems. The next section describes team stressors and support mechanisms.

Stressors for Teams

In the previous chapter, individual stressors were discussed in depth. Individuals can bring those same stressors to their team membership, which in turn, can cause problems for team functioning. There are also stressors that are unique to the team experience and arise as part of a group of people coming together to share common goals (Cairns, Thompson, and Wainwright, 2003). Some of these team-specific stressors include experiences when:

- Team members display a lack of trust, support, or respect for each other.
- The members are unclear about roles. This may include specialized skills and abilities, unique strengths, and overlap between roles.
- Team members have unrealistic expectations of one another.
- The members have conflicting beliefs or values about teamwork.
- Members work in isolation or with minimal communication. This can be particularly problematic for someone who has the mindset to work in a multidisciplinary team model but needs to change and adapt to a more interdisciplinary focus.

External stressors in the work environment can also affect team function. Important stressors to consider in this realm include:

- Inadequate resources to meet needs, including human, financial, and administrative
- Unrealistic expectations, especially around workload and schedules
- Conflicting beliefs about patient care and decision-making
- Poor communication at all levels of the organization
- Perceived lack of appreciation

Providing Support

Support comes from many levels, including the individual team members and the larger organizational structure. The latter is very important and can make a true difference in the long run. Organizational leaders must take a very broad view of support and provide it to their teams at every opportunity.

Box 4-7 ■   **SUPPORT PROGRAM PRINCIPLES**

1. Professionals, volunteers, and others who work with dying patients and their families, before death and during bereavement, require support to ensure that both their health and a high quality of care are maintained.
2. Primary responsibility for self-care lies with individual team members, with support from the organization.
3. Support programs must address the needs of the team, while being sensitive to the needs of the individual.
4. Support programs must be valued, encouraged, formalized, and funded by the organization.
5. Support must be embedded in an organizational culture that acknowledges the impact of working with death and bereavement, and that encourages open communication, shared decision-making, and risk taking.
6. An organization's commitment to support of health-care providers should be equivalent to its commitment to patients and families.
7. Support programs must be comprehensive, addressing various sources of stress and offering a continuum of strategies moving from prevention through crisis intervention, treatment, and rehabilitation.

Source: From Cairns, Thompson, and Wainwright (2003).

Box 4-7 identifies Support Program Principles. Likewise, it is important to realize that no single approach is likely to address everyone's needs and that peoples' needs change depending on the situation they are experiencing. For instance, an agency-wide exercise program will be supportive to some people and not others. Chapter 3 examines strategies for staying healthy within the context of organizational challenges.

Jones (2003) describes the practice of "clinical supervision" in the United Kingdom. With a trusted supervisor or supportive colleague, palliative care team members are able to examine different ways to help challenging patients and discuss troubling emotional and moral reactions to nursing situations. In sharp contrast to practice that is isolated and nonreflective, they ponder together the struggles of working at the end of life.

Other approaches for providing team support may include social events, educational workshops, and team involvement in problem-solving and decision-making. Activities may be planned or spontaneous and formal or informal. It is probably wise for some members of the team to engage in some activities that are specific to their discipline; for nurses, this may be attending continuing education conferences such as those sponsored by the

Hospice and Palliative Nurses Association (HPNA). Interdisciplinary activities are also important, however, and should not be ignored. Many hospices organize periodic memorials in which the entire team gathers to grieve recent deaths. Memorials may include music, candle lighting, solemn readings, and acknowledgment of each patient who has died. Taking time to honor the members of the team is also important. It is vital to recognize celebrations, plan transition rituals, and provide opportunities for renewal. It is important to remember birthdays, weddings, births, adoptions, and other life transitions.

WWW.   Internet Reference Box

At the highest level, hospice and palliative care professional associations model interdisciplinary teamwork with both individual conferences as well as jointly sponsored conferences among organizations. You can learn more about all of these activities at the following Web sites:

HPNA: *www.hpna.org* American Academy of Hospice and Palliative Medicine (AAHPM): *www.aahpm.org*

The National Hospice and Palliative Care Organization (NHPCO): *www.nhpco.org.*

To be effective, support programs must address the full range of activities of the team. Ongoing education and training are important for skill development and maintaining a high level of knowledge and expertise. Health-care professionals have a commitment to keep abreast of new knowledge, research, and innovations in their disciplines.

Communication is vital. Most interdisciplinary teams have regularly scheduled meetings, but other mechanisms for ongoing communication should also be explored. E-mail listservs among team members might be an option. If an agency does not have e-mail capabilities, broadcast voice mail might be possible. A newsletter or dedicated message board might be another way to keep communication flowing freely between meetings.

> *Taking time to honor the members of the team is also important. We should recognize celebrations, plan transition rituals, and provide opportunities for renewal.*

Team-building should not be ignored. Like a marriage, having a successful team takes commitment and time. It is helpful for team members to engage in those activities that help to build team cohesiveness and understanding. Examples include a retreat to explore the team mission, vision, and goals. Participation in activities like a "ropes course" may challenge the team in new and different ways.

CONCEPTS IN ACTION

At the local hospice, the volunteer coordinator and the director of nursing had planned a day-long retreat for the members of the agency, including nurses, physicians, the hospice pharmacist, social workers, volunteers, and other members of the program. Because time was short to plan the retreat, the coordinator and director had met with only a few people to get ideas for the day. Still, they were excited about the program and thought it would be a good opportunity for the staff to "take a break" and find some time for renewal. They planned a variety of activities, including continuing education sessions on pain and symptom management; a Native American leading a drumming session; and a humor consultant speaking on "Bringing Joy Into the Workplace." The program would be offered to staff at no charge, but it was scheduled for a Saturday. If staff wanted to be paid for their time, they had to take it as a vacation day.

In the days before the program, the planners received several angry e-mail messages. Some people complained about the program. One nurse wrote, "I am sick of pain management. That's all we ever hear." Another wrote, "What's with the drumming? That is tacky." A volunteer commented, "I think a discussion of 'humor' is completely unprofessional in the context of working with terminally ill and dying patients." There were also widespread complaints about the need to use vacation time to attend the conference and many staff members were threatening a boycott of the whole day.

The coordinator and volunteer met over coffee to discuss what had gone wrong in their planning. As they looked at each other, they said in unison, "We were only trying to do something nice for the staff. Can't they appreciate our efforts?"

- If you were a staff member, would you appreciate their efforts?
- What could they have done differently to plan the day?
- What do you think of the mix of topics on the agenda for the retreat?
- What is the level of organizational commitment to team support?
- In the days before the event, should the coordinator and director try to do anything to "put out the fires" that have arisen? List their possible options with pros and cons of each. What would you choose to do?
- What lessons can be learned from this for the future?

References

Ajemian, I. (1994). The interdisciplinary team. In D. Doyle, G. W. Hanks & N. Macdonald (Eds.), *Oxford textbook of palliative care* (pp. 17–28). New York: Oxford University Press.

Arter, S., & Berry, J. I. (1993). The provision of pharmaceutical care to hospice patients: Results of the National Hospice Pharmacist Survey. *Journal of Pharmaceutical Care, Pain and Symptom Control, 1*(1), 25–42.

Beresford, L. (1993). *The hospice handbook: A complete guide.* Boston: Little, Brown.

Berry, J. I., Pulliam, C. C., Caiola, S. M., & Eckel, F. M. (1981). Pharmaceutical services in hospices. *American Journal of Hospital Pharmacy, 38*(7), 1010–1014.

Cairns, M., Thompson, M., & Wainwright, W. (2003). *Transitions in dying and bereavement.* Baltimore: Health Professions Press.

Craig, E. L., & Craig, R. E. (1999). Prison hospice: An unlikely success. *American Journal of Hospice & Palliative Care, 16*(6), 725–729.

Crawford, G. B., & Price, S. D. (2003). Team working: palliative care as a model of interdisciplinary practice. *Medical Journal of Australia, 179*(Suppl 6), S32–S34.

Dalinis, P. (2004). Bioethics consultations. *Journal of Hospice and Palliative Nursing, 6*(2), 117–122.

Egan, K. A., & Labyak, M. J. (2001). Hospice care: A model for quality end-of-life care. In B. R. Ferrell & N. Coyle (Eds.), *Textbook of palliative nursing* (pp. 7–26). New York: Oxford University Press.

Evans, C., Herzog, R., & Tillman, T. (2002). The Louisiana State Penitentiary: Angola prison hospice. *Journal of Palliative Medicine, 5*(4), 553–558.

Fagin, C., & Diers, D. (1983). Nursing as metaphor. *New England Journal of Medicine, 309*(2), 116–117.

Fisher, C. (2003). The invisible dimension: Abuse in palliative care families. *Journal of Palliative Medicine, 6*(2), 257–264.

Foliart, D. E., Clausen, M., & Siljestrom, C. (2001). Bereavement practices among California hospices: Results of a statewide survey. *Death Studies, 25*(5), 461–467.

Fortner, B. V., Okon, T. A., Ashley, J., Kepler, G., Chavez, J., Tauer, K., et al. (2003). The zero acceptance of pain (ZAP) quality improvement project: Evaluation of pain severity, pain interference, global quality of life, and pain-related costs. *Journal of Pain Symptom Management, 25*(4), 334–343.

Gaydos, H. L. B. (2004). The living end: Life journeys of hospice nurses. *Journal of Hospice and Palliative Nursing, 6*(1), 17–26.

Hayes, C. (2004). Ethics in end-of-life care. *Journal of Hospice and Palliative Nursing, 6*(1), 36–45.

Jones, A. (2003). Clinical supervision in promoting a balanced delivery of palliative nursing care. *Journal of Hospice and Palliative Nursing, 5*(3), 168–175.

Letizia, M., Zerby, B., Hammer, K., & Tinnon, W. (2000). The development of a hospice junior volunteer program. *American Journal of Hospice and Palliative Care, 17*(6), 385–388.

Linder, J. F., Knauf, K., Enders, S. R., & Meyers, F. J. (2002). Prison hospice and pastoral care services in California. *Journal of Palliative Medicine, 5*(6), 903–908.

Lipman, A. (2002). ASHP statement on the pharmacist's role in hospice and palliative care. *American Journal of Health-System Pharmacy, 59*(18), 1770–1773.

Mazanec, P., Bartel, J., Buras, D., Fessler, P., Hudson, J., Jacoby, M., et al. (2002). Transdisciplinary pain management: A holistic approach. *Journal of Hospice and Palliative Nursing, 4*(4), 228–234.

Parker, G. M. (1994). *Cross-functional teams: Working with allies, enemies and other strangers.* San Francisco: Jossey-Bass.

Payne, S. (2001). The role of volunteers in hospice bereavement support in New Zealand. *Palliative Medicine, 15*(2), 107–115.

Steinhauser, K. E., Maddox, G. L., Person, J. L., & Tulsky, J. A. (2000). The evolution of volunteerism and professional staff within hospice care in North Carolina. *Hospice Journal, 15*(1), 35–51.

Swanson, R. W. (1990). Role of the family physician in treatment of cancer. *Canadian Family Physician, 36*, 389.

von Gunten, C. F. (2002). Secondary and tertiary palliative care in U.S. hospitals. *Journal of the American Medical Association, 287*(7), 875–881.

von Gunten, C., Ferris, F., Portenoy, R., & Glajchen, M. (Eds.). (2001). *CAPC manual: How to establish a palliative care program.* New York: Center to Advance Palliative Care.

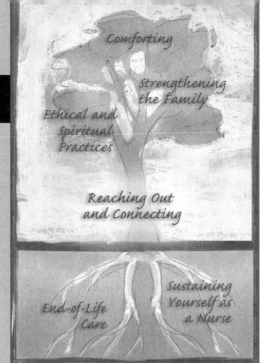

Comforting

Strengthening
the Family

Ethical and
Spiritual
Practices

Reaching Out
and Connecting

End-of-Life
Care

Sustaining
Yourself as
a Nurse

REACHING OUT AND CONNECTING

CHAPTER 5

Understanding the Dying Experience

INGE KLIMKIEWICZ AND JOYCE V. ZERWEKH

Philosophical Reflections

"A man may by custom fortify himself against pain, shame, and suchlike accidents; but as to death, we can experience it but once, and all are apprentices when we come to it."

MICHEL DE MONTAIGNE, ESSAYS, 1580–1588

Learning Objectives

1. Identify five different categories of awareness of dying.
2. Identify the types of small deaths that people experience at the end of life.
3. Explore the meaning of suffering at the end of life.
4. Explain how dying can be considered the final stage of growth.
5. Give examples of near-death experiences.
6. Describe interventions for the relief of four kinds of emotional distress commonly experienced at the end of life: depression, anxiety, anger, and powerlessness.

In order to develop relationships with dying patients, we must understand how dying changes living. In the family caregiving model, the trunk of the tree represents the process of developing connections or relationships with dying people. Connecting requires that the nurse develop a fundamental understanding of the human experience of dying. This chapter examines dying when it begins, personal awareness of dying, dying as a final stage of growth, and the experience of small deaths as death draws near. Then the chapter explores suffering at the end of life and some ways to alleviate selected kinds of psychological distress. Finally, the conclusion explores near-death experiences.

A TERMINAL PROGNOSIS

Once they are identified as terminal, patients live in a world apart from mainstream society. Their terminal status sets them apart from healthy and ill people alike. When an illness is identified as serious but not terminal, treatments exist. Regardless of how long the treatment takes, how uncomfortable it is, or how much it may change life goals and expectations, the patient with a nonterminal but serious disease still makes plans to celebrate another birthday, attend another wedding, and watch another sunset.

But when people come to understand their conditions as terminal, the picture changes dramatically. They begin to live with a stopwatch, counting the moments remaining before death. Dying is that ambiguous state of being during which both patient and family anticipate and await death. It is a period of waiting for a terminal event that will mark the beginning of a new life for the survivors, and the absolute end of mortal life for the patient. To quote the late Isaac Asimov, "Life is pleasant. Death is peaceful. It's the transition that's troublesome."

> When people come to understand their condition as terminal, the picture changes dramatically. They begin to live with a stopwatch, counting the moments remaining before death.

When Does Dying Begin?

Philosophers and poets (Box 5-1) have said that dying begins at the moment of birth. Practically, however, the final pathway at the end of life can be sudden and without warning, such as with a fatal heart attack or car crash. In such a case, there may be only seconds or minutes of dying before death occurs. Commonly today, there is a long period of chronic illness that eventually threatens life. But it is often difficult to discern when that serious illness can no longer be medically managed and the person is facing the end of life. Examples include chronic respiratory disease, cardiac failure, renal failure, and many neurological diseases. Finally, there are illnesses that have a clear downhill course despite the best medical interventions. At a certain point, the

---

Box 5-1 ■   PHILOSOPHERS ON DEATH

"The whole of life is nothing but a journey to death." Seneca, 64 A.D.

"Life follows upon death. Death is the beginning of life. Who knows when the end is reached?" Chuang-Tsze, 400 B.C.

"All the time you live, you steal it from death; it is at her charge." Montaigne, 1580

"All flesh weareth out like a garment. For the covenant from the beginning is that thou shalt die the death." Ben Sira, 190 B.C.

"The first breath is the beginning of death." Thomas Fuller, 1732

"Death borders upon our birth, and our cradle stands in the grave." Bishop Joseph Hall, 1608

Source: Stevenson (1965).

---

prognosis will be terminal despite the best resuscitative interventions. Examples are cancer with multiple metastases and end-stage neurological disease, such as Alzheimer's or Parkinson's, in which the person is immobilized and infections have developed. Although it is true that everyone must die, there is a moment when mortality becomes personal. The limitations of life "hit home" for the individual. Kalish (1981) identifies both the objective and subjective elements of dying. Objectively, dying begins when trained personnel have sufficient information to make an informed diagnosis and prognosis. Subjectively, it begins when people acknowledge their own impending death, with or without medical confirmation. The two do not necessarily occur at the same time. For example, dying individuals may continue to hold out hope or deny impending death long after medical prognosis clearly indicates that death is imminent. Test and biopsy results may be withheld from a terminal patient due to advanced age, cultural considerations, or mental state. Consider those suffering from senile dementia, cerebrovascular accident, or brain metastasis. In these cases, it is often family members who are ultimately given the physician's prognosis, and must make life-determining decisions on the patient's behalf. In such cases, the patient has no subjective awareness of dying.

On the other hand, the patient may know subjectively that he or she is dying before tests and health-care professionals confirm it. Many people know their bodies and are attuned to the internal messages they receive. The trip to the physician's office may be more for confirmation than consultation. Did the dying process begin when the patient scheduled the visit to the physician, or when the physician revealed the test results to the patient? Although the beginning of the dying interval may be ambivalent, physiological changes begin to manifest one-by-one. For instance, first there might be changes in bowel patterns, difficulties with digestion, tiredness, and weight loss. Then the side effects of treatment and unrelenting disease progression further impair physiological functioning. Everyday living becomes harder and harder to manage.

Awareness of Dying

Glaser and Strauss (1967) describe types of awareness of dying. In *closed awareness*, the patient is unaware of impending death while the staff and/or family engage in tactics to avoid disclosure. This occurs when the patient does not recognize the signs, the physician avoids the subject, the family guards the secret, and the entire staff keeps the conversation focused on a superficial level. Closed awareness prevents any choice or end-of-life planning for the patient and makes reconciliation with friends and family impossible. In many traditional cultures, speaking of death is believed to do more harm than good. For instance, Greek physicians and nurses fear that revealing the truth to patients will provoke unhealthy emotions (Georgaki, Kalaidopoulou, Liarmakopoulos, and Mystakidou, 2002). Only 11% of Greek physicians disclose the diagnosis of cancer to all their patients and 66% of nurses find it difficult to speak openly to a patient about death.

In *suspicion awareness*, the patient suspects his prognosis but the family and staff do not confirm this, and continue to use tactics to avoid the subject. This occurs because of fear that troubling emotions will be expressed. If the situation is not acknowledged, feelings are avoided.

In *mutual pretense*, all parties are aware of dying but agree to act as if the person is going to live. Neither wants to disturb the other with discomforting news. Tact and silence dominate the environment. Rituals focusing on wellness continue and discussion is about safe subjects. If a nurse or family member witnesses the person crying, he or she will avoid calling attention to the situation and attempt to change the subject. Many cultures, particularly non-Western cultures, place a high value on avoiding the awareness that death is coming closer. In 1886, Leo Tolstoy (1981, pp. 102–103) wrote about the lies required to maintain mutual pretense:

> Ivan Ilyich suffered most of all from the lie, the lie which, for some reason, everyone accepted: that he was not dying but simply ill, and that if he stayed calm and underwent treatment he could expect good results. Yet he knew that regardless of what was done, all he could expect was more agonizing suffering and death. And he was tortured by this lie, tortured by the fact that they refused to acknowledge what he and everyone else knew, that they wanted to lie about his horrible condition and to force him to become a party to that lie. This lie, a lie perpetrated on the eve of his death, a lie that was bound to degrade the awesome, solemn act of his dying to the level of their social calls. . . . He saw that no one pitied him because no one even cared to understand his situation.

Finally, *open awareness* occurs when both staff/family and patient acknowledge dying. The patient then has the opportunity to bring closure to his life, say good-bye, say, "I'm sorry," and state final wishes. Open awareness invites closure not only for the patient, but for loved ones as well.

One challenge to acknowledging death openly is that the terminal nature of many illnesses has changed and continues to change. Some diseases, once terminal, are now chronic, and innovative treatments that may postpone death are developed every day. Thus, patients may be told that their disease is life threatening, but then find that there is still another therapy. The resulting uncertainty yields an ambiguous situation for both patient and family, and postpones closure. The ambiguity often changes the focus from completing tasks at end of life to managing symptoms and anticipating invasive therapies. Rather than discussing dying wishes, a physician might say to someone who is imminently dying, "You're doing so much better. We've gotten your creatinine under control and your hematocrit is looking better, too." However, you might ask, if there are possible therapies, are these people truly "imminently" dying? As body organs fail, there is a limit to the rejuvenation capacities of modern medicine. Often a focus on tests or therapies ignores situations that have become increasingly futile. Understanding the course of terminal illnesses and the challenging art of prognostication will be discussed in Chapter 13. Contemporary physicians tend to avoid talking about terminal prognoses; professional norms favor maintaining an optimistic view (Christakis, 1999).

There is general philosophical agreement among American health professionals that open awareness is best. It allows the family and patient to support each other, and make important end-of-life decisions. Open awareness provides the vehicle for positive interaction between patient and caregivers, and while it may be difficult, it avoids the pain and suffering that accompanies deceit. All other forms of communication require ever-increasing lies and subterfuge to maintain a false sense of hope. Closed, suspicion, and mutual pretense awareness also rob all parties of important opportunities to complete important tasks, such as leave taking, atonement, and forgiveness.

> *Open awareness is best. It allows the family and patient to support each other, and make important end-of-life decisions. Open awareness provides the vehicle for positive interaction between patient and caregivers, and while it may be difficult, it avoids the pain and suffering that accompanies deceit. All other forms of communication require ever-increasing lies and subterfuge to maintain a false sense of hope.*

Planting the Seeds

It takes time to develop the skills of open communication. Begin by sitting beside a patient with life-threatening illness and asking him or her to tell you about thoughts and feelings. Slow down. Invite openness by your body language and tone of voice. Ask a question like, "How are you doing really?" Listen attentively. If the person has not heard a clear message about prognosis from the physician, arrange that. If family need to be brought together to listen to one another, assist as needed.

THE FINAL STAGE OF GROWTH

According to Erikson, the final task in human growth and development is "Integrity versus Despair" (Craven & Hirnle, 2003). During older adulthood, many people evaluate their lives, and develop a sense of peace and acceptance for the life they have lived, with all its perceived faults and shortcomings. Failure to find this peace can cause despair, and a perceived lack of meaning to life. As people age, they usually experience other losses—of friends, family members, and lifestyles. Many octogenarians may be heard lamenting the fact that their companions and peers have predeceased them, and that their world has become empty. For those who feel they have experienced life fully, the greater fear is dying, not death. They often have a sense of peace and acceptance about death itself, but they fear physical suffering.

Death in earlier developmental stages presents challenges of life unfinished. According to Erikson, the task of young adults is "Intimacy versus Isolation," which means that they are seeking relationships. Therefore, a dying 30-year-old man who wanted to marry and have children has to struggle with impending death because he did not fulfill one of his major goals in life. The developmental stage of middle adulthood is called "Generativity versus Stagnation." So it is that a dying 48-year-old mother has to face the prospect of death knowing that she will never return to finish college and that she will not live to meet her own grandchildren.

Recognizing the patient's developmental stage and the reality of what may or may not be accomplished before death, nurses need to understand that terminal patients have arrived at the final stage of life and growth. The dying process offers a rich opportunity for growth, one to be shared by all the participants. They may choose to focus on what is being lost or never accomplished, or reflect on the life lived. In this stage of growth, patients may open their hearts and minds to their loved ones, and share their uniqueness and personhood through meaningful dialogue and story, or choose to shut themselves off from those whose lives they have most touched, and languish in their own fear, anxiety, and suffering. This final stage of growth can be productive or nonproductive. For those willing and able, the final stage can be a transformative experience. It can be a final gift to self and others. For those individuals, dying becomes a final opportunity for awareness and development. "In the very shadow of death one's living experience can yet give rise to accomplishment, within one's own and one's family's system of values" (Byock, 1998, p. 32). Through an acceptance of death and dying, families can together grow and find accomplishment. Byock calls this process *dying well:*

As a dying person reaches developmental landmarks such as experienced love of self and others, the completion of relationships, the acceptance of the finality of one's life, and the achievement of a new sense of self despite one's impending demise, one's life and the lives of others is enriched" (p. 33).

WWW.   Internet Resource Box

See *www.dyingwell.com* to explore the Web site of Dr. Ira Byock and better understand this concept of "dying well."

Likewise, Jaffe and Ehrlich (1997) describe the growth that patient and families can share when they are willing to drop all pretense, and use their time together to garner as much understanding and intimacy as possible. Such honesty and involvement leaves each individual enriched and fulfilled. Although the family must ultimately experience the pain and grief of a loved one's death, the members come away with a sense of satisfaction from their participation in their loved one's final days.

Life Review

Providing patients with an opportunity to speak about their lives and reminisce can enhance growth during this final stage of life. By asking the patients to summarize their lives' important milestones, nurses can guide them to begin to see their lives as meaningful wholes. They are the only ones who can tell the story of their lives and consider what it means. They begin to see their strengths and contributions to both their family and community. Focusing on challenges they faced successfully in the past gives many patients the reassurance and resolve they need to face their current challenge. For terminally ill patients, such insight may provide a keener sense of acceptance and meaning for life.

Knowledge and understanding of the patient's past history help nurses to see the patient as whole and complete, and to provide better care. The patient is no longer a metastatic lung cancer, but has become a husband and father who watched his own father die of the same disease. Life review allows nurses to understand a patient with end-stage liver disease as a former sexually abused teenager who stayed in an oppressive marriage for the sake of her children. Seeing the patient rather than the disease improves patient care. Life review provides substance to the life and allows care of the patient as whole and complete, and not as a terminal illness. Story enhances personhood, and enhanced personhood improves the quality of life and care for terminally ill patients. Consider Hank's dying:

Hank had spent most of his life on merchant ships and squandered much of his adult life on drugs, alcohol, and fast living that resulted in abandoning his family. He had been estranged for many years from his only surviving daughter. Hank considered the telling of "his story" to be a gift to his daughter. His daughter considered the story a labor of love, which brought newfound understanding for the man who was her father. Rather than facing death alone and full of regret, life review aided Hank and his daughter to experience meaning, reconciliation, and accomplishment in their final days together.

> *Seeing the patient rather than the disease improves patient care. It provides substance to the life and allows care of the patient as whole and complete, and not as a terminal illness. Story enhances personhood, and enhanced personhood improves the quality of life and care for terminally ill patients.*

As we listen to each patient's story, we share a listening presence. Presence is putting aside all preconceived notions, all extraneous thoughts, all self-serving behaviors, and focusing all attention on the patient. It is making the patient the center of the universe. It is exposing oneself in order to allow the patient to put aside pretense. It is joining together in the moment. Genuine presence says to the patient, "You are important. Your needs are important. I am here to help, in whatever way I can. I do this because I care." Genuine presence allows patients to express their deepest fears and concerns, and to address their own mortality. Presence reminds the patient that they matter, and that their needs are being heard. The practice of presence is discussed further in the next chapter.

Mitch Albom, in his powerful book, *Tuesdays with Morrie,* describes presence through the words of his beloved teacher, Morris Schwartz. He tells us,

"I believe in being fully present," Morrie said. "That means you should be with the person you're with. When I'm talking to you now, Mitch, I try to keep focus on what's going on between us. I am not thinking about something we said last week. I am not thinking about what's coming up this Friday. . . . I am talking to you. I am thinking about you." (pp. 135–136).

Terminal patients require and deserve this caring presence, especially in light of the losses they continually encounter in the dying process.

SMALL DEATHS

One of the reasons that caring for the dying is so difficult is that dying patients often experience dying gradually, through a series of losses. Each dying patient feels each loss acutely and nurses should be sensitive to the unique experience of each individual. See the following summary of the "small deaths" that may be faced by a dying patient.

Loss of Health

As death draws near, symptoms become more apparent and bodily systems begin to fail. Kidney and liver function may slow, leaving the patient lethargic or ultimately, comatose. Cardiac function may become erratic, leading to poor circulation. Pulmonary function may become inadequate, compromising endurance and further straining the heart's ability to pump oxygenated blood throughout the body. Degeneration of nerve cells or tumor growth may affect cognitive ability. The daily tasks of life become more difficult and greater expenditures of energy are required to perform tasks previously taken for granted. The patient and the family witness bodily disintegration.

Loss of Self-Care Abilities

Activities of daily living (ADLs) will require personal assistance and supportive devices, such as walkers, bedside commodes, wheelchairs, and hospital beds. The patient may no longer be capable of bathing, dressing, or eating independently. Some patients are uncomfortable with their increasing dependence upon others, and issues of privacy may cause personal discomfort for patient and caregiver alike. Cultural and prior family dynamics concerning matters of personal hygiene and privacy are especially relevant.

Loss of Relationships

Feeling inadequate and uncomfortable with their own feelings, friends and relatives often distance themselves. The anticipated death may trigger personal fears concerning their own eventual death. With an extended course of terminal illness, loss of friends and loved ones can be quite pronounced to the point of social death, which involves no longer being acknowledged or seen in the eyes of other persons (Kastenbaum, 1995). People who are dying are "trapped in a diseased and protesting body and existing in a social order that has virtually no use for them" (Moller, 2000, p. 155). In response, those "in the world" find their response to the dying patient to be one of withdrawal and avoidance.

Jose, who was nursed by one author (Klimkiewicz) had endured a social death. Jose had been living in a nursing home for the past 2 years. He suffered from Parkinson's disease, and he was now incapable of speech or movement. He was fed via gastric tube as his body slowly but steadily curved into a fetal position. Though well cared for physically, the staff had stopped thinking of Jose as a complete person. Jose, who was once a major in the Marine Corps, and a graduate of West Point, was now turned and fed and washed and changed without so much as a "hello" or "good morning." Staff cared for the external body without caring about the man trapped within. It was so simple to forget Jose. It was so much easier not to bear witness to the suffering that this man endured. But those eyes! He had marvelous eyes that spoke of the pain of being forgotten.

During my first several visits, Jose looked blankly at me, as though he was unaware of my presence. Slowly he began to accept the fact that I was going to keep coming back, and I was going to give him all of my attention. I asked his permission before taking vitals, or giving him a bed bath. I spoke of current events, and asked his opinion. I asked how he felt, and if there was something he needed. We began to converse, Jose and I. I could tell from his eyes what type of day he was having, or whether he was comfortable. His eyes became his voice, and they laughed and cried. We spoke from the heart of things past and things to come. We marveled at a beautiful sunset and gentle breezes. I will never forget the beauty and clarity with which that man spoke. How sad that more people did not "hear" him. (The practice of nonverbal presence is discussed in Chapter 6.)

Even with patients who have been able to maintain strong family and community connections, the social world implodes as their illness progresses. All but the most essential aspects of living are given up to save strength and energy for essential areas of life. Participation in religious gatherings, such as church, temple, or mosque, may be curtailed or eliminated. Attending celebrations such as marriages, graduations, or promotion parties may be too difficult. Activities such as dining out, going to the movies or theatre, and participating in clubs will dwindle. Through choice or necessity, social interactions are replaced by treatment interactions. As prior social support systems slip away, the patient and family begin sharing their hopes and fears with members of the medical community instead.

> 66   *Even with patients who have been able to maintain strong family and community connections, the social world implodes as their illness progresses.*

Living in Isolation

Many people in America live a remarkably isolated life before their dying begins. Many individuals have chosen to be free of ties to committed relationships, family, and a religious community. Often we live far from those we love. We do this in the name of freedom and independence, but the consequence is often alienation and loneliness. We are left to carve out relationships and a sense of purpose from the transient environment in which we currently exist (Moller, 2000).

Isolation in living predicts isolation in dying. Even with a network of friends and family, the emphasis on privacy and individualism makes it difficult for concerned friends and family to find common experience with the person who is dying. They don't know how to act or what to say. Their friend or relative has become a stranger. Their preoccupation with activities or achievement is distant from the dying person's concerns. Likewise, most people have little experience with disability, illness, and dying because these experiences commonly occur behind closed doors in institutional settings.

However, nurses can guide them to stay connected with the dying person, rather than pulling way.

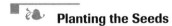

Planting the Seeds

You can play a major role in encouraging friends and family members to visit and maintain supportive connections to dying patients. Many withdraw because they don't know what to say or do. Offer to help them practice what they will say. Teach them to ask the patient what would be helpful. Remind them that actions are louder than words. Encourage them to offer what they do best. For instance, a dying fireman's partners from the fire station visited every day to play cards. He was never alone in the afternoon.

Loss of Intimacy

Knowledge that a life partner is dying often places a strain on the emotional and sexual intimacy shared by a couple. The healthy partner may not have had previous experiences with death and dying, or may be psychologically unable to continue a close relationship. He or she may move out of a shared bedroom, for fear that sleeping together might disturb their loved one's sleep. Likewise, he or she may withdraw as a result of fear or emotional discomfort with the manifestations of the patient's illness. Regardless of the underlying reason, the dying partner can be left feeling alone and betrayed by this loss of intimacy.

Loss of Roles

As health continues to wane, family members and friends may step in and begin to assume roles previously held by the patient. A spouse may begin to manage the household budget, as well as social and medical activities. Head of household duties may shift to the "living" partner, as may household chores. The role of disciplining minor children may shift as well. Adult children may begin asking questions concerning wills, estate planning, and the sale of property. They may begin to assume more dominant roles in decision-making. While the dying patient may still be employed, or attempting to manage an existing business, responsibilities will often shift to others in the organization. Business associates often begin deciding how best to "fill the gap," even before the patient has departed. Slowly but steadily, the patient's roles and responsibilities in all aspects of life will transfer to others.

66 | *Slowly but steadily, the patient's roles and responsibilities in all aspects of life will transfer to others.*

Loss of Identity

Identity and self-image are linked to life roles and responsibilities. People often allow society to define their worth. They identify with the position or titles they hold, the partner they have, the home or other personal belongings they have accumulated. For many people, the loss of vocation is more devastating than death itself. As the terminally ill watch their lives unravel, they may begin to lose a sense of self-worth or personal identity. "When the day comes that we're ill and can no longer be the banker, traveler, doctor or coach, we have to ask ourselves an important question, 'If I'm not those things, then who am I?' " (Kubler-Ross & Kessler, 2000, p. 33).

Loss of Independence

Declining health and needed assistance with ADLs limit a patient's independence. Activities need to be planned in advance, and timed to ensure adequate preparation and completion. As energy wanes, and dependence on both people and assistive devices increases, the more taxing areas of one's life are sacrificed in favor of the more essential elements.

Loss of Financial Security

Many patients recognize that their death has significant negative effects on the family's financial security, and feel responsible for the burden they feel they are causing. Death and dying may place significant monetary strain on family units. As the dying trajectory continues, paid help may be necessary to assist with ongoing family responsibilities, such as house and yard work, or babysitting. For families who are at the higher end of income and savings, disposable income begins to decline as family members provide additional support for the terminal patient at the expense of their own careers. Loss of a principal wage earner threatens future economic security. For those with lower income, paid help is out of the question. Families with dying or caregiving wage earners may find themselves without resources to pay for essentials like food, rent, and heating. After the death, traditional burial rituals can be expensive. In the United States, the costs of medical treatment at the end of life are poorly covered by Medicare and private insurance, and many families are without any insurance. The medical costs of dying and wages lost can heavily burden surviving family members.

Loss of the Future

The human race may be the only species that has a pre-awareness of personal death. By the time we are about 11 years old, we understand that death is permanent and realize the implications of terminal illness (see Chapter 12).

Nonetheless, in our daily lives, we generally assume that our death will not occur in the immediate future. We enroll in school, sign mortgages, purchase automobiles, and plan vacations with full intent of seeing our plans through to completion. The terminal patient, however, recognizes that such plans are tenuous, at best. He views the future in incrementally shorter periods. Shall I plan on a visit with a new grandchild? Will I live to graduate high school? Will I make it to my next birthday? Further, the anticipation of future events is marred by the knowledge that each will occur later in the disease process, and closer to death. Thus, events that would have evoked anticipation and joy may now cause sorrow and fear. Box 5-2 describes the multiple losses and gradual experience of gradual disengagement by a patient who has "Finished My Stay."

Box 5-2 ■

I'VE FINISHED MY STAY

By Inge Klimkiewicz

I know I must die; we all do some day.
But some day, not this day,
Not this day, I pray.

I can't go tomorrow, there are bills left to pay.
And soon will come weddings and babies, I pray.
And what of my husband and children? I say.
Who will hold them, and kiss them, and love them
As I do, only I do, only I should? I say.

I don't mind the pain; it's become an old friend.
But this friend makes me tired and weak at the end.
The things that now surround me don't concern me, I say.
I'm apart now, unattached now.
Soon to go now, I pray.

Time gone is time spent, no matter the way.
My life was my life, the price I did pay.
It was what I made it, and I made it my way.
It might have been different; but then who's to say.
And who would I be then? I ask and I pray.

I may not be ready to leave you today.
But it's time now, to go now.
I've finished my stay.

Go now. It's time now. I'm ready. I say.

Grief in Response to Multiple Losses

Each of these "small deaths" causes suffering and sorrow. The dying person, family, and friends grieve continually over their losses, and it is important that nurses recognize this and are supportive. Chapter 7 explores the nature of grief and ways nurses can care for people living with persistent grief.

EMOTIONAL SUFFERING AT THE END OF LIFE

In addition to sustained grief reactions, the extraordinary losses just detailed lead to a variety of other emotional reactions. Profound emotional suffering is caused by threat to the wholeness and continued existence of the self (Cassell, 1991). The sufferer becomes aware of the disintegration of identity and purpose. Suffering of seriously ill persons begins with their inability to achieve previously important purposes. The person recognizes what he or she cannot do and is conscious of a lost sense of possibility in the future. Initially, the sufferer feels alienated from self, others, and any sense of meaning (Younger, 1995). Working through such suffering requires an initial silent period when there are no words to express the despair, then an expressive phase when telling one's story is vital. As nurses, we are initially "dumbstruck" by the suffering, then we begin to listen and help the sufferers find the words to tell their stories and search for meaning.

66 | *Profound emotional suffering is caused by threat to the wholeness and continued existence of the self (Cassell, 1991). The sufferer becomes aware of the disintegration of identity and purpose.*

It is important that the nurse recognize that emotional suffering cannot be adequately addressed until physical suffering is relieved. Primal needs come first. Many patients enter the dying process after a series of tests, treatments, and hospitalizations in which symptoms were not managed. These earlier experiences with the medical community may have left patients fearing inadequate care and still further physical suffering. In a comprehensive national survey (Teno, 2004), 1578 family members were asked about the quality of care where their deceased relative spent the last 48 hours of life. Nearly one-quarter reported that their loved one did not receive adequate relief of pain or dyspnea; half reported that their loved one did not receive adequate emotional support.

Physiological needs such as physical pain and other symptoms will dominate consciousness until they are controlled. As overwhelming symptoms are managed, the patient becomes aware of emotional suffering. Emotional reactions are manifested as changes in appearance, behavior, or conversation, or as physiological responses to alterations in the autonomic nervous system. Emotional distress makes it difficult for the patient to experience joy in living, and to experience meaning and connection with others. Emotional turmoil causes significant suffering among terminally ill patients and seriously reduces quality of life. This section addresses how nurses can provide relief and comfort for the following emotional problems: powerlessness, anxiety, depression, suicidal ideations, and anger. Nurses are responsible for identifying these problems, providing therapeutic interaction to relieve distress, and collaborating with medical providers to administer medications that provide relief.

Powerlessness

Powerlessness is the state in which a person perceives a lack of personal control over his or her life. Powerlessness increases as dying progresses. Activities of daily living become monumental challenges. Responsibilities are being shouldered by others. Pain and other symptoms are often out of control. Nurses should attempt to help patients retain as much power and control as possible. "No caregiver would consciously or deliberately try to diminish a person's life during its final phases, but we often do so unintentionally: 'Here, eat just another spoonful of applesauce . . . Now take your pill dear; you know it will make you feel better . . . Oh here, I'll do that for you . . .'" (Smith, 1997, p. 1). To the extent possible, it is important to consult patients on their care. They should be asked when it is convenient for visits or assistance with activities of daily living, and consulted concerning treatment options. If patients are competent to make decisions, health-care providers must respect their treatment wishes. Chapter 6, Connecting and Caring Presence, discusses ways to encourage patients' making decisions at the end of life. Box 5-3 identifies empowering nursing strategies at the end of life.

Box 5-3 ■ EMPOWERING STRATEGIES AT THE END OF LIFE

Power through Attention: Listen so that the person feels truly heard.

Power through Identity: Foster self understanding. Ask patients who they are and how they have lived.

Power through Knowledge: Continually teach and explain to minimize fear of the unknown.

Power through Active Choice: Based on self understanding and knowledge, patients are encouraged to make choices. We then are able to advocate for their wishes.

Power through Sustained Network Support: Encourage patients to mobilize their support network and then encourage support network members to sustain their involvement.

Power through Imagination: Envision possibilities for quality of life at the end of life and guide the patient to see these possibilities for choice.

Power through imagination involves encouraging the terminally ill person who is still cognitively intact and functioning with minimal assistance to consider possibilities in the coming months. Does she want to travel? Would she like to live near her children? What does she want to eat that she has been denying herself for years? Chocolate perhaps? What creative decisions could be included in her will? For instance, one high-spirited patient living with metastatic breast cancer chose to re-write her will and gave fanciful vacations to her close friends, who worked too hard and seldom took holidays.

Control of Dying

Some terminal patients are aware of their imminent demise, and seem to be able to modify the timing of their death, either hastening or delaying the event. We don't know how this happens, but hospice team members witness this again and again. An expert hospice nurse describes her mother's dying:

> She knew she was going to be dead by Friday. She was working through her list of things to do before she went. The last thing she wanted was to meet her cousin who was living in her mother's home. So he got there at six o'clock in the evening and she sat up and had a cup of tea with him. She visited and talked about every family member who existed from the time of her birth all the way through her life. About eight o'clock, I was standing at the end of the bed, and she sat forward, and she handed the cup to him. And this look came over her. It was a shadow that traveled from the top of her head all the way down. I said to her, "Mom, is this it?" And she said, "Yes." She lay down and within 30 minutes was in a coma. We called the whole family. When everybody was there, her head fell to the side and within probably 20 minutes she was gone. It was Friday night.

For those who have lost the will to live, surrender and death often proceed quickly. Others, especially those with an especially strong will to live, can and do survive beyond reasonable survival estimates. Patients may cling to life in order to complete important goals, or participate in rituals or events, such as anniversaries or holidays. Once the focus of attention takes place, death comes quickly.

Anxiety

Anxiety at the end of life can be defined as fear of what is both known and unknown (Spencer, 2002). The physiological response to fear involves neurohormone release, including cortisol, epinephrine, norepinephrine, and serotonin. Emotional symptoms of anxiety include feelings of fear and dread, worrying, apprehension, nervousness and irritability, and difficulty concentrating. The physical effects of epinephrine and norepinephrine include trembling, tachycardia, hyperventilation, shortness of breath, sweating, dizziness, nausea, diarrhea, and severe panic reaction. There are many

causes of anxiety in dying patients: the small deaths discussed earlier, anticipated loss of self, fear of death, fear of the unknown, fear of dying in pain,
and physiological changes. Keep in mind that anxiety often has physical
causes in the terminally ill. Anxiety can be an adverse reaction to drugs prescribed to promote comfort. For instance, corticosteroids (prednisone,
dexamethasone) are commonly prescribed at the end of life and can sometimes
precipitate severe anxiety reactions. Likewise, benzodiazepines prescribed for
anxiety can sometimes paradoxically cause anxiety. Organic causes of anxiety
at the end of life include hypoxia, dyspnea, fever, hypoglycemia, and brain
tumor (AAHPM, 2003).

Interpersonal Relief Measures

Connecting and human presence are essential nursing responses when
patients are anxious. Listening to their human experience is the beginning. In
cases of mild anxiety, supportive relationships with health professionals and
loved ones are highly effective to alleviate recurrent distress. Nursing interventions designed to relieve anxiety include the following:

- Naming the underlying cause of fear
- Encouraging expression
- Explanation and anticipation of physical events
- Promoting patient control
- Encouraging physical presence of support persons
- Relaxation and deep breathing
- Imagery and visualization
- Relaxing music
- Interdisciplinary referral for counseling
- Anti-anxiety medication

Consider Amanda, who had been battling cervical cancer for several
years when she was admitted into a hospice residence. Her cancer had
recently infiltrated her abdominal cavity, and her husband, also in failing
health, could no longer manage her pain and distress.

By 1 month after admission to hospice, Amanda's weight had dropped
to 80 pounds. She found it difficult to eat more than a spoonful of pureed
food at a time, and often did so only to please her husband or family.
Metastatic bone pain in her hips and vertebrae had started to become a
problem, and she became more and more nervous and irritable. She had
many physical signs of anxiety, such as tachycardia and trembling, but it
was difficult to distinguish whether the cause was a consequence of cancer
or emotional distress. Amanda's nurse decided to see if she could *name* the
cause of her apparent anxiety and asked her directly, "You seem troubled
with something. Are there some particular things troubling you?" Amanda
replied, "I'm so afraid the pain is going to get worse and worse and I just
can't stand the thought. I feel panicky." This was an opportunity for the
nurse to *explain* the effectiveness of pain relief for metastatic bone pain and

how the hospice team would keep it in check. She emphasized that Amanda would be *in control* of how much medication she took. Amanda's anxiety about pain control was noted on the care plan and in the change of shift report with a recommendation that staff visit her frequently to be a *supportive presence* at her bedside, as well as to ascertain her level of pain and medicate accordingly. One hospice nurse taught Amanda to use imagery *to relax* when she recognized a growing feeling of dread. She learned to imagine herself lying on soft sand with the warm sun heating and comforting her back and hips. She visualized herself at the ocean, feeling the soft breeze and hearing the regular rhythms of the waves. She frequently listened to tapes with the rhythm of the ocean waves in the background. As a result of these interventions, Amanda's anxiety diminished significantly.

Then about a week before Amanda died, the nursing staff still saw new evidence of anxiety. They brought their concerns to the *interdisciplinary* team meeting and the attention of Amanda's chaplain and social worker. Working together, it was discovered that Amanda had been raised Catholic, but converted to Judaism when she married. Now her devout Roman Catholic sisters were concerned about Amanda's eternal soul and regularly shared their concerns with her. Amanda was very close to her sisters, and she had become preoccupied with their worries. She was terribly conflicted. She considered her husband the love of her life, and had embraced Judaism out of her love for him. Together, the staff helped Amanda come to terms with her spiritual distress, and she, with her husband's blessings, received the Catholic Church's Sacraments of the Sick. Long-acting pain medications kept Amanda comfortable and alert for her constant visitors. She was free of pain and anxiety. She had decided that any day early in January would be all right to die, as it wouldn't interfere with her niece's birthday at the end of that month. She died quietly on January 5th with her husband by her side.

Pharmacological Relief of Anxiety

Anti-anxiety drugs should complement interpersonal measures when anxiety intrudes significantly on quality of life. The staff nurse brings the symptoms to the attention to the prescribing provider. There are four categories of anti-anxiety drugs (anxiolytics). By far the most commonly used are the benzodiazepines (such as diazepam, clonazepam, alprazolam, lorazepam). Common side effects are drowsiness and sedation. Depressant effects are aggravated in the presence of other depressant drugs, such as antidepressants and opioids (Damron, 2001). Respiratory suppression is always a risk as doses are initiated or increased. Lorazepam (Ativan) can be considered a prototype benzodiazepine and is very popular in hospice care. It has a rapid onset and is short acting. It can be administered by mouth, through the oral mucosa (sublingual), rectally, intramuscularly, and intravenously. A common dosage is 0.5 to 2 mg, three to four times daily by mouth, but dosage and scheduling must be adjusted to individual differences. It is often used for multiple purposes beyond relief of anxiety. For example, it also can be used to manage muscle spasm, nausea, shortness of breath, and seizures.

Other medications used to relieve anxiety include buspirone (BuSpar), which takes 5 to 10 days to become effective; neuroleptics (major tranquilizers) such as haldoperidol (Haldol) when psychotic symptoms accompany anxiety; hydroxyzine (Vistaril), which also has a direct analgesic effect; and antidepressants when depression accompanies anxiety (Damron, 2001).

Depression

Sadness is a normal human response at the end of life. However, profound sadness can progress to the point of clinical depression. Study by Breitbart and Heller (2003) has revealed that less than 20% of people with a month to live were clinically depressed. Depressive disorders are usually characterized by changes in energy, anorexia, weight loss, fatigue, and disturbances in sleep. However, these symptoms also characterize advancing illness and are of little use in identifying depression in the dying. Therefore, nurses should recognize depressive disorders when such patients demonstrate significant disinterest in activities and loved ones, inability to experience pleasure, expression of worthlessness, persistent guilt and hopelessness, poor concentration, indecisiveness, and wishing for death including suicidal thinking (Abrahm, 2000). Because the person is dying, health professionals often dismiss these symptoms as inevitable. They are not. Quality of life can be improved through treatment; the nurse must be tuned into the patient and refer to the interdisciplinary team. Some clinical scholars are looking beyond the diagnostic label of clinical depression to identify the components of despair specific to those at the end of life. See Box 5-4.

Interpersonal Interventions

How can nurses intervene to relieve this troubling level of depression and despair? We can make interpersonal connections, behavioral interventions, meaning-centered interventions, and cognitive interventions. We can also

---

Box 5-4 ■ COMPONENTS OF DESPAIR AT THE END OF LIFE

- Demoralization
- Loss of dignity
- Loss of meaning
- Hopelessness
- Desire for a hastened death

Source: Breitbart & Heller (2003).

propose complementary therapies, such as music and imagery. The following chapter, Connecting and Caring Presence, examines the essential relationship skills to develop a rapport with patients. Making that connection is the foundation of all interpersonal interventions. Behavioral interventions reinforce positive self-care behaviors and small achievements so that the depressed patient, whose physical abilities are quite impaired, can remain functional for as long as possible. Meaning-centered interventions focus on helping patients identify the sources of meaning that remain in their lives (Breitbart & Heller, 2003). For instance, a patient who has always found meaning in his career can be invited to consider other sources such as love, family, nature, creativity, responsibility, positive deeds, and spiritual growth.

Cognitive interventions are grounded in helping the depressed patient change negative false assumptions that are aggravating depression (Pascreta, Minarik, and Nield-Anderson, 2001). First, the patient is helped to identify self-defeating automatic thoughts, to stop those thoughts, and to consider instead the truth of his or her life. Obviously, there are negative experiences that cannot be changed by substituting positive thoughts. Here are some examples of nurses guiding thought:

> Mr. J. laments, "My life has been worthless."
> The nurse replies, "Tell me about your greatest moments. What has given your life meaning?" The nurse then helps the patient develop this positive line of thinking.
> Ms. A. asserts, "My children all turned out bad."
> The nurse responds, "Tell me about them. What are they doing now?" The nurse then helps the patient restructure preoccupations based on reality, facing the difficult but bringing out the positive.
> Ms. J. sadly states, "I'm nobody now. I was a nursing supervisor in this hospital for 33 years and now I'm just one more complaining patient."
> The nurse replies, "You're nobody? You nursed here for 33 years! Tell me about your career! I bet you've done an awful lot."

Pharmacological Interventions

Antidepressants should be used with interpersonal measures when depression significantly impairs quality of life. The bedside nurse clearly documents symptoms to the prescribing provider. Norepinephrine and serotonin are reduced in depressive disorders, and drug therapy seeks to elevate these neurotransmitters. Thus, depression is treated with tricyclic antidepressants, serotonin-specific reuptake inhibitors (SSRIs), and psychostimulants (Damron, 2001). Tricyclics potentiate serotonin and norepinephrine activity. The first generation of tricyclics includes amitriptyline (Elavil) and doxepin (Sinequan). They are the most studied group of antidepressants. They may take weeks of gradually increasing dosage until a desire effect is attained. Most worrisome side effects include sedation, anticholinergic effects (dry mouth, constipation, delirium), orthostatic hypotension, and cardiac arrhythmias. Given at bedtime, they are highly effective to treat insomnia. Tricyclic antidepressants are known to reduce the pain due to nerve involvement (neuropathic pain).

The SSRIs increase circulating serotonin. The SSRIs cause less sedation and fewer anticholinergic effects than the tricyclics. Representative drugs include citalopram (Celexa), sertraline (Zoloft), and paroxetine (Paxil). Their benefit for neuropathic pain remains uncertain. There are also some newer antidepressants in a class by themselves, such as bupropion (Wellbutrin), which also work to enhance energy. Cost can be a consideration in the use of both SSRIs and newer miscellaneous agents.

The psychostimulants include dextroamphetamine (Dexedrine), methylphenidate (Ritalin), and pemoline (Cylert). They elevate epinephrine and norepinephrine levels and act quickly to energize patients and can significantly promote a feeling of well-being, reduce fatigue, stimulate appetite, and improve attention and concentration (Damron, 2001). Dosage must be carefully adjusted to the individual. Anxiety, restlessness, and insomnia are unwanted side effects.

Sometimes depression leads to thoughts of suicide in those nearing death.

Suicide Risk

Suicidal ideation, or thoughts of suicide, may be due to mental illness or to feelings of profound despair. It may be triggered by the multiple losses previously discussed, particularly loss of control. Physical pain, real or anticipated, may also lead to thoughts of suicide. Box 5-5 identifies Risk Factors for Suicide by Dying Patients.

Box 5-5 ■ RISK FACTORS FOR SUICIDE BY DYING PEOPLE

- Suicidal thinking and planning
- Previous suicide attempts
- Family history of suicide
- Preexisting psychiatric disorder
- Social isolation
- Substance abuse
- Recent death of loved one
- Uncontrolled pain or other symptoms
- Exhaustion and fatigue
- Impulsiveness; loss of inhibition
- Fear of being a burden
- Being an older male
- Severe existential distress

Source: From AAHPM (2003); and Damron (2001).

Nurses working with dying people need to be alert to the risk of suicide, particularly when patients begin to talk about it, plan for it, and have the means to succeed (for instance, drugs or guns). Other risk factors include a previous history of suicide attempts, suicide history in the family, preexisting mental illness, social isolation, substance abuse, and recent death of someone close. Nurses should never shut down the topic when the patient brings it up. Rather, we must be willing to acknowledge the issue and ask questions. For example, Damron (2001) proposes the kind of questions nurses should ask to assess each risk:

- Acknowledging. "Most people living with a terminal illness have passing thoughts of suicide. Do you ever think about it?"
- Planning. "Have you ever thought about how you would do it?"
- Bereavement. "Has someone one close to you died recently?"

Every effort should be made to control depression and resolve underlying calls for help, as discussed earlier. Suicidal thinking and planning need to be reported to the interdisciplinary team to develop a collaborative and supportive individualized plan of care. A major ethical dilemma presents itself today as many patients ask for assistance with suicide. Does the nurse respect patient choice or refuse to participate in any way? This dilemma is explored is Chapter 9 on Ethical and Legal Issues.

Although only a small proportion of terminal patients act on suicidal thoughts, many terminally ill patients do consider suicide at one or more times preceding death. Block (2000) reports as high as 45% of all terminal cancer patients report such thoughts at one or more times during their illness. This is one reason why Humphrey's (2002) do-it-yourself suicide book has become a best seller. *Final Exit* is a self-help book for the terminally ill that describes, in detail, various chemical and physical methods with which terminally ill patients can take their own lives.

In 1997, Oregon became the first state to legalize physician-assisted suicide. This law allows terminally ill patients to request a prescription from their physician for medication that, when taken as prescribed, will cause death. The law does not invite direct physician participation in the terminal event. From 1998 to 2002, 129 patients in Oregon died by physician-assisted suicide. Patients sought suicide as a response to loss of autonomy, reduced ability to participate in enjoyable activities, and lost control of bodily functions.

WWW.   **Internet Resource Box**

The Oregon Department of Human Services maintains a Web site (*www.dhs.state.or.us/publichealth/chs/pas/pascdsum.cfm*) that details the provisions of their Death with Dignity Act and provides an annual report.

What has not been adequately documented are the number of terminally ill patients, nationwide, who deliberately choose to stop eating and drinking. Decreased food intake is common for many patients during the dying process. Many suffer from nausea or difficulty swallowing. Dying persons naturally may experience a period of "terminal withdrawal" during which they lose all interest in food. Some terminal patients, however, simply choose to stop eating and drinking as a way of hastening death. Death normally occurs days to several weeks after the decision is made, depending on the patient's physical state when the decision is made (Quill & Byock, 2000). Death brought about by the voluntary cessation of food and liquid is not reported as suicide, and is only known through anecdotal report.

Planting the Seeds

Never accept anxiety and depression as natural symptoms of dying that cannot be relieved. Learn to recognize their signs and consider whether interpersonal or pharmacological measures should be offered to enhance quality of life. We can disperse the clouds a bit so that the light can penetrate the darkness.

Anger

Why me? What have I done to deserve this! How could life/God/fate be so cruel? According to Kubler-Ross (1969), anger is often "displaced in all directions and projected onto the environment at times almost at random" (p. 64). Family members, God, health and social service agencies, and health-care personnel are frequent targets. Often nurses become the targets of this anger. Some anger is normal. People who have lived a chronically angry life are likely to die as they have lived, angry. Box 5-6 identifies constructive nursing responses to angry dying patients. Imagine yourself responding to a patient who becomes angry when you bring in her medications late. She begins to shout obscenities and proclaims, "You are all torturing me. You're a bunch of sadists who just don't care!" Your initial response might be to defend yourself. Your body might be tense. You might feel a headache threatening and tears welling up. You might be imagining angry words in return. We are all different, but it is critical to be in tune with one's own feelings and not reject the patient. However, you need never passively accept a verbal attack. You might want to give yourself and the patient a "time out" and make a clear statement like "I feel terribly hurt when you call me a sadist. I am going to leave the room to calm down and check on some other patients. When I come back, let's talk about what you are going through."

Many terminal patients have been living with chronic conditions for some time. Illness and the continual cycle of tests and hospitalizations may have been a way of life for months, if not years. The following excerpt from an essay written by a nurse and cancer survivor (Hall, 2003, p. 4)

Box 5-6 ■ CONSTRUCTIVE NURSING RESPONSES TO ANGRY DYING PATIENTS

- Understand one's own response and do not reject the patient because of his or her behavior.
- Accept anger as a natural manifestation of the grief process.
- Do not accept anger that is abusive to you or another person.
- Leave the room or home if the patient cannot control emotional or physical aggression. Explain that you will return when the patient is under control.
- Help the patient name the underlying causes of anger and identify changes that can be made to alleviate the problem.
- Guide the person to explore more constructive ways to express feelings and solve problems.
- Advocate for the person when misunderstanding or injustice can be righted.
- Guide the person to recognize negative consequences of angry behavior.

Source: From Kemp (1999).

bears witness to the anger of many cancer patients as a consequence of being medicalized:

> As cancer patients we are . . . encouraged to live our lives in fear and trepidation from what might get us if we are not ever-vigilant, and having long ago lost the ability to decide for ourselves that we are safe for a few months longer. . . . Fear of death is constantly reinforced as it is thrown in our faces at every turn in the road. Nobody says, "Go out and live your life with abundant energy and joy. Life is short for all of us. Make every day count." Instead we are encouraged to live from scan to scan.

Planting the Seeds

Dying is fraught with fears, losses, and suffering. Patients respond to pressures and change in their unique way. What may seem commonplace to one may be anxiety-producing in another. It our task to be aware of all cues presented to us, and respond in the most beneficial manner possible. We must put aside our preconceived notions of a "good death" or a "good life," and accept our patients, their view of the world, and their methods of coping. We cannot change our patients. They will die using many of the defense mechanisms that aided them throughout their lives. They will die in the extended family in which they live. We can discover the patient's unique personhood, and try to make their dying a time of growth and final accomplishment.

NEAR-DEATH EXPERIENCES

Near-death experience is marked by an altered state of consciousness. It generally results from severe trauma, oxygen deprivation, or any number of sudden, life-threatening conditions that normally result in death. The most common causes of near-death experiences are near-drowning, heart attacks, self-asphyxiation, and wounds. Individuals who have had near-death experiences often do not fear death. Jansen (1996) describes near-death experiences as a five stage continuum:

- Feelings of peace
- A sense of detachment
- A transitional period of darkness
- Emerging into light
- Movement into another realm of light and awareness.

Jansen, a psychiatrist, has looked for a neurophysiological explanation for these age-old phenomena. He believes the causative agent is a neurochemical called ketamine, and is currently exploring methods to support this theory. Regardless of cause, the outcome often includes a changed perception of death. According to Elisabeth Kubler-Ross and David Kessler (2000), people who have a near-death experience are no longer afraid of death. They see death as "a shedding of the physical body, no different than taking off a suit of clothes one no longer needs" (p. 82). Further, they experience a feeling of "wholeness" during the near-death experience, and report feeling as though they were never alone or abandoned during that time. They return with reports of bright lights, welcoming spirits, or deceased friends and relatives beckoning them to another realm. The experience often leaves the person permanently changed.

Terminally ill patients may have similar experiences. Callahan and Kelley (1997) describe a number of interviews with terminal patients who report visits with a spirit, or to an "other" world. Experiences generally occur later in the dying process, as the patient's physical systems are shutting down. Experiences are generally brief. They may have meetings with deceased loved ones, or find themselves in a serene, beautiful setting. The experience may not be very specific, but generally leaves the patient feeling peaceful and anticipatory. This type of experience often marks a turning point for terminal patients, and death usually follows shortly thereafter.

Dreams of terminal patients may be symbolic of unexplored needs and feelings. Callahan and Kelley believe that caregivers can help terminally ill patients recognize and understand those needs and feelings by being alert and carefully listening to what the patient shares concerning dreams. Asking the patient what the dream may mean may provide an opportunity for closure, forgiveness, or acceptance.

CONCEPTS IN ACTION

June was a dynamic, 69-year-old widow. She was financially secure, and had a well-developed circle of close and caring friends. June valued her independence, and maintained the home she had shared with her husband of 36 years, before his death. Always a physically able woman, June rode her bicycle 10 miles each day, and volunteered her time at several community agencies. Then June started to suffer from gastric upset and became jaundiced.

Within 36 hours of her visit to the doctor, June was hospitalized, biopsied, and diagnosed with cancer of the liver and spleen. She was given a life expectancy of 6 to 12 months. Upon arriving home, June set about preparing for her death. She reviewed her will, power of attorney, and living will. She began deciding who should receive what after her death, and saying good-bye to her friends and neighbors. Two weeks later, she had mentally completed a distribution of her worldly belongings. June called her daughter, and requested that she come and stay with her.

Her daughter has arrived and the community hospice has been called. You are the nurse making the initial home visit. You find a thin, jaundiced woman with strong circulation and healthy breath sounds. Her mind is clear. She has very little to say but reports, "I just want to die." Her daughter is distressed that June refuses to eat, is no longer interested in visits with her friends, and takes no pleasure in anything that used to bring her delight. She will not watch movies or go outside to the garden. She refuses to see any family members. She can walk but is refusing to get out of bed. Since her heart and lungs are strong, June is likely to live a while. Her daughter states, "I want my mother back for her last few weeks."

- What is the likely diagnosis for her psychological distress?
- In collaboration with the physician, what class of drugs would you recommend?
- What interpersonal approaches would be helpful?

After several weeks of visiting, June's mood lifts considerably and she is able to experience some quality of life. However, she is quite hostile to you during one visit and abruptly inquires, "Aren't you the angel of death? Why am I not dead yet?" How should you respond to her anger? June becomes completely bedridden and is overwhelmed with her lack of control. What could you do to reduce her feeling of powerlessness?

References

AAHPM (2003). *Pocket guide to hospice/palliative medicine.* Glenview, IL: American Academy of Hospice and Pallative Medicine.

Albom, M. (1997). *Tuesdays with Morrie.* New York: Random House.

Abrahm, J. L. (2000). *A physician's guide to pain and symptom management in cancer patients.* Baltimore: Johns Hopkins.

Block, S. (2000). Assessing and managing depression in the terminally ill patient. *Annals of Internal Medicine, 132*(3), 209–218.

Breitbart, W., & Heller, K. (2003). Reframing hope: Meaning-centered care for patients near the end of life. *Journal of Palliative Medicine, 6*(6), 979–988.

Byock, I. (1998). *Dying well.* New York: Riverhead Paperback.

Callahan, M., & Kelley, P. (1997). *Final gifts.* New York: Bantam Books.

Cassell, E. J. (1991). Recognizing suffering. *Hastings Center Report, 21*(3), 24–31.

Christakis, N. (1999). *Death foretold: Prophecy and prognosis in medical care.* Chicago: University of Chicago Press.

Craven, R., & Hirnle, C. (2003). *Fundamentals of nursing: Human health and function.* Philadelphia: Lippincott Williams & Wilkins.

Damron, B. (2001). Depression and anxiety. In R. Gates & R. Fink (Eds.), *Oncology nursing secrets.* Philadelphia: Hanley & Belfus.

Georgaki, S., Kalaidopoulou, O., Liarmakopoulos, I., & Mystakidou, K. (2002). Nurses' attitudes toward truthful communication with patients with cancer: A Greek study. *Cancer Nursing, 25*(6), 436–441.

Glaser, B., & Strauss, A. (1965). *Awareness of dying.* Chicago: Aldine Publishing.

Hall, B. (2003). An essay on an authentic meaning of medicalization: the patient's perspective. *Advances in Nursing Science, 26*(1), 53–62.

Jaffe, C., & Ehrlich, C. (1997). *All kinds of love: Experiencing hospice.* Amityville, NY: Baywood Publishing Co.

Jansen, K. (1996). Neuroscience, ketamine, and the near death experience: the role of glutamate and the NMDA receptor. In L. Bailey & J. Yates (Eds.), *The near death experience.* New York: Routledge.

Kalish, R. (1981). *Death, grief, and caring relationships.* Monterey, CA: Brooks/Cole Publishing.

Kastenbaum, R. J. (1995). *Death, society, and human experience.* Boston: Allyn & Bacon.

Kemp, C. (1999). *Terminal illness: A guide to nursing care.* Philadelphia: Lippincott.

Kubler-Ross, E. (1969). *On death and dying.* New York: Simon & Schuster.

Kubler-Ross, E., & Kessler, D. (2000). *Life lessons.* New York: Touchstone Publishing.

Moller, D. W. (2000). *Life's end: Technocratic dying in an age of spiritual yearning.* Amityville, NY: Baywood Publishing.

Pasacreta, J., Minarik, P., & Nield-Anderson, L. (2001). Anxiety and depression. In B. Ferrell & N. Coyle (Eds.), *Textbook of palliative nursing* (pp. 269–289). New York: Oxford.

Quill, T., & Byock, I. (2000). Responding to intractable suffering: the role of terminal sedation and voluntary refusal of food and fluids. *Annals of Internal Medicine, 132*(5), 408–414.

Smith, D. C. (1997). *Caregiving: Hospice proven techniques for healing body and soul.* New York: Macmillan.

Spencer, P. (2002). Anxiety. In D. Kuebler & P. Esper (Eds.), *Palliative practices from A–Z for the bedside clinician.* Pittsburgh, PA: Oncology Nursing Society.

Stevenson, B. (Ed.). (1965). *The Macmillan book of proverbs, maxims, and famous phrases.* New York: Macmillan.

Teno, J., Clarridge, B., Casey, V., Welch, L., Wetle, T., Shield, R., & Mor, V. (2004). Family perspectives on end-of-life care at the last place of care. *Journal of the American Medical Association, 291* (1), 88–93.

Tolstoy, L. (1981). *The death of Ivan Ilyich.* New York: Bantam Books.

Younger, J. (1995). The alienation of the sufferer. *Advances in Nursing Science, 17*(4), 53–72.

CHAPTER 6

Connecting and Caring Presence

Philosophical Reflections

"Compassion challenges us to cry out with those in misery, to mourn with those who are lonely, to weep with those in tears. . . . Compassion means full immersion in the condition of being human."

NOUWEN, MCNEILL, AND MORRISON, 1982, P. 4

Learning Objectives

1. Define caring, compassion, connecting, and responsive use of self.
2. Describe five dimensions of listening at the end of life.
3. Identify ways to speak truth about difficult subjects at the end of life.
4. Explain ways to encourage patients' decisions at the end of life.
5. Define the practice of presence and its dimensions.
6. Describe the practice of connecting with disenfranchised populations.
7. Evaluate nursing interactions to identify ways to strengthen the practice of connecting and caring presence.

As has been discussed, competency in caring for patients at the end of life is rooted in keeping ourselves healthy and working collaboratively. In the End-of-Life Caregiving Model, the trunk of the tree visually represents the development of the nurse-patient relationship through connecting and caring presence. The trunk connects the roots to the branches. When strong connections are not developed with patient and family, end-of-life care is limited to technical tasks that are out of touch with the human being. This chapter explores caring, the dimensions of connecting in relationships, the challenges of connecting, and caring presence.

CARING

Human beings survive and thrive through caring for each other. Caring affirms the dignity and preciousness of human life (Roach, 1984). The commitment of nursing to human caring, relationships, and human community contrasts with social trends that emphasize materialism, individualism, and competition. The capacity to care has been repressed, so nursing often is practiced within a society that does not care. "We are constantly being asked to turn our faces away from our own internal images of what is right, true, and most of all alive for us" (Whyte, 1994).

Boykin and Schoenhofer (1993) propose that all relationships are opportunities to draw forth caring, to reinforce the value of each person. Relationships are chances to celebrate humanness by appreciating others as whole persons. Through caring we seek to know the uniqueness of persons and to support, strengthen, and sustain them in their processes of suffering and growth.

Compassion is the foundation for caring. The word *compassion* is rooted in the Latin words *pati* and *cum,* which mean *to suffer with.* Compassion requires more than kindness. It requires us to "walk in the shoes" of those who are hurting and afraid, to feel the strong connection between their experience and our own. Sometimes in our lives we are not able to offer compassion because of our own pain and fear. We are so preoccupied with our own suffering that we are not able to attend to the suffering of another. Staying healthy, as discussed in Chapter 3, is the root of compassion. By caring for ourselves emotionally and physically, we are able to sustain compassion. Connecting is the outward expression of compassion.

CONNECTING

In the End-of-Life Caregiving Model, connecting involves the nurse joining or linking in partnership with the patient and family. Connecting begins with the nurse having a strong sense of shared humanity. Feeling those common bonds, she chooses to establish a connection by developing a caring relationship. The partnership with patient and family is built through the practice of responsive use of self, listening, speaking truth, encouraging choice, building trust, and practicing human presence.

By caring for ourselves emotionally and physically, we are able to sustain compassion. Connecting is the outward expression of compassion.

Responsive Use of Self

SmithBattle, Drake, and Diekemper (1997) define "responsive use of self" as the process that expert nurses use to come to understand the lives of vulnerable clients. These nurses are not passively hearing their clients' stories. Instead, they continually reflect and respond with growing insight as they discover the other person's life. The authors vividly describe nurses "situating themselves in the worlds of their clients" to understand how their clients live, to discover their beliefs, and comprehend their social connections. "They learn to see clients as members and participants of families and communities and begin to appreciate how this social embeddedness shapes and organizes clients' beliefs, actions, choices, and possibilities" (p. 82). Assumptions and stereotypes are overturned as the nurses come to know families very different from their own. A highly experienced nurse describes her responsive use of self in coming to know and appreciate people who lived in very difficult circumstances:

Survivors

Being able to be in that shabby environment with my dying patient and her husband, who lived a life that was totally foreign to me, people who drew knives on each other, was remarkable. I was able to find truly great things about them and recognize who they were. I don't think these people ever had much validation. People had always criticized their shack and their drinking and saw everything wrong. They had not heard any validation about being the survivors they were.

Responsive use of self is an important component of connecting; another key element of connecting is listening.

Listening

Listening is vital to connection. Effective "listening is the art of developing deeper silences in yourself, so you slow your mind's hearing to your ear's natural speed, and hear beneath the words to their meaning" (Briskin, 1996). Active listening involves continual decoding of the thoughts and emotional messages of others (Craven & Hirnle, 2003). It involves quieting the mind and totally focusing on the patient's words and nonverbal cues. "Listening creates a holy silence. When you listen generously to people, they can hear truth in themselves, often for the first time. And in the silence of listening, you can know yourself in everyone" (Remen, 1996, p. 220).

| Box 6-1 ■ | GUIDELINES FOR LISTENING |

1. Create a physical environment that fosters listening. Eliminate physical barriers. Reduce distractions. Take time.
2. Place yourself at the same level as the other person, not standing above.
3. Speak in a normal tone of voice or as needed if the person is hard of hearing.
4. Maintain eye contact and use touch unless culturally inappropriate.
5. Do not ask questions that can be answered with a simple "yes" or "no." Instead, ask those that are open-ended and encourage expression.
6. Restate and summarize the essence of the messages you hear to indicate that you understand what is being said and to encourage elaboration.
7. Listen for underlying feelings and then reflect them back to verify these emotions with the patient.
8. Continue to seek clarification of the patient's thoughts and feelings.
9. Allow time for silence when the patient needs time to think or is having difficulty expressing himself. Sometimes there are no words truly adequate to respond to the suffering described. Silence without physical withdrawal may be the best response.

There are a number of guidelines nurses should follow to learn the art of listening (see Box 6-1). For example, nurses should sit at the same level as patients. Being at the same physical level eliminates the physical intimidation or power division represented by standing over or sitting higher than a patient. Eye contact, where culturally appropriate, is also critical to foster trust and to let patients know you are with them listening. Listening at the end of life has five dimensions: hearing what is being said, believing what is said, understanding their story, opening up difficult subjects, and discovering truth.

Hearing

An expert nurse explains her focus: "I want to be able to hear people. I want to be able to hear what's not said so I watch body language and eye contact with me and with each other." Frequently people talk, but no one hears the message. We must seek to pay attention, even though the words may be difficult. A hospice expert explains how she developed her ability to hear:

I was never around swearing and early on I used to let those words interfere with my ability to hear. So if someone said "f___" to me, I didn't hear the pain and frustration. It was a real challenge to move beyond the words to the feelings that were behind them and to help people express them by saying the words "hurt" or "angry" or "frustrated."

This ability to hear is particularly helpful to patients when others cannot hear what they are saying. For instance, a husband may not be able to hear his wife's feelings and fears because of his own emotional distress. Likewise, a physician may not be able to hear a patient's complaint of pain because of his or her own denial and fear. The nurse often becomes the sounding board for upsetting words like "I am so afraid."

 Planting the Seeds

Sometimes patients tell us things that upset us so much that we tend to screen out their words. Hearing a patient's fear and pain requires being aware of our own feelings and quieting them.

Believing

If you seek to believe what patients say, you will build a strong bond with them. Many times, dying people make statements that others doubt. They may describe experiences or symptoms such as pain or dyspnea that family or other professionals refuse to believe. We may not believe them because we don't want to face their suffering; it is too painful, so we discount it. We may not believe them because we fear being deceived; we see ourselves as experts on their disease and they don't fit the usual pattern. Here are two examples of believing patients' report of symptoms:

I Didn't Discount

Every time he told me how bad it hurt and how much medication he had to take, we would talk about his options and I encouraged second opinions. He often had problems with the technological management not working. His report was very important. I didn't discount him at any time.

The Pest

She was old and needy and would talk your leg off. Others told her she was a pest when she said that her oxygen wasn't working right. Before I came to her home and believed her, she had not had enough oxygen for two days.

In addition to believing reports of physical distress, we must also respect that people know what is best for their own living and dying. A nurse explains, "I always believe in him. I always let him take the lead." This approach can be quite different from the paternalistic one that health providers often take, assuming they know what is best for patients' lives.

> 66 | *If you seek to believe what patients say, you will build a strong bond with them.*

Understanding Their Story

Discover who the person is. From the first visit, you can ask people to tell you their stories. Initially, that might be their medical journey from diagnosis through treatment, and now, palliation. Over time, invite stories of their lives, victories, and disappointments. You might ask to see family pictures. Encourage friends and family members to reminisce together and with the patient. Even when the person is comatose or just after death, you might ask, "What was he like?" Often, people need a little prompting to tell stories about their lives. Reminiscence and life review are great gifts of listening to people at the end of their lives.

> 66 | *Reminiscence and life review are great gifts of listening to people at the end of their lives.*

Whenever we listen to peoples' stories, we are likely to build trusting relationships. For people with many trusted loved ones and little societal conflict, trust may come readily. On the other hand, patients who have encountered betrayal and mistrust may be quite resistant to letting nurses into their lives. Here is an example of initial mistrust, which the nurse was able to relieve by listening and emphasizing patient choice:

Be Patient with Me

She lived without furniture in her roach infested apartment and she wouldn't talk to me. She wouldn't answer anything. We just spent a long time together. I knew that she basically was waiting to find out what I would say. Finally, I told her, "You know, I might make some mistakes. I want you to be patient with me. I'm here to listen and to make sure you don't have pain. And I'll do everything I can to keep you at home and to hold your children next to you." And she started crying and said that's all she wanted.

Opening Up Difficult Subjects

At the end of life we can create strong connections with patients by inquiring about matters that no one else has the courage to bring up. It is such a relief to many patients to able to speak about their difficulties. Of course, if you ask

---

Box 6-2 ■	**QUESTIONS TO OPEN UP DIFFICULT SUBJECTS**

- What are your greatest concerns?
- What is it like for you right now?
- You're really sick. What do you feel is happening?
- How are you doing with this?
- How are you within yourself?
- I hear you're having a bad time.
- What did the doctor actually tell you?
- What do you think is happening? What are they telling you?
- What really matters for you right now?

---

about difficult matters, then you must listen to what they say. A nurse explains how rewarding this is: "You are just so thankful that you are able to say the words to the patient to help her talk about it." Byock (1997) proposes asking, "How are you within yourself?" Consider the following words as openings:

- "I hear you're having a bad time."
- "What's it like for you right now?"
- "What do you feel is happening?"

See Box 6-2, Questions to Open Up Difficult Subjects, for some examples of questions that might work to open up difficult subjects. Consider the words that you would choose to encourage a patient to express worries and concerns. By asking these difficult questions, and by listening to and validating the responses, you can connect to patients at the end of life on a deeper level, which will not only make the patient's end-of-life experience better but will also enrich your relationships with patients.

■
WWW. **Internet Resource Box**

See www.dyingwell.com to explore the Web site of Dr. Ira Byock, who recommends certain conversations that are important to have with people at the end of their lives.

Speaking Truth

Listening is critical at the end of life, but it is also important to speak the truth about what is happening in a person's life. Dying people and those who love them are adjusting to and coming to terms with what is really going on, and you can be there to help them. When people are enduring life-threatening illness, the health team focus is usually on encouraging them to comply with treatment. We feel obliged to point out the positive and to reassure patients that everything is going to be all right. Friends and family members feel obliged to do the same. The result can be that no one speaks the truth or ever approaches the topic of life ending.

Nurses should speak honestly about what is happening. A hospice nurse explains, "Usually people are just grateful, grateful to hear truth. Truth sets people free. It sets families free, sets patients free. They no longer have to keep secrets. Then that truth can empower them to make choices." Hospice and palliative-care programs in the United States have strongly emphasized speaking the truth about terminal prognoses and issues related to treatment. However, it is important to recognize that many traditional cultures around the world forbid telling the patient that he or she is dying. Terminal news and end-of-life decisions are left to families and those with traditional authority. The chapter on cross-cultural caring addresses the nurse's challenges when speaking the truth is forbidden by cultural traditions.

Speaking truth begins with opening up difficult subjects, as previously discussed. We need to say the words that permit honesty. Timing this is quite challenging. Knowing when to push and when to back off is not easy. You need to open up the difficult subject, then pay attention to verbal and non-verbal responses. If you receive signals that a patient does not want to talk, you must never force the conversation. Such a situation is illustrated in the case of nurse Jamie Nguyen visiting 45-year-old Martha Bixler, a home hospice patient. After the third home visit, Jamie sits down with Martha and explains his assessment and the meaning of the symptoms she is experiencing. Martha is living with metastatic cancer, which has metastasized to multiple organs. Following a moment of silence, Jamie asks Martha, "How are you *really* feeling now?" Martha shoots back, "Really awful, what do you think? What's going to become of my children! They need me!" Jamie remains silent and then asks, "Are you able to talk to your husband about it?" Martha turns away and mumbles, "Whatever. I'm too tired to talk about this. Would you leave now?" Jamie responds, "Of course. We'll talk more on Wednesday," and lets himself out the front door. Jamie has learned to open up difficult subjects, but then to back off and not push when the patient cuts off further discussion for the time being. We welcome discussion, but we never force it.

Although we seek to speak the truth when patients and families choose, the truth is ever changing. In the 21st century, people with end-stage illness are successfully pulled back from the brink of death over and over again. Everyone has become treatable. No one can say with certainty when they will die. Nevertheless, when death hovers closely, nurses can offer an opportunity to speak truthfully about that. If the physician has not recently given prognostic information, then we can help patients and family members to ask the necessary questions of the physician about what is going on. "People are getting in touch with what's really going on and we're there to help them with that" (Zerwekh, 1994, p. 31).

DENIAL

Some patients are unable to recognize or acknowledge when the end of life is near. Nurses should be mindful of this perspective and should not force upfront conversations. In the following two examples, both patients want to avoid speaking about their true conditions, but for different reasons. Connecting involves speaking the truth, but only to the extent that patients have an ability or desire to incorporate it.

Zest

> I was impressed with their zest for life. I told them that I would answer their questions honestly, always tell the truth. But we rarely talked about death and dying. We talked about the moment-to-moment things that were happening. Whenever I visited, they would take only a couple of minutes out of each visit to focus on reality. We had to talk gently around it.

Even when death is close, some people never let go their zest for life. We must respect their denial and follow their lead about what in the moment is vital in their lives.

Miracles

> I have seen Ruth perhaps four times. We talk about Bernie Siegel's Love, Medicine, and Miracles and about her holy water from a sacred place in Yugoslavia. She prays continually for a miracle. She tells me, "I know I am sick and I don't want to talk about it." The air is fragrant with Secret Garden spray failing to cover the odor from her draining lesions. Ruth's power of positive thinking is keeping her alive as malignant melanoma consumes her lower body. I go into the kitchen and speak to her daughters as they ask me what is really happening. With them I can speak the truth. They ask me what is happening.

Connecting with patient and family involves speaking the truth if they choose. Decisions at the end of life are made possible when we are able to speak truthfully about life ending.

Encouraging Decisions

"When the truth is being told, people can make informed decisions about how they will live and die" (Zerwekh, 1994, p. 33). You can promote self-determination at the end of life by assessing what people want, fostering communication about decisions, respecting those decisions, and advocating for their decisions when the social or medical system puts up road blocks.

Once the truth has been opened up for discussion, assessing decisions involves attentive listening and questioning. First, a dying person needs to become aware of possible decisions to be made. Such decisions include final

| Box 6-3 ■ | **EXAMPLES OF END-OF-LIFE CHOICES** |

- How will the patient relate with friends and family? Are there matters to be resolved? Is there need for thanks or forgiveness? Are there people who should be seen?
- How will the patient resolve financial matters? Is there a will documenting what he or she desires?
- Will the patient seek aggressive treatment until the end of life? Does he or she understand the consequences? What are the limits of what he or she wishes to be done? Has a durable power of attorney been designated to make medical decisions when the person is no longer capable?
- Where does he or she want to die? Who should be there?
- Does he or she desire spiritual counsel? What would be helpful to find spiritual peace?

family matters and business matters as well as options around dying itself. Patients and family members usually need assistance to reflect, make up their minds, and express their choices. You can promote communication about decisions. At the end of life people need help to realize all of the choices they have. Box 6-3 lists Examples of End-of-Life Decisions.

Treatment Decisions

Each medical intervention at the end of life should be chosen by patients and families, rather than imposed by health-care providers. Remember that patients have a right to informed consent before treatments are initiated. The doctrine of informed consent proclaims that a mentally competent person has a right to make an informed decision about treatment alternatives. See Box 6-4, Principles of Informed Consent. Nurses can help people understand treatment choices and make treatment decisions by translating medical information into lay terms. Patients often feel more comfortable asking nurses for the critical information needed to make difficult treatment decisions. As each treatment option presents itself, nurses should inform patients that they can choose to accept or reject the treatment. Often, proposing a trial period for the treatment or its withdrawal may be useful. For instance, a young woman with total bowel obstruction is vomiting fecal material. You might suggest that she could choose a trial period of slowing her TPN infusion to see if the vomiting is diminished. Suppose an opioid naïve patient is hesitant to begin taking long-acting morphine for pancreatic cancer because it is important to him to remain alert and communicate with his family. You can explain the drug action and that initial side effects may include some nausea and sedation, which then usually disappear. You might encourage a

| Box 6-4 ■ | **PRINCIPLES OF INFORMED CONSENT** |

The person giving consent must:

1. Be capable of understanding the relevant facts. This requires that the person is mentally competent.
2. Be given a translator if necessary.
3. Be provided with all of the information on treatments, risks, benefits, and alternatives necessary for a reasonable person to render an informed decision.
4. Be more than 18 years old or emancipated.
5. Not be coerced to make the decision.
6. Be granted the right to have all questions answered to ensure understanding.
7. Be given the right to have the consent in writing.

5-day trial period before the person makes the decision to reject or accept the medication.

❝ *Each medical intervention at the end of life should be chosen by patients and families, rather than imposed by health-care providers.*

Sometimes family members' decisions are in conflict. For instance, a dying husband may want no code and hospice care. His wife may want "everything done" so he can stay with her. The nurse's role in that circumstance is to encourage them to talk to each other. Nurses frequently guide loved ones who are unable to discuss difficult subjects to speak to each other. The nurse may be the one who brings the conflict into the open.

Even though informed choice is strongly emphasized in the United States, many individuals because of their personal, family, or cultural history may not wish to make a choice. They may delegate decisions to family members or the health-care team. If someone other than the patient is the decision-maker, nurses are often in the role of advocating for the patient's best interests. You may be the one who brings the patient's suffering, concerns, and opinions to the attention of decision-makers.

Some choices must be limited because patients are cognitively impaired due to mental illness, developmental disability, alcohol, drugs, or terminal pathophysiology. You may have to make a difficult judgment call to deny patient choice when that choice may be self-destructive. Because we are in the home or present at the bedside in hospital and nursing home, nurses are continually setting limits when we observe self-destructive behavior due to cognitive impairment. For example, in the home we may advise families that their loved one is no longer able to drive or cook or get out of bed or take medicines or live alone without help. We identify patients' risk of injury due to cognitive impairment. Likewise, in hospital and skilled nursing facilities, nurses protect patients from countless threats, such as falls and skin breakdown, by taking charge when patients can no longer think clearly.

Respecting decisions that we would not choose ourselves is a great challenge. The ethical principle of autonomy, however, requires nurses to put aside their own feelings and respect the end-of-life decisions that competent patients render. Troubling choices are wide ranging and include decisions that contradict traditional medical practice, challenge mainstream social values, or go against what we usually consider "common sense." For instance, patients may make risky choices involving drugs and alcohol or staying with abusive family members. Even the most broad-minded nurse can be unsettled by choices that include suicide or active euthanasia, decisions to go through extraordinary suffering without symptom relief, or decisions to withdraw from outside assistance and die alone.

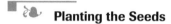 **Planting the Seeds**

You need to balance respect for individual self-determination with your responsibility to do no harm and protect the suffering. Turn to the interdisciplinary team to explore troubling situations. Sometimes you may need to withdraw from the case rather than witness the effects of self-destructive behavior.

Advocating for Choice

Often, agency policies or individual professionals do not want to make exceptions to their usual ways of doing things. Consequently, nurses often advocate for patient choices amidst system resistance. After the truth has been spoken and the patient has decided on a course of action, you may have to run interference with a resistant medical or social system. You may need to explain patient preferences to physicians, hospitals, community agencies, and reimbursement sources. You might say to the physician, "The patient has told me and his family that he wants to stop chemotherapy." Or, you might explain to the hospital administration, "This patient wants to have chanting and prayers at his bedside until he dies. He's going to need a private room." Another example would be speaking for the patient about to be discharged from a home-health agency, "He is at great risk of injury if we discharge him now. He is too weak to care for himself." Sometimes the nurse may be called upon to stop aggressive resuscitative interventions if the family has called 911 or if the patient is brought to the emergency room or intensive care unit. Patients should be encouraged to complete living wills and set up durable powers of attorney. In the absence of explicit legal documents, the nurse should articulate the patient's choices by recording them and speaking out.

For instance, a hospice nurse might explain to the emergency room physician, "He is a hospice patient and he has repeatedly told me he didn't want to go on the vent again. He has liver, bone, and brain mets." When the patient and family are unable to speak, we become their voice, and that is at the essence of connecting.

Practicing Caring Presence

The practice of caring presence can be defined as the intentional authentic responsiveness of the nurse to another human being. The nurse is sincere and expresses genuine caring feelings. The practice of caring presence is also known as *healing presence, practicing presence, being present, presencing,* and *being there* (Zerwekh, 1997). This concept is founded in the thinking of existential philosophers and theologians. The concept of the I-Thou relationship instead of an I-It relationship is central. As first explained by Martin Buber in 1923, we can come into a sick person's presence either by treating her as an *It* whom we are investigating and probing, or as a fellow human being or *Thou*. Sr. Madeline Clemence Vaillot (1966) was the first to apply existential philosophy to nursing. She invited nurses to see patients as presences instead of objects. She believed that practicing presence would result in growth of nurse and patient. Practicing presence requires deliberate, focused attention; receptivity to the other person; and persistent awareness of the other person's shared humanity. When we focus our attention on another person, we deliberately let go of the distractions. We are aware of our mind's chatter, and we consciously clear our mind. Our only thoughts are focused on that person. By practicing receptivity, we are willing to take in that person's words and feelings. Box 6-5 contains quotations from the *The Art of Being a Healing Presence* (Miller & Cutshall, 2001) about how to practice presence. Interviews with the expert hospice nurses revealed four ways of practicing presence with those close to death:

- Being without words
- Paying attention
- Being physically present
- Being "where they are" emotionally

Being without words is a deep level of connection. The nurses describe silent, wordless connections: "The essence of me is sharing with the essence of them beyond the words we're talking about." "She couldn't talk anymore. She was looking at me. This was like hell being trapped. She knew that I knew." "You look at each other's eyes and you know whether the night went well or not." A simpler indication of human-to-human communication beyond words involves shared experience, "We shared the first dandelion of the spring." "We sat silently and sipped the tea."

Paying attention is integral to every nursing action, and is certainly a way to connect. The nurse practicing presence is attuned to the entire patient and

| Box 6-5 ■ | QUOTES FROM *THE ART OF BEING A HEALING PRESENCE* |

"Healing presence is the condition of being consciously and compassionately in the present moment with another or with others, believing in and affirming their potential for wholeness, wherever they are in life." p. 12

"You have to stay awake to each unfolding moment." p. 15

"We will have to persist in quieting our mind's chatter if we want to really hear what another person has to say." p. 17

"As you become more clear about who you are and why you do what you do, you will become more receptive to whomever you're with." p. 23

"Consciously create a space for another that feels welcoming, quieting and secure." p. 27

"Let go of what was happening just prior to this time you have together. . . . If you don't have much time to prepare, perhaps you can simply stand for a moment and take a deep breath or two." p. 32

"Honor the others' significance." p. 36

"Sitting in silence with others can be deeply healing." p. 40

Source: From Miller & Cutshall (2001).

family situation. A nurse explains, "I pay attention to what is going on. I go in and read the situation." Nurses follow the patient's lead. Paying attention is holistic and surveys all that is happening. Some nurses describe it as "having your antennas out" or "detecting what's really going on." "First of all you get a baseline assessment in terms of physiological, psychosocial, and spiritual issues. From that baseline you get some understanding of what they've gone through, what their understanding is, who their supports are, what their beliefs are, why they're here in this life."

Being present so they are not alone is quite challenging in today's health-care system. This is the most literal way to practice presence and includes being physically nearby, frequently at the bedside to respond to needs, and available during crises. The greatest fear of dying people is abandonment (Byock, 1997). The health-care system ideally would ensure dying people 24-hour availability of skilled nursing at home, but currently this is only the case in hospice programs. Nurses should make efforts to mobilize a dependable back-up caregiving system for patients dying at home. Nurses who can be so available describe the satisfaction of continuing presence through hard times. "We promise them we will keep being there. We are there in a way that they don't have to do it alone." If you are in an inpatient setting, it is important to arrange schedules so that dying individuals are seldom alone. In skilled nursing facilities, it is often the nursing assistants who guarantee physical presence at the end of life.

Being where they are emotionally involves tuning into the person's emotional world through responsive use of self. People are accepted and validated. An expert nurse explains, "Meet them where they are. Just be present. Let them talk. Don't force your ideals." Nurses need to connect with the person at that person's level. Every person is different and calls for an individualized response. To do this, one nurse calls herself "a chameleon" as she modifies her approach based on where each person is emotionally. Here is one expert nurse's story of the kind of flexibility required by nurses caring for patients at the end of life and their families. The nurse describes tuning into the emotional world of a patient's only caregiver:

Totally Macho

He has been her pimp and misused her for years. But he loves my dying patient and their kids are all she has. So I don't start putting value judgments on him just because he's a louse and totally macho. Their caregiving system is working right now. This man and I just sit on the front step of the house in the middle of summer heat and talk and talk and talk. We get up and walk. He shows me the neighborhood bars and talks and talks about how his heart is breaking because he is losing her. Without him, she could not stay at home to die with her children around her.

CHALLENGES OF CONNECTING WITH PEOPLE LIVING ON THE MARGINS

The "Totally Macho" story illustrates one of the real challenges of connecting. Sometimes we find ourselves greatly conflicted about reaching out to certain people. They may live in ways that challenge our deepest values. They may hold cultural or religious beliefs very different from our own. Caregivers may not provide safe and humane care. Patient and family members may be abusive to each other or to us. Their housekeeping skills may be terrible.

Sometimes "the truly broken overwhelm us; when by the time they reach us, they are physically unappealing, disturbed, abusive, confused, unreachable, and often visibly ungrateful. . . . The gulfs of class, race, economics, experience, and expectation separate us—then it is little wonder that we are ready to declare them beyond our caring" (Hilfiker, 1994, p. 179). In such situations, it is important to be aware of our own reactions, consider our own capabilities and limits, and make every effort to reach beyond these preconceptions and judgments to connect. Sometimes we will need to find other caregivers rather than impose our judgment and anger on vulnerable patients.

Some nurses are particularly skilled at working with clients living on the "ragged edge of society," people who are marginalized and living in difficult circumstances. Patients such as those with chronic mental illness, criminal histories, stigmatizing physical illnesses, and poverty can be characterized as separated from human community and living in fear as well as causing us to fear (Zerwekh, 2000). "Disenfranchised people are defined by their own fear and by the avoidance of others because they are afraid of their behavior or afraid of encountering their intense level of hardship and suffering" (p. 51). Nurses who persistently care for people living "on the ragged edge" find meaning in their work through belief in shared humanity, through experiencing their work as a religious or philosophical calling, by the gratification of overcoming great challenges, and often by perceiving disenfranchised people as similar to members of their own families. Caring on the ragged edge emphasizes the practice of connecting, with particular focus on honoring mutual humanity and knowing patients' life stories; it involves connecting the disconnected with community resources. This may require a type of relentless effort, which one nurse has described as "haunting the case." Nurses often find themselves mediating with bureaucracies to obtain needed services and to request exceptions to bureaucratic rules. For instance, a client may need electricity turned back on, requiring countless phone calls. A client may be hungry and the visiting nurse may buy food and bring it to the home, against agency rules. Nurses caring on the ragged edge make patient self-care possible through teaching and respecting choices. They specialize in working with people who are living in intense emotional turmoil, often alternating between anger and fear. One nurse describes how she connected with a paranoid woman suffering from metastatic breast cancer:

> She didn't trust anybody and didn't want to do anything. . . . She would throw things and curse and have fits. . . . I sat many, many hours with her to discover what it is she needed to know. And I finally realized that she needed everything explained . . . and then re-explained. She had a very hard time understanding. If she didn't understand, it angered her. . . . I agreed to answer her questions as many times as she needed as long as she gave me a little leeway and time.

The challenging practices of connecting and human presence support the branches and leaves of the End-of-Life Caregiving Model. The stronger the trunk, the stronger our ability to provide care. Understanding of grief and loss, covered in the next chapter, is an essential dimension of being able to connect.

CONCEPTS IN ACTION

In each of the following three stories, the nurse is challenged to listen and respond effectively. Apply the guidelines discussed in this chapter to Gretchen and Todd, Joseph, and Sally.

Denial and Fear: Gretchen and Todd

Todd is 27 years old and worked as a bartender at Harry's Hideaway until his diagnosis with metastatic colon cancer. He has had a colostomy and also suffers with a perineal fistula draining a large amount of bloody mucus. He's strikingly handsome, green eyes, freckles, and red hair. He loves boats, fast cars, liquor, and girls. His latest girlfriend, Gretchen, is 19. You find them in bed together in the hospice unit where he is dying. Todd is lying in a fetal position and Gretchen is curled around him, crying softly. When you enter the room, Gretchen moves to the chair beside the bed. You introduce yourself and ask Todd how he is doing. He replies, "We're fighting hard. I'm gonna lick this thing, whatever it takes." How should you respond?

You ask Gretchen how she is. She looks at you sadly, wordlessly. You suggest she join you for a cup of coffee in the family lounge. Alone there, she says, "I'm so afraid." What do you say?

Anger: Joseph

Joseph has had a lot of shoulder and back pain. Over 3 years, he has gone through many diagnostic procedures but no effective treatment. Several times, doctors told him the "pain is all in your head" and "you're becoming addicted to these narcotics." Finally, his debilitating pain was diagnosed as lung cancer, metastasized to the right scapula. By the time you meet him on the oncology unit, he is receiving continuous subcutaneous morphine infusions and has an inoperable bowel obstruction. Joseph is 70 but appears to be 55. He is described in report as angry, resentful, and frustrated. He has been rude to the entire nursing staff. You walk into his room and sit down, explain you are a nursing student who will be caring for him, and ask how he is feeling. He immediately responds, "What do you want with me? Am I a guinea pig or what?" How might you best respond?

Independence: Sally

Sally proudly describes herself as a Mountain Lady, fiercely independent, and she wants to return home to her isolated house in a rural county. She proudly asserts that she has always been self-sufficient. Now she has end-stage heart failure and has been treated for pulmonary edema, which is becoming refractory to treatment. She is breathless walking from bed to

(continued)

> ### CONCEPTS IN ACTION   (CONTINUED)
>
> bathroom. You are discussing discharge plans and the physician's hospice referral. When you suggest that a nurse will come to the house, she angrily responds, "I don't want anyone messing in my business." How can you best respond?

References

Boykin, A., & Schoenhofer, S. (1993). *Nursing as caring: A model for transforming nursing practice.* New York: National League for Nursing.

Briskin, A. (1996). *The stirring of soul in the workplace.* San Francisco: Jossey-Bass.

Byock, I. (1997). *Dying well: The prospect for growth at the end of life.* New York: Riverhead Books.

Craven, R., & Hirnle, C. (2003). *Fundamentals of nursing.* Philadelphia: Lippincott.

Hilfiker, D. (1994). *Not all of us are saints: A doctor's journey with the poor.* New York: Ballantine Books.

Miller, J., & Cutshall, S. (2001). *The art of being a healing presence.* Fort Wayne, IN: Willowgreen.

Nouwen, H., McNeill, D., & Morrison, D. (1983). *Compassion: A reflection on the Christian life.* New York: Image Books Doubleday.

Remen, R. (1996). *Kitchen table wisdom: Stories that heal.* New York: Berkley Publishing.

Roach, M. S. (1984). *Caring: The human mode of being, implications for nursing.* Toronto, Canada: University of Toronto.

SmithBattle, L., Drake, M., & Diekemper, M. (1997). The responsive use of self in community health nursing practice. *Advances in Nursing Science, 20* (2), 75–89.

Vaillot, M. C. (1966). Existentialism: A philosophy of commitment. *American Journal of Nursing, 66,* 500–505.

Whyte, D. (1994). *The heart aroused: Poetry and the preservation of the soul in corporate America.* New York: Currency Doubleday.

Zerwekh, J. (1994). The truth tellers. *American Journal of Nursing, 94*(2), 30–34.

Zerwekh, J. (1997). The practice of presencing. *Seminars in Oncology Nursing, 13*(4), 260–262.

Zerwekh, J. (2000). Caring on the ragged edge: Nursing persons who are disenfranchised. *Advances in Nursing Science, 22*(4), 47–61.

CHAPTER 7

Grief and Mourning

Philosophical Reflections

Courage is the letting go
Of things that are familiar.
Choosing paths where no one else has gone.
And though the fear can freeze your soul in woe
The only way to go is letting go
To give up the familiar.

LYRICS BY FOLKSINGER LINDA ALLEN (1988), "WOMEN'S WORK." CHICAGO: FLYING FISH RECORDS, INC.

Learning Objectives

1. Explain current understanding of grief as not occurring in a predictable sequence.
2. Recall common emotional, cognitive, physical, and behavioral manifestations of grief.
3. Explain the manifestations of unhealthy or complicated grief.
4. Explain the effects of sudden death on survivors.
5. Define disenfranchised grief, anticipatory grief, and chronic sorrow.
6. Explain the value of mourning rituals.
7. Summarize current research on the value of emotional disclosure to promote resolution of grief.
8. Develop a plan of care that includes normalizing and emotional support.

One of the keys to reaching out and connecting with people who are dying, as visualized by the trunk of the tree in the End-of-Life Caregiving Model, is understanding grief and caring for those who are grieving. Life involves a continual rhythm of coming and going, achieving and failing, loving and losing, mourning and recovering. This chapter explores current understandings of grief, and caring for those who grieve. Initial sections define grief-related terminology, frameworks for understanding grief, healthy grief, and complicated grief. The chapter continues by examining the unique aspects of dying suddenly, anticipatory grief, and chronic sorrow. The chapter concludes by considering how grieving individuals may find comfort in the rituals of mourning and by caring nurses.

INTRODUCTORY DEFINITIONS: LOSS, BEREAVEMENT, GRIEF, AND MOURNING

Many terms referring to the grief process are used interchangeably and have overlapping meanings. *Loss* occurs when something or someone is missing. *Losses* associated with death and dying include loss of health and accompanying normal physiological functions, diminishing energy, loss of ability to work at a job or in the home, loss of relationships, loss of hope for the future, and loss of life itself. *Bereavement* is defined as the experience of loss of a person to whom one has a significant attachment. Bereavement occurs when a valued person dies. Bereavement is the loss itself, whereas grief is the intense emotional response to that loss.

Grief is a universal human response that floods life when security is shattered by loss. Grief reactions are automatic, like a reflex, and are expressed according to cultural expectations. For example, a Northern European may be expected to grieve only in private, whereas a traditional Greek public response might include loud weeping. The grief process involves letting go of life and facing the unknown. Grief is experienced emotionally and is accompanied by changes in thought, behavior, social interaction, physical well-being, and ability to go about everyday life. For survivors, grieving ultimately involves the process of re-engaging in life. *Mourning* is the outward expression of grief with other people and in public. For instance, grief expressed through weeping at funerals and memorials is referred to as mourning.

WWW. Internet Resource Box

See *www.growthhouse.org*, which offers "best of the net" sites to understand grief and loss.

FRAMEWORKS FOR UNDERSTANDING GRIEF

Whenever we are attached or bonded to another person, activity, or object that we lose, grief is a normal response. Sigmund Freud published *Mourning and Melancholia* in 1917; he introduced the term *grief work* and proposed that healing occurs when individuals face painful realities. He believed that healing occurred when the individual was able to break ties with those who had died. Freud's ideas were applied to soldiers living with post-traumatic stress syndrome from their fighting in the First World War (Parkes, 2001).

Then, in 1944, Erich Lindemann published his study of 101 survivors of a nightclub fire in Boston where 500 people died. He vividly described acute grief responses and distinguished between normal and pathological grief, which he attributed to repression of memories of the experience. Like Freud, he believed that therapy should focus on facing painful realities.

Many models and theories of grief were proposed in the second half of the 20th century. Grieving as a step-wise process and grieving as a transition process are discussed later. Nevertheless, today we recognize that no two individuals experience grief in the same way and that no single process can accurately describe grief for all people.

Stages of Grief

In the past, the grief response to one's own impending death was explained as proceeding through stages until the person accepted death. This classic explanation was proposed by Elisabeth Kubler-Ross (1969), who observed five stages often experienced when people are grieving: denial, anger, bargaining, depression, and acceptance. See Box 7-1, Grief According to Kubler-Ross. These psychological reactions made a great deal of sense then and now, and are understood today to be common grief responses. Kubler-Ross depicted these responses as proceeding systematically from one stage to another until acceptance. Although this step-wise process has not been confirmed over the years since she first described it, there are predictable dimensions of grief, just as she described. In 1970, Bowlby and Parkes described four different stages through which people move back and forth: numbness, yearning and searching,

---

Box 7-1　■　GRIEF ACCORDING TO KUBLER-ROSS

Denial—Conscious or unconscious refusal to accept or believe prognosis.

Anger—Strong feelings of resentment or blame that are expressed as rage toward family, health-care system, God, or other external forces.

Bargaining—Trying to strike an agreement with God or fate to postpone death in return for a change in behavior.

Depression—Deep sadness when the person believes that life will soon be over.

Acceptance—A sense of peace and calm that death is imminent.

disorganization and despair, and reorganization. (Parkes, 2001) They use different words from Kubler-Ross, but describe the same underlying processes.

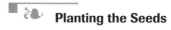

Planting the Seeds

Grief does not progress in one direction through predictable stages. People move into and out of various emotions in a far more unpredictable way. For instance, a dying person might on Monday morning demonstrate acceptance by writing his will and planning his funeral. That same night he might demonstrate denial by talking about returning to his job.

Transition Process of Loss

Bridges (1980) described a transition process that holds true for all losses, including bereavement. The transition from endings to new beginnings has three phases: Ending, The Neutral Zone, and Beginning. To visualize this, see Box 7-2, Bridge's Transition Process. Consider the relevance of his framework to the end of life. "Ending" alone has four aspects: (1) Disengagement involves separation from the familiar and breaking old connections; (2) Disidentification involves losing old ways of identifying oneself; (3) Disenchantment means losing assumptions about how the world works, losing an understanding of "the way things are;" and (4) Disorientation involves feeling lost and disoriented. Thus, a 56-year-old woman married for 30 years, and newly bereaved, experiences separation intensely, has lost her sense of identity around which she has built her view of the world and herself, and feels disoriented and without direction for her present and future life.

After the Ending stage, the woman in our example enters The Neutral Zone as described by Bridges. This is an empty space between endings and beginnings, a gap between old life and new life. In The Neutral Zone, the world is dark and the bereaved is no longer sure that the sun will rise. The woman wakes up in the morning, but has no direction for her day. She is no longer a wife; what meaning is left? How can she organize her time? Her old life plan is gone and she has not yet developed a new plan. In The Neutral

---

Box 7-2 ■	**BRIDGE'S TRANSITION PROCESS**	
ENDING	THE NEUTRAL ZONE	BEGINNING
1. Disengagement	Darkness and confusion	Re-engagement
2. Disidentification		New identity
3. Disenchantment		New meaning
4. Disorientation		Reorientation

Zone, the bereaved cannot make sense of these experiences of disengagement, disenchantment, and disidentification.

Beginning again after loss, Bridge's third stage involves re-engagement, new identity, a resurgent sense of meaning, and re-orientation. Making a beginning is gradual and may be incomplete, particularly following death of a lifelong partner. The woman in our story ventures back to church, begins to invite friends over for meals, sits down with her adult son to consider her financial future, moves to a smaller apartment, and eventually decides to finish a college degree in nursing. She is developing a new identity and sense of meaning.

Through most of the 20th century, psychologists and therapists believed that beginning again required severing bonds with the deceased in order to make new attachments. It is now understood, however, that it is normal for mourners to hold onto a sense of connection with the deceased (Klass, Silverman, and Nickman, 1996). Some survivors hold onto continuing bonds through inner conversations, memories, dreams, and even a sense that the deceased remains present or occasionally visits. As a result, new beginnings may involve the paradox of letting go of life as it was formerly known yet feeling an enduring connection to the deceased as the bereaved person re-engages in a new way of living. Complete detachment is not necessary for a healthy new beginning.

TYPES OF GRIEF

Grief is an individual manifestation of loss and takes many paths. It is important for nurses to recognize what types of grieving behaviors are healthy and what types are not.

Healthy Grief

Grief is determined by a wide range of factors, including the grieving person's age, sex, mental health, coping skills, relationship to the person who has died, religion, previous losses, current stressors, and quality of support system. Again, cultural rules govern all expression of grief, including feelings, behaviors, and bodily complaints. For instance, among Puerto Ricans, normal grief reactions may include seizures or stupor (Eisenbruch, 1984).

Regardless of culture, attachment theory is now considered to be the best predictor of healthy or unhealthy grieving (Shapiro, 2001). Parent-child attachment predicts subsequent bonds to that child throughout life. Adults who had secure and comforting bonds to their parents have the healthiest adult relationships and healthy bereavement in adulthood when those they love die. Adults whose parents were highly anxious, avoided the child, or were disorganized in their parenting have been shown to have more troubled adult attachments and more troubled bereavements. "Grief . . . is rooted in the attachments that we make to the people and objects around us" (Parkes, 2001, p. 41)

> ❝ *Grief . . . is rooted in the attachments that we make to the people and objects around us (Parkes, 2001, p. 41).*

Box 7-3 ■   NORMAL EFFECTS OF GRIEF

EMOTION	COGNITION	BEHAVIOR	PHYSICAL EFFECTS
Denial of feeling	Disbelief	Crying, sighing	Insomnia
Numbness	Disorientation	Screaming	Excessive sleeping
Anger	Lack of concentration	Reduced activity	Anorexia; nausea
Guilt	Difficulty problem solving	Withdrawal	Exhaustion
Blame	Reduced ability		Trembling
Bitterness	Preoccupation with deceased	Can't complete tasks	Muscle aches
Despair	Disorganization		Muscle weakness
Depression	Search for meaning	Restlessness	Palpitations
Loneliness	Moments of experiencing presence of deceased	Increased or decreased sexual drive	Chest pain Shortness of breath
	Disinterest in daily life		Headache

Normal grief affects emotions, thinking, behavior, and the physical body. In North America, manifestations that can be predicted in each category are summarized in Box 7-3, Normal Effects of Grief. Each category is described in more detail in the three subsections that follow. Healthy grief does not usually resolve quickly. Its duration is determined by the strength of attachment to the loved one who has died. Many people experience painful memories, distressing symptoms, and diminished quality of life for years.

■ ⸎ **Planting the Seeds**

Grief affects how we feel and think and behave, and how our body functions. Always consider grief as a possible underlying etiology for distressing symptoms that patients describe.

Emotions of Grief

The initial emotion is commonly an absence of emotion, a sense of numbness or denial. This denial of emotion is a natural buffer from overwhelming news and commonly occurs immediately after hearing a terminal prognosis or experiencing loss of a loved one. Denial frequently returns throughout the grieving process. As a short-term coping style, denial protects individuals from overwhelming emotions they may not be equipped to handle. Denial permits engagement in normal, everyday living without continual awareness of death. As a prolonged coping style, denial immobilizes feelings and blocks energy to go forward. Many people deny their own impending death, as do their relatives.

Beyond denial of feeling, anger, guilt, and depression are the most common feelings expressed. Anger is a common emotion of grieving. People frequently become bitter and seek to blame someone, including God, loved ones, and caregivers. As anger becomes prolonged, human beings may become estranged from one another. Some people resolve their anger over time, while others never let go of their rage. Anger persists for many reasons. For some people, anger and blame have been a life-long coping style. Others have not been able to recover from abusive relationships, and the death is just one more betrayal. Remember, anger is not rational or reasonable. Guilt is another typical emotion, as angry grieving people turn blame on themselves. Guilt can emerge when an individual has intense regret over past interactions with the deceased person. The individual remembers and finds fault internally. Only now, there is no longer a way to right the perceived wrong.

Depression and despair are predictable dimensions of grief. Briefly, intermittently, or for prolonged periods, a grieving individual may become immobilized in sadness, withdrawn, and without pleasure, hope, or meaning. Many people discover inner resources to move beyond depression and despair to develop a sense of peacefulness in the face of death. For both the dying and the bereaved, acceptance involves the achievement of emotional tranquility, letting go and trusting that all will be well. Death totally interrupts our sense of control. Acceptance of dying requires "relaxing into the process. . . . At the time of death, we may be forced to deal with surrender and trust. . . . We reach the end of our need to control" (Smith, 1998, pp. 164–165).

Thoughts and Behaviors of Grief

Cognitive manifestations of grief may include initial disbelief, confusion, and an inability to concentrate and problem-solve. "Everyone knows they're going to die, but nobody believes it" (Albom, 1997, p. 80). For survivors, disbelief usually does not last long because of the striking physical absence of the deceased. However, alterations in thought processes are common. For instance, a survivor may be preoccupied with the deceased while trying to do work. Survivors may encounter sleepless nights, dream of the deceased, or experience his or her presence. Behavior may become restless, withdrawn, hyperactive, disorganized, or absentminded, and crying is common. Survivors may also have a difficult time focusing on everyday tasks. Those in mourning may try to avoid all reminders of the deceased or, in the converse, may actively seek out reminders of the deceased. Particularly in teens or young adults, behavior associated with grief may also include hostile acts directed inward (drinking, drug use, dangerous sex) or outward.

> *Everyone knows they're going to die, but nobody believes it (Albom, 1997, p. 80).*

Effects of Grief on the Body

Grief can be somatized in a wide range of bodily complaints. Physical symptoms experienced during bereavement include disturbed sleep, exhaustion, appetite changes, changes in activity, changes in sexual drive, trembling, shortness of breath, heaviness in the chest, pounding heart, headaches, and muscle weakness or aches. Bereaved people are at greater risk of death and diminished physical health in the period immediately after the death. Heart disease is the most frequent cause of higher mortality in the bereaved; thus, there is a literal risk of dying from "a broken heart" (Parkes, 1999). Research has clearly documented an increased secretion of cortisol, epinephrine, and norepinephrine associated with bereavement. Likewise, immunity is depressed and, in particular, natural killer cell activity diminishes (Hall & Irwin, 2001). These neurological and immunological mind-body effects contribute to the development and progression of disease, particularly cardiovascular.

Complicated Grief

Grief is normal when individuals are able to acknowledge their loss and feel emotionally connected to and trusting of others (Prigerson & Jacobs, 2001). It is normal if they still feel that life holds meaning and are not consumed by anger. Likewise, the grief process is normal if they continue to have a sense of themselves and their own ability to function at work and home. For individuals grieving normally, sadness diminishes over time and they are capable of adjusting to new circumstances and gradually reinvesting in life.

Grief is considered complicated when individuals isolate themselves from others, have lost a sense of meaning, are consumed by anger, and fail to invest in life and adjust to new circumstances. Complicated grief can also be called traumatic, dysfunctional, pathological, morbid, abnormal, or unresolved. Grief is considered complicated when the person is so disturbed that function is impaired at home or work or in other social roles. In general, complicated grief is diagnosed when symptoms have lasted for two or more months.

Symptoms of Complicated Grief

Prigerson and Jacobs (2001) have described the results of an expert consensus conference on traumatic grief. The symptoms fall into two categories:

- Preoccupation with the deceased that impairs function
- Marked and persistent symptoms, including feelings of futility or loss of meaning, absence of emotional response, feeling dazed, difficulty acknowledging the death, self-destructive behaviors, and excessive bitterness or anger

Consider how Martha, age 37, is grieving following the sudden death of her twin sister, Maria, 3 months ago. Although both sisters married, they have always lived within one block of each other. Martha's grief is complicated. Her affect is flat; she expresses no feelings. Her words and behaviors indicate severe dysfunction. She has stopped bathing and dressing, and she stays in bed most of the day. She has lost her job as an administrative assistant due to absenteeism. Her bitterness and hopelessness are evident in expressions such as, "God has taken Maria from me. I hate him. There's no reason to get out of bed. I'm only half a woman now." See Box 7-4, Complicated Grief Assessment, and notice how it applies to Martha. She is angry and bitter, believes life is meaningless, feels that she does not deserve to live, and is not able to function at home or work.

One complication of grief that is particularly damaging to the bereaved and to the bereaved person's relationships is called "ruminative coping." Literally, to ruminate is to chew over and over. A person who has adjusted to grief through ruminative coping is unable to stop musing about grieving, persistently and repetitively engaging in thoughts and behaviors that maintain a focus on negative emotion (Nolen-Heoksema, 2001).

Complicating Factors

Grief is more likely to become complicated in the following circumstances, several of which are discussed in more detail:

- Preexisting mental illness
- Multiple losses
- Lack of social support
- Absence of sustaining spiritual beliefs
- When dying involved great suffering
- When coping with multiple other struggles
- When relationships have been extremely dependent and intertwined
- When a child has died
- When death is sudden, particularly from homicide or suicide

SUDDEN DEATH

Sudden deaths are one of the clear predictors of complicated grieving. Nurses commonly encounter sudden death. Sudden death encompasses

| Box 7-4 ■ | COMPLICATED GRIEF ASSESSMENT |

Although there are vast individual differences, experienced therapists have identified patterns across populations that are indicators of unhealthy coping. Determining frequency of troubling feelings and thoughts is vital to the assessment. **For each item, does the experience occur several times daily, once a day, several times weekly, or less than once a week?** All of these experiences are normal initially and should gradually diminish over time. Thus, it is important to determine how many months have passed since the death. Two months after bereavement, the nurse should refer bereaved people who are experiencing severe impairment of everyday functioning (Question No. 18) and at least six of the following symptoms daily, to professional counselors.

1. Overwhelmed or devastated
2. Preoccupation with deceased making it hard to do daily activities
3. Memories of the deceased upsetting
4. Trouble accepting the death. Can't believe it
5. Longing and yearning for deceased
6. Drawn to things connected with deceased
7. Angry about death
8. Feelings of shock and numbness since the death
9. Difficulty trusting people
10. Feeling distant from others including loved ones
11. Having same symptoms as the deceased
12. Avoiding reminders that the person is gone
13. Feeling life is empty or meaningless
14. Feeling don't deserve to live now that deceased is dead
15. Feeling bitter since the death
16. Feeling the future holds no meaning
17. Lost sense of safety and control since the death
18. Difficulty with functioning at work or home
19. Feelings of being on the edge or easily startled
20. Problems sleeping.

Source: Modified from Prigerson, Kasl, and Jacobs (2001).

short illnesses and trauma, as well as cardiac arrest or sudden infant death syndrome—any death where there is little warning. The most traumatic are deaths from murder, suicide, or natural disaster. Survivors of violent death are left feeling profoundly vulnerable, helpless, and angry.

Although survivors avoid the burdens and struggles leading up to anticipated death, therapists repeatedly find that sudden death is hard on survivors who may suffer a variety of dysfunctional symptoms. When a loved one dies suddenly, survivors are deprived of anticipatory grieving, which would have allowed them an opportunity to prepare emotionally and to say good-bye. Survivors of sudden death are more prone to the whole range of persistent symptoms seen in complicated grieving, and are more likely to need counseling to resolve their traumatic grief reactions. Survivors are likely to continue worrying about what really happened, to have many questions and regrets. The suddenly dead individual also has had no opportunity to bring closure to his or her life (Lynn & Harrold, 1999). Sudden death leaves practical matters unsettled; relationships, property, and financial concerns are left to survivors with the desires of the deceased person often unknown. Many people hope that their own death will be sudden rather than prolonged, but it is particularly difficult for the survivors who have had no chance to say good-bye. "While sudden deaths are attractive among the healthy, in reality they leave many things undone, and they are often the hardest deaths for families to accept" (Byock, 1997, p. 53).

> 66   *While sudden deaths are attractive among the healthy, in reality they leave many things undone, and they are often the hardest deaths for families to accept (Byock, 1997, p. 53).*

DEATH OF A CHILD

We do not expect to outlive our children. In a society where most children live to adulthood, it is particularly difficult for survivors to find meaning in the death of someone so young. Feelings of guilt and blame are predominant (Warden & Monahan, 2000). Parents may believe that they should have done something different to prevent the child's death. They may feel that God is punishing them for past sins. Frequently, they look for someone to blame for the great wrong they have experienced. Relatives and friends may blame the parents for failing to protect their children. The grief of parents and children is discussed further in Chapter 12.

Disenfranchised Grief

Many deaths and other losses cannot be acknowledged or mourned openly, which creates serious difficulties for survivors (Parkes, 1999). To be enfranchised is to have rights or privileges. Disenfranchised grief occurs when people die and we cannot publicly declare our attachments; we have no public right to grieve. The relationship might have been an extramarital one, for example. Similarly, when nurses and physicians lose patients, there is no place for us to mourn. Our grief is also disenfranchised. Other losses that cannot be fully acknowledged include fetal deaths, abortions, giving up children for adoption, death of a pet, or loss of a loved one to severe cognitive impairment. In the last situation, for example, the person is still alive but poor cognitive function prevents continuing recognition and relationship. In such cases, grief is usually minimized or ignored, there are few publicly acceptable rituals of mourning, and there may be little, if any, social support. This means the bereaved are not permitted any social expression of mourning. They are compelled to grieve alone.

In disenfranchised grief, an individual is likely to suppress his feelings rather than acknowledge them. When grief and mourning are denied, physical and emotional symptoms can persist and turn into complicated grief. Grief as the underlying cause of symptoms, however, is often not acknowledged by the bereaved or recognized by health-care providers. The following alternatives may help those living with disenfranchised grief:

- Small ceremonies with close friends and family to acknowledge the loss
- Shared meals of commemoration
- Symbolic burials or burning of clothing or object associated with the one lost, accompanied by prayer, poetry readings, and/or personal statements by survivors
- Writing journals or letters to the loved one
- Lighting candles and praying for the one lost

🌱 Planting the Seeds

Nurses need to find ways to grieve the deaths of so many patients who die in our care. Some agencies have monthly ceremonies that might involve reading names, lighting candles, tolling bells, or other rituals that have meaning to participants.

Anticipatory Grief

Anticipatory grief is a process that occurs in response to forewarning of life-threatening illness in oneself or a significant other. It involves recognizing the loss, reacting to the loss, reviewing and remembering, and letting go of life as it has been known. It is not a process that can fully reconcile a person to loss because it occurs before the reality of death. For survivors, anticipatory mourning can often promote healthy bereavement after their loved ones' death (Rando, 2000). In fact, for some people, the mourning after death may be less intense due to mourning that precedes death. The benefits of anticipatory mourning include open communication between the dying person and the grieving person, and resolution of unfinished business. Nevertheless, it is difficult and confusing for some individuals to mourn when the person they are mourning is still alive.

Anticipatory mourning may be beneficial in moderating actual mourning, but if it goes on for a prolonged period, it may create additional complications for the bereaved. For example, the burdens of prolonged anticipatory mourning for the survivor may include emotional exhaustion, guilt, anger, and withdrawal from the person who keeps on dying but is not yet dead. The mourning persons may feel guilty because they have thoughts about wishing their loved one dead. They may express anger toward the dying person because their own life is being consumed by caregiving without relief. They may withdraw emotionally when they can no longer face the close encounter with their love one's suffering. Edgar Allan Poe described the impact of his wife's repeated cerebral hemorrhages (Corr & Corr, 2000, pp. 224–225):

> Her life was despaired of. I took leave of her forever and underwent all the agonies of her death. She recovered partially and I again hoped . . . the vessel broke again . . . then again. Each time I felt all the agonies of her death . . . and at each accession of the disorder I loved her more dearly and clung to her life. I became insane . . . I drank. . . . I had indeed nearly abandoned all hope of a permanent cure when I found one in the death of my wife.

During the process of anticipatory mourning, those who are dying and those who anticipate their death walk a fine line between denial and acceptance. It is common for patients and those who love them to live in two realities so that they might be planning funerals while planning holidays.

People with similar experiences may vary dramatically in terms of how much they let in reality and mourn. Denial contravenes anticipatory mourning; it does not allow for saying good-bye, reconciling, and completing final arrangements of all kinds. The period before death offers many possibilities for human growth and meanings that are lost when denial dominates. However, it is important to try not to force anticipatory mourning. Some people lack the internal resources and do not have the interpersonal support to confront in advance their own death or the death of a loved one (Connor, 2000). Likewise, for many people, family, religion, or culture prohibits overt expression of anticipatory mourning. Box 7-5 contains some fundamental guidelines for support of those who are experiencing anticipatory mourning. When nurses work over time with dying people, they are often able to guide the process of letting go during the period of anticipatory grief. This is discussed in the final section of this text.

Chronic Sorrow

Many people live in chronic sorrow, living losses that are never-ending without death being imminent (Roos, 2002). Chronic sorrow involves recurring grief reactions when there is a significant loss of crucial functions in oneself or in another to whom a person has a deep attachment. The loss is never-ending as long as the person lives. Examples of persons coping with chronic sorrow are those living with disability and those caring for them. Chronic sorrow was first identified in parents with developmentally disabled children.

Consider the example of 80-year-old Hannah, who has all of her mental faculties but is gradually declining physically. Diminishing vision due to macular degeneration has led to the loss of her ability to drive. She can no longer read and must now rely on tape-recorded books. A fine tremor of her

> **Box 7-5 ■   ANTICIPATORY MOURNING: CARING GUIDELINES**
>
> 1. Affirm the value of the person living with dying.
> 2. Be sensitive to multiple sources of stress and loss.
> 3. Realize that losses and challenges will change over time.
> 4. Recognize that dying is experienced in a complex social network, with many people suffering various degrees of anticipatory mourning; help them help each other.
> 5. Listen actively and pay attention to nonverbals to determine priorities for assistance.
> 6. Pay attention to losses that are being grieved at the moment.
> 7. Consider emotional, cognitive, behavioral, and physical effects of grieving and work with an interdisciplinary team.
> 8. Use the experience to learn about your own humanity and the human condition and to grow in sensitivity to your fellow human beings.
>
> *Source:* Adapted from Corr & Corr (2000).

hands is preventing her from enjoying her former hobbies of knitting and embroidery, and is making cooking very difficult. Despite joint replacements, walking any distance has become too painful so that outside of her small apartment she must rely on a wheelchair. Despite attendance at an elder activity program and active engagement with her nieces and nephews, she lives in chronic sorrow with the accompanying emotions ranging from denial to anger to sadness to acceptance.

Although we as nurses are expected to focus persistently on restoration and maximizing function in those living with such losses associated with disabling illness, it is important to acknowledge the degree of loss experienced and to open the door to expression of grief. We need to listen.

 Planting the Seeds

As nurses, we also are living with chronic sorrow over our patients' suffering and dying. We need to find ways to mourn and ways to maintain our own well-being through healthy life-affirming choices.

RITUALS OF GRIEF AND MOURNING

Rituals are customary procedures or ceremonies expected within cultural and religious traditions. Rituals of mourning guide the preparation and disposal of the body, ceremonies after death, and obligations of the community and family after death. Death rituals prescribe words, symbolic actions, and appropriate behavior of the bereaved (Rosenblatt, 2001). In many cultures, rituals of mourning extend for months or years after the death. To compare just how different death rituals can be in two different cultures, see Box 7-6, Contrasting Funeral Rituals: Vietnamese Buddhist and African American Protestant.

In North America, death rituals within the mainstream culture are subdued and less visible than in many places around the world. Historically, North Americans donned black clothing and specified a period for mourning. In America today, survivors are expected to attend a funeral or memorial and then quickly return to business as usual.

Box 7-6 ■ CONTRASTING FUNERAL RITUALS: VIETNAMESE BUDDHIST AND AFRICAN AMERICAN PROTESTANT

AFRICAN AMERICAN PENTECOSTAL AND MISSIONARY BAPTIST FUNERALS

Death is believed to involve God calling the person home to the afterlife. The funeral service celebrates "crossing over" or going home to dwell in heaven. The sermon is likely to call upon sinners to repent and to praise the redeeming qualities of the deceased. Hymns, solos, and choir music reflect the rich tradition of black funeral music. Lyrics might include words such as "Going home, going home, I am going home" or "She's not dead; she's resting in the bosom of Jesus" (Irish, Lundquist, and Nelson, 1993). Traditionally, all are invited to a final viewing of the body in the casket, accompanied by much weeping and expression of distress.

Source: From Abrums (2000); Irish, Lundquist, and Nelsen (1993).

VIETNAMESE BUDDHIST FUNERALS

Death is an opportunity for reincarnation, to be reborn into another life cycle. The bereaved wear white clothing, or perhaps simply white headbands or armbands. Services may be at a temple or funeral home. Family members are expected to perform specific rituals. The room is filled with incense and chanting. Traditionally, a large picture of the deceased is on a stand near the casket. Expression of strong emotions is considered inappropriate during prayers, but weeping and wailing are common during the burial itself.

Source: From Dinh, Kemp, and Lasbridge (2000); Irish, Lundquist, and Nelsen (1993).

ADVANCE PLANNING FOR FUNERALS

North Americans generally attend funerals, which are ceremonies accompanying burial. The funeral "parlor" or "home" and the funeral director figure prominently in determining the nature and cost of the funeral and burial. Funeral homes are establishments that have one or more rooms that can be rented for funeral services, including "viewings" of the deceased in open coffins. Funeral directors are managers of the funeral home, but their roles have expanded to provide religious counsel regarding these matters. Sometimes funeral directors recommend expensive caskets and ceremonies to demonstrate the person's value or relieve the guilt of those who have been emotionally cut off during the person's life. Planning in advance of the death increases the chance of making affordable decisions.

The benefits of funerals have been demonstrated over the centuries. Funerals enable survivors to reflect on the meaning of the decedent's life, draw caring people together in support of each other, and provide a tribute to the deceased. Within a religious setting, funerals or memorials unite everyone in worship and search for meaning.

Memorials are formal or informal ceremonies held after the burial or cremation to remember the deceased. In contemporary America, many people reject the notion of a formal service as an appropriate bereavement ritual. In these cases, survivors may hold gatherings that serve as informal memorials intended to draw people together to speak of the deceased and to support each other. A memorial may occur in an apartment with survivors enjoying beer and pizza, in a garden with champagne as survivors spread ashes on beloved roses, or in any other setting where loved ones can gather comfortably and remember.

WWW.   **Internet Resource Box**

See *www.growthhouse.org* for information on funeral and memorial planning.

CARING FOR GRIEVING PEOPLE

Understanding the bereavement process is crucial for nurses who frequently come into contact with grieving patients and loved ones. Not only will such information assist you in comprehending physical and emotional problems that your patients may be having, but it will also help you in your interaction with family members at the end of life. But simply understanding bereavement is not enough. Nurses must also learn practical ways to care for grieving people. Nursing responses to the bereaved include the following:

- Normalizing the grief process
- Supporting disclosure while allowing for individual differences
- Making referrals for complicated grief

Normalizing the Grief Process

In North American society, there are few norms or standards for grieving to help people understand that their symptoms of grief are normal. In the past, and in traditional cultures today, mourning customs permitted the bereaved to suspend everyday obligations for prolonged periods. It was understood that grief prevented full functioning. However, the pace of modern day life simply does not allow for this. People are expected to return to business as usual in 3 days or less, yet they often are emotionally and cognitively impaired by grief and do not realize that their condition is normal. *Normalizing* is the process of assuring people that their experiences are indeed normal, within the range of what human beings in similar circumstances experience. Refer to Box 7-3 again to reexamine symptoms of healthy grief.

&. **Planting the Seeds**

It is comforting to explain to grieving people that certain disturbing thoughts, feelings, and physical symptoms are normal during grief.

Consider the situation of Thomas, a graduating senior nursing student at City Community College. During the beginning of Tom's final term, his performance evaluation was grim. He was often late for clinical. He couldn't explain the basic rationale for the procedures he was performing and couldn't identify clear nursing goals for his patients. As the instructor was standing by his side while he was preparing an antibiotic for intravenous infusion, she noted that his hands were shaking. This was not the first time she had noticed this. Stopping him in the middle of the procedure, she asked someone else if she could please complete the task and took Tom into the quiet corner of the report room where they both sat down. Then she inquired, "Tom, nothing is going right for you. What is wrong?" Tom was hesitant initially but then after awhile blurted out, "I think I'm going crazy. I can't do anything right any more." She asked Tom to consider if anything had happened since last term, when he was a capable student. In time, he revealed that his twin brother had died in a boating accident about 1 month ago. He hadn't let anyone in the School of Nursing know because "I just want to get through school." He revealed that he kept missing interstate highway exits, couldn't sleep, and had a constant ache in his chest. He was worried that he might have angina. In response to these revelations, the instructor took time to normalize Tom's symptoms. She explained Tom's trembling, chest pain, and insomnia as common manifestations of grief. Likewise, she reassured him that his disorientation and inability to prob-lem-solve were normal signs of grief. She referred him for immediate counseling.

Another example is that of Madeline and her father. Madeline's 58-year-old mother died suddenly of cardiac arrest. Her father Fred awoke one morning to find his wife of 33 years deceased at his side. In addition to grieving his wife's sudden death, Fred encounters Madeline's great fury. She blames him for not performing CPR on his wife and repeatedly states, "You didn't love her enough Dad. You just let her go." Every time she says this, he feels heart-broken and walks out of the room. Normalizing involves helping Fred and Madeline understand that anger is a normal response to grief. The nurse sits down with Fred and explains, "You know, Fred, Made-line is grieving, and anger is a normal emotion for her to express." Fred responds, "I know she's just upset with her Mom's leaving us, but I feel like she's stabbing me every time she says these things." Fortunately, the nurse also has an opportunity to speak to Madeline. She begins, "I know you're really angry about your mom's death." Madeline acknowledges this and explains that she feels her father caused her mother's death by not perform-ing CPR. The nurse reflects the reality that myocardial infarction caused the death and explains that CPR cannot revive someone who has been dead for hours. Again, she normalizes the anger that Madeline is expressing, yet expresses her concern that if it is prolonged, serious estrangements can occur.

Supporting Disclosure of Emotions

The latest research on grief and bereavement emphasizes that there are enormous variations in healthy grief expression. As previously discussed, we now understand that there are no predetermined stages through which a person must pass. However, throughout the 20th century, since the writ-ings of Freud, psychotherapists have asserted that a grieving person must directly confront feelings and face the reality of loss, review memories, and work toward detachment. These assumptions that "grief work" is essential have been unquestioned until recently by those working in bereavement therapy.

In fact, contemporary research is repeatedly demonstrating that sharing of thoughts and feelings with others does not necessarily reduce the level of distress or facilitate adjustment following bereavement. Likewise, there is no certainty that withholding of feelings is unhealthy. (Stroebe, Stroebe, Schut, Zech, and van den Bout, 2002; Schut, Stroebe, van den Bout, and Terheggen, 2001; Pennebaker, Zech, and Rime, 2001). Strongly encouraging people to

---

Box 7-7 ■   BEREAVEMENT MYTHS AND TRUTHS

MYTH	TRUTH
1. It is always good to talk about your feelings.	1. It may or may not be good to talk about your feelings.
2. Confronting feelings after death is better than avoiding those feelings.	2. Confronting feelings should not be forced. The value of expression is determined by individual personality, family values, and religious beliefs.
3. You cannot heal following bereavement unless you express intense feelings.	3. Healing from loss proceeds over time whether you express intense feelings or not.
4. Bereaved individuals who continue to feel a connection with their deceased loved ones require therapy for their pathological grief.	4. It is common to feel a continued connection with loved ones who have died.

Source: Adapted from Wortman & Silver (2001).

"open up" about their grief can actively contradict personal, family, and cultural rules. The 21st century nurse who cares at the end of life and after death cannot continue to practice according to the bereavement myths of the 20th century. See Box 7-7, Bereavement Myths and Truths.

Although sharing feelings does not appear to hasten recovery from acute grief, many people do perceive sharing as comforting and helpful (Pennebaker et al., 2001). Disclosure of feelings enhances memories of the deceased and fosters interpersonal connection. Each individual processes and recovers from grief in a different way.

Planting the Seeds

People who choose to share their feelings and experiences of grief often perceive this as helpful. However, research indicates that sharing of feelings cannot be predicted to lessen the intensity of grief. The effective nurse offers to listen, but does not push the bereaved to ventilate emotions.

Nurses offering emotional support for grieving people are best guided to practice presence and active listening. Nurses should acknowledge the impending or actual loss and invite expression without forcing it in any way. Here are beginning words that may be helpful with the newly bereaved:

- "I understand you just lost your husband. Would you like to talk about it?"
- "I'm truly sorry for your loss. How are you doing?"
- "I hear you have gone back to work. Have you been able to grieve?"
- "You've been caring for him for years. Have you been grieving all that time?"

We open the door to expression by naming the grief and being willing to listen. Those grieving choose what and how much to share.

Making Referrals

When grief is uncomplicated, time is the healer, as symptoms gradually subside over months or years. Professional counseling is not needed. Some individuals will benefit from sharing through bereavement support groups, which are offered by most hospices as well as other community agencies.

WWW.   Internet Resource Box

See *www.rivendell.org* for information on Internet e-mail support groups.

In contrast to those enduring normal grief, evidence demonstrates that individuals with complicated grief reaction benefit from intervention. Bereavement counseling after a sudden traumatic death such as suicide, for instance, and counseling for children who are dealing with sibling or parental deaths has consistently been demonstrated to be beneficial. The more complicated the grief process, the more likely referral for therapeutic intervention will be helpful (Schut et al., 2001). Therefore, skilled nursing assessment of grieving individuals is essential. Take another look at Box 7-4, Complicated Grief Assessment. Therapists with grief counseling expertise include social workers, individual and family counselors, psychiatrists, clergy, and those specifically trained as grief therapists. The local hospice is usually an excellent source for names of those with the best reputation in the community.

Loss and transitions in life cause great suffering, but also provide opportunities for individuals to emerge stronger. New coping skills developed through the bereavement experience can include renewed meaning, enhanced problem-solving, stronger relationships with family and friends and within the community, and enhanced personal resources such as greater self-esteem, independence, compassion, and appreciation of everyday life (Schaeffer & Moos, 2001). Grief can be devastating but it is possible to rise out of it stronger and more resilient.

CONCEPTS IN ACTION

Amy has been the sole caregiver for her 47-year-old husband Tom, who is in the final stages of a progressive neurological disorder (ALS). He is short of breath and having great difficulty swallowing. Tom has chosen not to have a feeding tube or a ventilator. Amy has presented at the clinic with anorexia and weight loss, nausea, and headaches. The work-up for underlying disease is negative. When you sit down with her to understand her personal circumstances, she tells you about Tom's circumstances. She confides to you that she is really angry at Tom for being a very demanding patient, and that her caregiving skills are slipping. She describes herself as growing more and more disorganized. She perceives herself as deteriorating mentally. Every time he has an acute episode of respiratory distress, she becomes agitated and forgets what medicine to give him.

- Identify the name of the grief-related nursing diagnosis for Amy. What evidence supports this diagnosis?
- What words would you use with Amy to normalize her symptoms?
- What words would you use to encourage her to express emotions, if she chooses?
- Imagine that Amy and Tom live in your community. What resources are available in your community to help with the caregiver role strain that Amy is experiencing?
- What are the limits of the resources available in your community?
- If Amy's grieving becomes complicated (dysfunctional), what grief counseling resources are available in your community?

References

Abrums, M. (2000). Death and meaning in a storefront church. *Public Health Nursing, 17*(2), 132–142.

Albom, M. (1997). *Tuesdays with Morrie.* New York: Doubleday.

Bridges, W. (1980). *Making sense of life's transitions.* Reading, MA: Addison-Wesley.

Byock, I. (1997). *Dying well: Peace and possibilities at the end of life.* New York: Riverhead Books.

Connor, S. R. (2000). Denial and the limits of anticipatory mourning. In T. Rando (Ed.), *Clinical dimensions of anticipatory mourning* (pp. 253–266). Champaign, IL: Research Press.

Corr, C.A., & Corr, D.M. (2000). Anticipatory mourning and coping with dying: Similarities, differences, and suggested guidelines for helpers. In T. Rando (Ed.), *Clinical dimensions of anticipatory mourning* (pp. 223–252). Champaign, IL: Research Press.

Dinh A., Demp, C., & Rasbridge, L. (2000). Vietnamese health beliefs and practices related to the end of life. *Journal of Hospice and Palliative Nursing, 2*(3), 111–117.

Doka, K. J. (2000). Re-creating meaning in the face of illness. In T. Rando (Ed.), *Clinical dimensions of anticipatory mourning* (pp. 103–114). Champaign, IL: Research Press.

Eisenbruch, M. (1984). Cross-cultural aspects of bereavement: II. Ethnic and cultural variations in the development of bereavement practices. *Culture, Medicine and Psychiatry, 8*(4), 315–347.

Hall, M., & Irwin, M. (2001) Physiological indices of functioning in bereavement. In M. Stroebe, R. Hannson, W. Stroebe & H. Schut (Eds.), *Handbook of bereavement research: Consequences, coping, and care* (pp. 473–492). Washington, D.C.: American Psychological Association.

Irish, D., Lundquist, K., & Nelsen, V. (1993). *Ethnic variations in dying, death, and grief.* Washington, D.C.: Taylor & Francis.

Klass, D., Silverman, P., & Nickman, S. (Eds.). (1996). *Continuing bonds: New understandings of grief.* Washington, D.C.: Taylor & Francis.

Kubler-Ross, E. (1969). *On death and dying.* New York: Macmillan.

Lynn, J. L., & Harrold, J. (1999). *Handbook for mortals: Guidance for people facing serious illness.* New York: Oxford University Press.

Nolen-Hoeksema, S. (2001). Ruminative coping and adjustment to bereavement. In M. Stroebe, R. Hannson, W. Stroebe & H. Schut (Eds.), *Handbook of bereavement research: Consequences, coping, and care* (pp. 545–562). Washington, D.C.: American Psychological Association.

Parkes, C. M. (1999). *Bereavement: Studies of grief in adult life.* Madison, WI: International Universities Press.

Parkes, C. M. (2001). A historical overview of the scientific study of bereavement. In M. Stroebe, R. Hannson, W. Stroebe & H. Schut (Eds.), *Handbook of bereavement research: Consequences, coping, and care* (pp. 25–45). Washington, D.C.: American Psychological Association.

Pennebaker, J., Zech, E., & Rime, B. (2001). Disclosing and sharing emotions: Psychological, social, and health consequences. In M. Stroebe, R. Hannson, W. Stroebe & H. Schut (Eds.), *Handbook of bereavement research: Consequences, coping, and*

care (pp. 517–544). Washington, D.C.: American Psychological Association.

Prigerson, H. G., & Jacobs, S. C. (2001). Traumatic grief as a distinct disorder: A rationale, consensus criteria, and a preliminary empirical test. In M. Stroebe, R. Hannson, W. Stroebe & H. Schut (Eds.), *Handbook of bereavement research: Consequences, coping, and care* (pp. 613–646). Washington, D.C.: American Psychological Association.

Rando, T. (2000). *Clinical dimensions of anticipatory mourning.* Champaign, IL: Research Press.

Roos, S. (2002). *Chronic sorrow: A living loss.* New York: Brunner-Routledge.

Rosenblatt, P. C. (2001). A social constructionist perspective on cultural differences in grief. In M. Stroebe, R. Hannson, W. Stroebe & H. Schut (Eds.), *Handbook of bereavement research: Consequences, coping, and care* (pp. 285–300). Washington, D.C.: American Psychological Association.

Schafer, J. A., & Moos, R. H. (2001). Bereavement experiences and personal growth. In M. Stroebe, R. Hannson, W. Stroebe & H. Schut (Eds.), *Handbook of bereavement research: Consequences, coping, and care* (pp. 145–163). Washington, D.C.: American Psychological Association.

Schut, H., Stroebe, M., van den Bout, J., & Terheggen, M. (2001). The efficacy of bereavement interventions: Determining who benefits. In M. Stroebe, R. Hannson, W. Stroebe & H. Schut (Eds.), *Handbook of bereavement research: Consequences, coping, and care* (pp. 705–738). Washington, D.C.: American Psychological Association.

Shapiro, E. R. (2001). Grief in interpersonal perspective: Theories and their implications. In M. Stroebe, R. Hannson, W. Stroebe & H. Schut (Eds.), *Handbook of bereavement research: Consequences, coping, and care.* Washington, D.C.: American Psychological Association.

Smith, R. (1998). *Lessons from the dying.* Boston: Wisdom Publications.

Stroebe, M., Stroebe, W., Schut, H., Zech, E., & van den Bout, J. (2002). Does disclosure of emotions facilitate recovery from bereavement? Evidence from two prospective studies. *Journal of Consulting and Clinical Psychology, 70*(1), 169–178.

Warden, J., & Monahan, J. (2001). Caring for bereaved parents. In A. Armstrong-Dailey & S. Zarbock (Eds.), *Hospice care for children*. New York: Oxford University.

Wortman, C., & Silver, R. C. (2001). The myths of coping with loss revisited. In M. Stroebe, R. Hannson, W. Stroebe & H. Schut (Eds.), *Handbook of bereavement research: Consequences, coping, and care* (pp. 405–429). Washington, D.C.: American Psychological Association.

CHAPTER 8

Cross-Cultural Competency at the End of Life

Philosophical Reflections

"We must go beyond the familiar Golden Rule, which requires that we treat others as we would want to be treated, and instead treat others as they would like to be treated."

McGee, 2001

Learning Objectives

1. Understand the importance of culture and values in patients' perceptions of dying, death, and mourning.

2. Learn ways to perform cultural assessments in order to provide culturally competent care.

3. Identify practical strategies for bridging cultural gaps in providing end of life care.

4. Explain specific needs of selected cultural groups with whom nurses have frequent contact.

5. Explore challenges, such as poverty and informed consent, that are exacerbated by the obstacles posed by cultural variation.

6. Identify ways to overcome barriers to providing culturally competent care for marginalized populations.

Cross-cultural competency is an essential part of the End-of-Life Caregiving Tree; it is essential to connecting with patients and their families. The crown and the trunk reach upward to make connections with an American population that is becoming more and more culturally diverse. As you know, a primitive response to insecurity and unpredictability is to fight or flee. Tragically, this happens too often between nations and between neighbors of different ethnicities. As nurses, however, we can't fight or flee. In fact, we often must assist people who come from backgrounds that are very different from our own. Rather than fighting against beliefs, fleeing from calls for help, and opposing actions that we perceive as wrong, each of us needs to find ways to impart comfort. We can offer care more effectively to people of different cultures by sharpening our curiosity so that we can realize "the wholeness of other ways of living or seeing" (Bateson, 2000, p. 11). Although each of us may think that our own cultural beliefs define universal truth, our professional obligation is to listen, to respect, and to try to understand other ways. We must discover what others believe and how that affects the way they would like to be treated. Without losing our own center, we move outside our familiar circle and learn about other truths that define lives different from our own. We will discover many other ways of living and dying, and through that process we will be able to make better connections with our patients and their loved ones. This chapter addresses cultural identity, the practice of cultural competence, selected end-of-life beliefs of prominent ethnic groups, and cross-cultural issues at the end of life.

IMMIGRATION AND CULTURE

All Americans, except those who are 100% Native American, have ancestors who emigrated from other countries seeking freedom and economic opportunities. Immigration continues in large numbers today. The largest numbers arrive from Mexico, Central America, and South America. In addition, a large proportion of new immigrants were born in Asia, primarily Vietnam, China, India, Korea, and the Philippines. The number of immigrants from the Caribbean and from Eastern Europe is also significant. All of these groups have different ideas of truth and behavior (Spector, 2000).

Culture comprises the beliefs, practices, norms, likes, dislikes, customs, and rituals that we learn from our families and transmit to our children. Much of what we believe and do is determined by culture. Leininger and McFarlane (2002) assert that culture is the blueprint that predicts human motivation and action. *Socialization* is the process of growing up to acquire characteristics of culture. *Acculturation* involves identifying with one's traditional ethnic culture while, at the same time, learning about mainstream culture in order to survive. It is important for nurses to determine the degree to which people of a particular ethnic group identify with that group. To what extent is a person tied to traditional heritage and culture? Consistency with one's own ethnic heritage is determined by the degree to which a person has

> **Box 8-1 ■   FACTORS DETERMINING ETHNIC IDENTITY**
>
> The degree of identification with an ethnic "minority" group is determined by whether you:
>
> - Were raised in another country or in America.
> - Were reared in an extended family.
> - Presently stay in contact with extended family.
> - Marry someone of the same ethnic background.
> - Were educated in ethnic or mainstream environments.
> - Reside in an ethnic community.
> - Maintain traditional religious and cultural activities.
> - Interact primarily with people of similar ethnicity.
> - Speak the native language or have limited or no knowledge of it.

been socialized into ethnic or mainstream culture (Spector, 2000). See Box 8-1 to examine factors that determine ethnic identity.

■
WWW.   Internet Reference Box

To learn more about Leininger and Transcultural Nursing, log onto

www.tcns.org/documents/pdf/infopack.pdf.

Consider the majority mainstream American culture, largely white and of European background. Mainstream culture, and therefore values, dominates American politics, medicine, and nursing. Mainstream values emphasize personal control, individualism, self help, direct communication, action, and focus on future goals (Wurzbach, 2002). In contrast, many traditional cultures emphasize fate, group well-being, working as a group to help one another, indirect communication, being instead of doing, and the present or the past. Consider the clash of cultures that would take place trying to convince a new immigrant from a traditional culture to: take charge of her symptom management, help herself rather than always relying on her husband's decision, talk to you about her feelings and worries, and actively plan for what the family will do when her symptoms progress and she becomes bedridden. Cultural assessment is the groundwork for understanding.

Nurses are challenged in practice: bridging the cultural gaps between their own culture, each patient's culture, and mainstream health-care culture. A growing number of American nursing students and nurses are coming from cultures other than the mainstream European American culture. Nurses and nursing students who have strong ethnic identities may have already learned to bridge between their own backgrounds and mainstream social and health-care values.

> 66 | *Nurses are challenged in practice: bridging the cultural gaps between their own culture, each patient's culture, and mainstream health-care culture.*

CULTURAL COMPETENCE

Cultural competence involves having an attitude and developing behavior that permits effective work in cross-cultural nursing situations. Cultural competence at the end of life will increase trust and foster a comfortable, dignified death for the patient. Cultural competence requires a basic understanding of the different cultures that the nurse most commonly encounters.

Cultural Assessment

It is essential to complete individualized assessments of the cultural influences on a person's life. A cultural assessment guides individualized care planning. Standardized interventions may not be useful and could contradict deeply held cultural convictions. Cultural misunderstanding is a major barrier to providing emotional, spiritual, and physical comfort at the end of life. Box 8-2 outlines major questions that nurses should keep in mind as they interact with clients. Use this outline to assess your own background and to understand other members of the health-care team. Keep these questions in mind as you care for every patient whose cultural background differs significantly from your own. It will seldom be helpful to ask the questions directly in one session; usually the information will be gathered gradually and indirectly by several members of the health-care team. As you consider the need for cross-cultural assessment, it is important to realize that dying patients and their families may return to cultural values and behaviors of their youth.

Communication style varies dramatically between different cultural groups. See Box 8-3. It is very easy to get into trouble through ignorance of cultural rules about greetings, personal space, eye contact, and touch. In traditional cultures, for example, formal greetings, such as Mister, Reverend, and Doctor, are essential to respect. Younger North Americans may be more comfortable with casual first names. Different cultures have different rules about how far away or close to stand or sit. Some cultures will consider standing close as a threatening invasion of personal space, whereas other cultures consider maintaining distance as an impersonal indication of not caring. Eye contact is forbidden as rude and disrespectful by some cultures, and as essential to developing trust by others. Some cultures strictly prohibit touch between unrelated men and women; others consider a handshake as an essential mark of trust. Clearly, grasping even the most basic cultural mores can make the difference between offending someone and building trust.

Box 8-2 ■   **CULTURAL ASSESSMENT**

- Where was the person born? How long has the person lived in the United States? Where was the person's family born?
- How strong is the person's ethnic identity?
- Who are the person's support people and what is their ethnic identity?
- How does culture affect decisions regarding treatment? Who makes decisions?
- How will gender issues affect decision-making and caregiving?
- What languages are spoken and read? What is the person's educational background?
- How would you characterize communication style?
- What does the person believe about the cause and meaning of the illness? What language do they use to discuss it?
- What can be discussed openly and what cannot?
- How would the traditional culture treat the illness? How is this consistent with and conflicting with mainstream medicine?
- What foods are chosen and prohibited?
- What is the role of religion and spirituality at the end of life?

Source: Adapted from ELNEC (2000).

Spiritual beliefs and religious practices are often inseparable from end-of-life cross-cultural practices. A brief spiritual assessment is discussed here because it is integral to cultural understanding. Use the mnemonic "FICA" (Mazanec & Tyler, 2003) to remember to ask about the following concerns:

- *Faith.* Ask whether faith plays a significant role in the person's life. A fundamental question is "What gives your life meaning?"
- *Influence.* Ask how faith influences the person's thoughts about experiences with the current illness. "How is your faith influencing the way you are living?"
- *Community.* Determine whether the person is a member of a faith community and whether the community is supportive.
- *Address.* Inquire whether the person has spiritual concerns that she would like to discuss. To whom would she like to speak?

Building Bridges

After performing a thorough cultural assessment, the next step to care effectively across cultures is to bridge the gaps between cultures. Building bridges

Box 8-3 ■   CROSS-CULTURAL DIFFERENCES IN COMMUNICATION STYLE

GREETING

Always begin by using last name with Mr. or Ms. until further instructed. Inquire as to how the person wishes to be addressed.

PERSONAL SPACE

Observe the person's reactions to people standing close to them. For some cultures, a certain distance must be observed or the professional is considered to be aggressive. For others, a person who is not close enough might be perceived as uncaring.

EYE CONTACT

Watch the person's reactions. In some cultures, eye contact is essential for communication to be considered sincere. In other cultures, direct eye contact is seen as rude and disrespectful. The latter view is espoused by most Asian Americans, Native Americans, Arab American women with men, and sometimes Hispanic Americans. Among African Americans, eye contact indicates trust and looking away may signal distrust.

TOUCH

Observe the person's reaction. In some cultures, handshakes are respectful, and comforting touch of the shoulder or arm is reassuring. In other cultures, touch by strangers is invasive. Touch between men and women is often governed by strong cultural rules.

CONVERSATIONAL STYLE

Mainstream American style is often frank and straightforward about emotionally sensitive matters such as the symptoms of illness and need for end-of-life discussion. Many traditional cultures require indirect communication about difficult matters. Sometimes difficult issues must be referred to family. When patients look down, smile politely, or nod without speaking, the nurse cannot assume they understand or agree.

Source: Adapted from ELNEC (2000).

> ## Box 8-4 ■ CROSS-CULTURAL NEGOTIATION STRATEGIES
>
> - Ask the patient and family for their understanding of illness and prognosis.
> - Provide clear biomedical explanations in lay terminology.
> - Develop a plan that incorporates both traditional and biomedical approaches.
> - Incorporate helpful and neutral beliefs as patient and family wish.
> - Work collaboratively with traditional healers.
> - Acknowledge any continuing conflict between the heath-care team approach and that of patient and family.
> - Keep working toward compromise.
> - Refer the patient if no compromise can be reached and harmful practices continue.
>
> *Source:* From Tripp-Reimer, Brook, and Pinkham (1999).

between cultures requires sensitive negotiation (Tripp-Reimer, Brink, and Pinkham, 1999). See Box 8-4, Cross-Cultural Negotiation Strategies. The negotiation process involves a continual effort to find common understanding between medical and cultural approaches to the illness. Negotiation to find common ground requires time for mutual listening and shared decision-making. You will need to be patient and appear unhurried in order to understand and negotiate. Many traditional cultures, for example, require indirect communication about emotionally sensitive matters. Therefore, people who do not believe in straightforward communication are not going to say to you immediately, "It is forbidden to speak about dying in front of a dying person!" One major role of nursing is to recognize that great diversity exists in beliefs and expected behaviors around illness and dying, to openly address those differences, and to discover ways that beliefs can be incorporated into a palliative plan.

Often the nurse can serve as a broker between the patient and other health professionals, interpreting the system to the patient and the patient to the system. For instance, the nurse might explain to the physician that her patient will not complain of pain because he believes that suffering is essential to stay in control, but that the nurse observes his pain to be so severe that he cannot move out of the fetal position. Likewise, a nurse might explain to that patient that his severe pelvic pain can be controlled with opioids and that she has seen other patients with his kind of pain get out of bed and even go to church.

Nurses should be searching constantly for mutual understanding and common values. Many traditional customs can be incorporated into the plan of care. Such customs may prove beneficial, like singing and chanting that have a calming effect on the patient. They may have a neutral effect, such as the use of amulets (a charm worn around the neck, wrist, or waist as a protection against evil). Sometimes you might perceive them as harmful, in which case you need to work with team members to assess the degree of harm and exclude them from the plan of care. For instance, some traditions may practice aggressive use of laxatives and enemas. Will the family accept that this practice is creating more suffering than relief? If not, there may come a time when you have to withdraw from providing care. Most of the time however, sensitive negotiations can lead to compromise and comfort.

Planting the Seeds

Cultural ignorance has the potential to cause major mistakes in the provision of care. The culturally competent nurse becomes an invaluable player on the health-care team. The ability to translate patient values to the team and to translate medical values to the patient is a scarce but highly sought-after resource. By focusing on and perfecting skills of cultural competence, nurses become not only indispensable to the health-care team, but trusted partners with patients and families.

Practical Tips on Bridging Cultural Differences

Here are some suggestions for applying cross-cultural sensitivity to your practice:

- Consider each patient as an opportunity to learn. Take every opportunity to discover the person's world.
- Sit down with people and ask them what they believe and want. Be patient with indirect communication.
- Realize that dying patients may have little energy or ability to be cultural informants. Family and friends may be your major resources for understanding.
- Develop your ability to explain health-care practices in simple English.
- Develop your ability to explain the client's world to other members of the health-care team.
- Incorporate significant cultural practices into the plan of care.

ISSUES COMPLICATING CROSS-CULTURAL CARE

Several specific issues plague nurses trying to provide culturally competent care: poverty; trust and discrimination; expression and perception of pain; and truth telling and consent.

Poverty

A disproportionate number of African American and Hispanic families are poor. Immigrant families likewise suffer from higher rates of poverty and unemployment than mainstream Americans. As a result, those with strong ethnic identities are less likely to have health insurance. Throughout the nation, health services for those who cannot afford them are poorly financed. People with little money commonly endure poor health until problems severely disrupt their lives so that they are compelled to present themselves to the emergency department, which treats the immediate symptoms and sends them on their way. Continuity of care to manage a chronic problem like hypertension or diabetes is very rare. Therefore, when a poor minority person presents with end-stage disease, it is often the result of inadequate treatment earlier when cure or good management was possible (Crawley, Payne, Bolden, Payne, Washington, and Williams, 2000). Generally, he or she will have no familiar provider and may be referred to multiple specialists, who are difficult to access and do not communicate with each other. Patients may deliberately stay away because of fear of humiliation and discrimination. They may actually be denied specialist care because they lack insurance that will cover it. Is it any wonder that many poor people of color distrust the health-care system when they are finally told "nothing more can be done"?

At the end of life, nurses have the opportunity to listen compassionately to the stories of impoverished patients who tell us that the health-care system has been of little help to them and now they are dying. At the end of life, we cannot alter the cruelties of the past, but we can do everything in our power to foster respect and quality of life in the last days and months. We can work to build trust with those who have not felt that they could previously trust the health-care system.

Trust and Discrimination

Patients who lack trust and have endured discrimination form a cultural subgroup all their own. Nurses need to be aware of qualities that characterize patients who do not trust us because they have endured significant discrimination. African Americans, and other minorities who have lived with discrimination throughout their lives, may believe, for example, that withdrawal of aggressive treatment is a way to legalize neglect and abandonment. Having at times been denied the benefits of full participation in society during their lives, they are likely to fight for long life even if it means suffering. Therefore, they often refuse Do Not Resuscitate orders, hospice referrals, and advance directives. Refer to Box 8-5 listing African American barriers to palliative care. Fortunately, the Initiative to Improve Palliative End-of-Life Care in the African American Community has been launched to overcome these barriers in the coming years (Crawley et al., 2001).

> ### Box 8-5 ■　BARRIERS TO EFFECTIVE END-OF-LIFE CARE IN THE AFRICAN AMERICAN COMMUNITY
>
> - Lack of accurate knowledge about hospice and palliative care.
> - Lack of communication with health-care providers.
> - Believing that giving up aggressive treatment is giving up hope.
> - Avoidance of end-of-life planning as a dimension of the need to sustain hope.
> - Fear of racism and discrimination in health-care system that leads to inadequate care and premature death.
> - Unsympathetic, blunt health-care providers.
> - Fear that they will not be heard.
>
> *Source:* From Jackson, Schim, Seely, Grunow, and Baker (2000).

The sufferings of a minority person are compounded if they are living with a stigmatizing disease such as mental illness, drug or alcohol abuse, or AIDS. Issues around trust and discrimination are further compounded if they are homeless or living in a neighborhood perceived as dangerous, if they are survivors of war or torture in their native country, if they have few friends and are estranged from family, and if they have a history of violent behavior or have been associated with criminal activities. They may have deep emotional wounds worsened by whatever is now causing them to die. Working with people living on the "ragged edge of society" (Zerwekh, 2000) requires breaking through fear to connection with the humanness of the person who has often been forgotten and despised. A nurse describes one such patient:

> We have HIV patients who are economically challenged. . . . So many people prejudge them based on their economics or culture and so I make sure there are no biases. . . . They still come in with the expectation that they are going to be treated as a lesser class of society. J.J. had a history of substance abuse. He had gained weight, was clean-shaven, was looking for work, was stable, and then he fell hard and went back on the streets. Eventually he was arrested and thrown in jail. His mom called and said, "I am afraid he is going to die in jail." I got in touch with the jail and he had developed so many illnesses as a result of not being on therapy for 8 months. . . . He had lesions from head to toe. His hair was falling out everywhere. I put my hand on him for awhile, and he said it's so nice to have somebody just touch me because people have been afraid to touch me. . . . Even if it's just having my head on their shoulder while I listen to their heart, there is an expression of

caring that I believe is essential for anybody to be successful. My patients give back to me as much as I give to them. (Condensation of interview with Christopher Saslo, FNP, MSN)

Following are suggestions for work with patients who have severe problems with trust and much experience with discrimination (Hughes, 2001):

- Address them as Mr. or Mrs. unless they request otherwise.
- Shake hands unless culturally contraindicated (Muslim and Orthodox Jewish men).
- Make eye contact unless culturally prohibited or the patient reacts negatively.
- Realize physical contact may be either threatening or comforting.
- Put yourself in their shoes to try to understand behavior.
- Do not take insults personally. Do insist on basic respect.
- Ask for the person's story. Listen.
- Follow through on promises.
- Expect noncompliance and do not reject the person.
- Provide direct material assistance like food and hygiene kits if you are nursing in the community.
- Never forget your shared humanity.
- Celebrate small nursing victories.

For example, a nurse is working with Fred, a terminally ill alcoholic patient, who is living on the sofa in Harry's trailer. She has come to expect that Fred will not always follow through on medical appointments, that he does not take medication for symptom relief as prescribed, and that he asks for help finding housing and food whenever he has an argument with Harry. She recognizes the need to provide direct material assistance by working closely with the social worker to find subsidized meals and housing acceptable to Fred, who is used to living alone. She never forgets their shared humanity and states, "After all, we're all human beings. I treat him like I would my brother." Whenever Fred has a stable living situation and is taking medication regularly to relieve his suffering, she celebrates that small nursing victory.

🌱 Planting the Seeds

When our patients have lived with poverty and discrimination, it's a small nursing victory when they are gracious enough to open the door to us. It's a small victory when they laugh with us. It's a small victory when they are patient with all our paperwork and let us come back again. It's a small victory when they begin to tell us about their lives and worries. It's a small victory if they follow through on one suggestion we have made. It's a small victory when they tell us that the suggestion worked. It's a small victory when they tell us truthfully that our great advice didn't work. It's a small victory when they continue to listen to our suggestions and make one more effort to see if that might work to ease their suffering. Such victories should never be taken for granted.

Pain

Pain experience and pain expression are often determined by culture. Depending on one's culture, pain and other symptoms may be perceived as punishment, as a way to build character, as an indication that the body is fighting back, or perhaps as a spiritual necessity (Mitty, 2001). For some people, eradicating the pain may eradicate an experience that is considered spiritually and culturally necessary at the end of life. For other groups, expression of pain is expected and encouraged. For some, quiet endurance is highly valued.

> 66   *Depending on one's culture, pain and other symptoms may be perceived as punishment, as a way to build character, as an indication that the body is fighting back, or perhaps as a spiritual necessity (Mitty, 2001).*

It is useful to contrast pain beliefs and expression among some of the most common American ethnic minorities (St. Marie, 2002). As always, such generalizations risk stereotyping and are affected by degree of ethnic identity, age, education, sex, and individual uniqueness. African Americans are generally expressive of pain and may be particularly worried about the dangers of addiction. By contrast, Native Americans often do not report pain and seldom ask directly for pain relief. They respect silent endurance. Likewise, Chinese Americans are stoic and may not complain; they fear side effects of drugs. Although Hispanic Americans usually have an expressive style, there can be an expectation of stoicism in the face of suffering (Kemp, 2001). Pain may be perceived as punishment. Hispanics also likely fear addiction.

Whenever nurses are working with ethnic minority patients, we need to anticipate differing cultural perceptions and ways of handling pain. We should not stereotype, but should be aware that some people expect themselves to endure quietly whereas others expect to be able to express it loudly when they are suffering. Our pain assessment must be systematic and deliberate before we come to conclusions based on initial assumptions.

Truth and Consent

The United States health-care system values telling the truth about medical diagnosis and prognosis. We believe that people have a right to all pertinent medical information in order to render the most informed decisions about their care. However, the doctrine of informed consent causes many cross-cultural dilemmas because not only do views of telling the truth about medical diagnoses vary dramatically, but decision-making practices differ as well across cultures (Crow, Matheson, and Steed, 2000).

In some cultures, telling the truth is considered harmful, and the degree of truth-telling is the responsibility of family, not nurse or physician. Some Korean and Mexican American patients, for example, are unlikely to want to be told that they are dying and do not want any role in end-of-life decisions. Many cultures assert that speaking about death can bring it closer; this is true across continents in countries ranging from South Africa to Mexico, Italy to China (Mitty, 2001).

Consent is a critical issue at the end of life, and presents dilemmas at every turn. Many elders from mainstream and ethnic backgrounds want to have medical authorities make all decisions. Many ethnic people of all ages also defer to authority figures for decision-making. That authority, however, may be traditional leaders and healers rather than the health-care system. For most traditional people, the family is responsible for major decisions. Patient autonomy is not considered liberating; it is perceived as an unnecessary burden that causes loss of hope (Mitty, 2001).

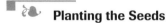 **Planting the Seeds**

Patients should always be asked whether they want to make decisions about their care, or whether they wish to defer to others in authority.

END-OF-LIFE BELIEFS AND BEHAVIORS ACROSS CULTURES

One distinguishing feature between cultures is how they approach dying, death, and mourning. When mainstream Americans are hurting from bereavement, they are expected to move toward greater autonomy and self-reliance. Many nurses possess this orientation, which explains why it is important to be aware that patients come from many different perspectives. Box 8-6 summarizes beliefs and behaviors before and after death of mainstream Americans and seven distinct traditional groups living in the United States. Such summaries can only be snapshot simplifications about each group. No matter what the culture, keep in mind that individualized assessment is essential and that stereotypes are dangerous. Cultures are continually evolving and there are many variations among groups and within groups. Moreover, people living within the United States have experienced varying degrees of acculturation, influenced by age, education, socioeconomic status, employment, and community connections. The following sections describe the experiences of individuals with strong ethnic identities from three cultural traditions: African American, Mexican American, and Chinese American.

An African American Man at the End of Life

Mr. Earl Roberts is a 65-year-old African American married man employed 31 years by the steel industry. Four years ago the plant in his town, employing

Box 8-6 ■ END-OF-LIFE BELIEFS AND BEHAVIORS

BELIEFS ABOUT DEATH	BEFORE-DEATH BEHAVIOR	AFTER-DEATH BEHAVIOR
MAINSTREAM		
Christian and Jewish	Reliance on technological answers	Funeral industry prescribes behavior
Increasing diversity	Nuclear families often isolated from	Limited expression of feelings
Significant number of atheists	extended family and community	Bereaved expected to go back
	Patient makes decisions	to work as soon as possible
HISPANIC		
Afterlife and resurrection	Family makes decisions	Prolonged wakes
Primarily Roman Catholic	Extended family care	Open displays of emotion
	Prayer and folk remedies	Families may want to prepare body
	Amulets common	Extended grieving
AFRICAN AMERICAN		
Primarily Protestant or Muslim	Elders may make decisions	Open displays of emotion
Believe in afterlife and	Caribbean and Louisianan	
Judgment	heritage may use voodoo rituals	
	May ask for help from lay healers	
	Family oriented	
	Fear of addiction with analgesics	
CHINESE		
Primarily Buddhist	Traditional Chinese medicine	Family stays with and prepares body
of many sects	Reluctance to complain	Controlled emotion
Belief in life as cycle	End-of-life issues not discussed	Ritual prayers
of suffering and rebirth	Family makes decisions	Relatives gather every 7 days
	Family provides care	
	Maintain harmony and balance	
	May use traditional therapies	
	such as acupuncture	

Group	Religion/Beliefs	Care/Customs	Death Practices
INDIANS FROM INDIA (From Bhungalia & Kemp, 2002)	Hindu Soul reincarnated on 12th day after death	Ayurvedic medicine Belief that suffering inevitable Family members gather Chanting and prayer at bedside	Family prepares body Organ donation prohibited Preference for cremation May control or express emotion
WEST AFRICAN: NIGERIANS (Henry & Kemp, 2002)	Muslim or Christian blended with pantheistic indigenous religion involving many gods and spirits	Extended family decisions May withhold or openly discuss Traditional healers including herbalists.	Burial at death Highly expressive funerals May be complex rituals to prepare the body Widow does not inherit material goods
EAST AFRICA: SOMALIANS (From Kemp & Rasbridge, 2001)	Muslim Belief in afterlife	Strong family commitment to caregiving Turning the body toward Mecca and ritual prayers as death imminent Outside family, strong rules keep men and women apart. No touching Women veiled Traditional healers; herbal remedies	Public and family funeral Cremation forbidden Family prepares body
NATIVE AMERICAN	Beliefs vary with tribe Christian acculturation	Families make decisions Avoid eye contact and aggressive questioning May not report pain Likely to avoid discussing death Herbs and traditional healers	Christian practices May incorporate traditional chanting

1300 workers, closed. He was recently diagnosed with advanced multiple myeloma and suffers from confusion, nausea, anorexia, and severe bony pain. He is receiving IV fluids for his hypercalcemia. He refuses all morphine but will accept an occasional Percocet when he cannot sit or stand due to the pain. His 41-year-old son, Matthew Roberts, a defense attorney in a neighboring state, has arrived at the hospital bedside as you are preparing for his father's transfer to the local hospice program. The son tells you to leave the room and loudly proclaims, "They are not going to give up on Dad! He's getting every test and treatment they have here! They just want to shove him out of here because he doesn't have any money. They just don't want to be bothered with him."

Consider the context of Mr. Roberts's circumstances. He and his wife Irna are life-long Bible-based church members. They believe in a better life where they will be going in Heaven and have attended many "home going" services for friends and relatives.

They have a long history of struggle in their own lives. Mr. Roberts's ancestors lived in slavery; his family expects him to endure through much physical pain in the battle against death. They are very unsure about accepting hospice care. They perceive entering a hospice as giving up hope, maybe even hastening his death. Mr. Roberts quietly explains, "Only Jesus can decide when I go. I've got to go through the fire until he takes me home."

Like many African Americans, the Roberts mistrust the medical system. It is true that black Americans are less likely to receive technological interventions for cancer, heart disease, and kidney failure (Crawley et al., 2000; Crawley, Marshall, Lo, and Koenig, 2002; Kagawa-Singer & Blackhall, 2001). They die earlier than mainstream Americans. However, they fight hard to live. They are more likely to request aggressive life-sustaining treatment because they believe that economic or racist motivations are behind clinicians' decisions to discontinue aggressive therapy. And sometimes they are right. Their pain relief is worse than relief of mainstream Americans (Crawley et al., 2000; Crawley et al., 2002; Kagawa-Singer & Blackhall, 2001). Refer to Box 3-6, which outlines frequently reported barriers to African American patients receiving comforting end-of-life care.

An experienced hospice nurse sits down with Earl and Matthew Roberts. She is familiar with the barriers African Americans experience. She understands that Matthew is opposed to hospice care and knows that she must plan time to listen to this family's story. She knows that she cannot hurry. She asks about Mr. Roberts's past and listens attentively, sincerely affirming who he is as a person and his many strengths in the face of difficulty. She goes over Mr. Roberts's physical condition and interprets the signs and symptoms of disease progression. She explains the limited capability of medicine to alter the course of disease. She goes over the hospice benefit and the relief it would provide for Mr. and Mrs. Roberts. She describes the extensive support network offered by hospice and she constantly emphasizes their right to choose. Even if Earl and Matthew Roberts decide to seek more aggressive interventions, they will remember the connection they made with the nurse and perhaps seek hospice care eventually.

A Mexican American Woman at the End of Life

Sandra Garcia is a 71-year-old immigrant from Mexico who speaks limited English. Two married sons and a widowed daughter live within three miles of her apartment. She has seven grandchildren. Sandra is receiving care through a hospice program connected with a county hospital. She has no health insurance and no doctor. All of her life, she has relied on curanderos, folk healers in her neighborhood, who have been making regular house calls to prescribe her a mix of spiritual and herbal remedies. Two days ago, she presented to the emergency room for severe shortness of breath. Now she has newly diagnosed metastatic breast cancer that has spread to her lungs, liver, ribs, and hips. She will be receiving palliative radiation to the bony lesions and corticosteroids to improve her breathing. She is alert and oriented. Upon entering her room, you find her wearing a religious medal, fingering Rosary beads, and looking at a large picture of the Virgin Mary on her bedside table. Pictures of nieces, nephews, and grandchildren are also prominently displayed. A consulting surgeon has recommended a right mastectomy to remove the disfiguring tumor covering her right breast. You, as the nurse, have been trying to talk to Mrs. Garcia about her situation, whether to focus on comfort only or to accept more aggressive treatment, which would have only limited benefit. You ask her whether she wants the surgery and she smiles and tells you, "My son will talk to the doctor." Her fingers are continually moving along her Rosary beads and she seems distracted. However, you are very conscious of her rights and emphasize, "It's your body Mrs. Garcia. You have a right to make the decision!" She nods and looks down. You feel frustrated. The next day, her son Juan Garcia has a brief opportunity to speak to the surgeon on the phone. He comes into his mother's room and explains to you that his mother will not have the operation. He explains, "The doctor told me it won't help so much." Several family members are visiting. When you ask her about pain, she smiles and says "good, good." You are puzzled because you heard from report that she was often overheard moaning during the night.

In Hispanic culture, patients often defer to the father or oldest male relative to make decisions that are perceived to be too burdensome for patients themselves. Men are usually the key decision-makers. Extended families gather for support at times of difficulty; women are expected to be the primary caregivers. For instance, Juan hopes to take his mother home and his wife Cynthia will be expected to care for her mother-in-law, as well as their three young children. Respect for status and authority often leads families to follow the recommendation of physicians. Health beliefs have strong religious associations and illness is often seen as the consequence of supernatural forces, sometimes punishment from God. Illness is often managed through prayer, religious rituals, herbal remedies, and foods understood to be healing. Lay healers in the community are frequently consulted. The physical and spiritual world are strongly linked. Many Mexicans will deny physical and psychosocial pain, especially in the presence of relatives. Fortunately, Mrs. Garcia's family has accepted hospice care. As with African Americans, there are significant barriers that prevent many Hispanics from using hospice services: limited English, value placed on not expressing suffering, expectations that family will assume all responsibility for care, providers' ignorance of Hispanic culture, lack of health insurance, recent immigrant status, and lack of program outreach (Kemp & Rasbridge, 2001). A cross-cultural nursing plan of care for Mrs. Garcia should begin with the goals and interventions identified in Box 8-7.

Box 8-7 ■ PLAN OF CARE FOR MRS. GARCIA

GOALS	INTERVENTIONS
Control dyspnea and pain although patient denies both when asked directly.	Frequent attention to shortness of breath and nonverbal pain expression such as moaning. Around-the-clock medication rather than waiting for patient to request medication. Encourage patient to acknowledge distress.
Foster verbal communication despite patient's poor English skills.	Arrange for interpreters. Use assessment tools and other communication devices translated to Spanish. Ensure informed consent.
Reduce conflict between mainstream belief in patient decision and patient belief in family decision.	Serve as bridge between family and health team to interpret patient's desire for family to make all decisions. Be sure that patient is given continual opportunity to express preferences. Actively involve family in all decisions. Interpret the family to the health-care system and the health-care system to the family.
Prevent spiritual distress.	As patient and family request, actively involve hospice chaplain and church priest or other pastoral ministers. Ensure that comforting religious objects are at the bedside.
Prevent caregiver role strain.	Daughter-in-law will need extensive teaching. Ensure hospice home visiting. Interpret anticipated caregiver burdens to Juan and other male decision-makers. Encourage mobilization of extended family.
Foster healthy anticipatory grief.	Respect traditional grieving behavior and explain to rest of health-care team.

A Chinese American Woman at the End of Life

Lillian Chin is a 79-year-old Chinese American woman who emigrated from Hong Kong when she was 19. She is confined to bed and wheelchair at home, with severe chronic obstructive pulmonary disease. Mrs. Chin has been repeatedly hospitalized with pneumonia and twice placed on a ventilator. Your physical examination reveals that Mrs. Chin has bilateral coarse crackles and wheezing throughout her lungs; her apical pulse is 122 and irregular; she has pitting edema toe-to-knee; and there are multiple round red bruises over her back. Her son and his wife, Jim and Alice, are providing care for her in their home. She has said, "I never, never will go back to that hospital. Don't let them take me again." A hospice referral has been made and you are completing the paperwork with the Chins. To obtain her consent to services, you read the statement about hospice being provided for people who are dying. The daughter-in-law interrupts mid-sentence and urgently proclaims, "Come into the kitchen. I need to talk to you in the kitchen right now."

In the kitchen, Jim explains to you, "We can't talk about that. Mother understands that this is the end, but we can't speak it out loud. She'll sign the paper but she doesn't want to talk about it. I'll make any decisions that need to be made. That is her wish. Actually, we're not sure about hospice. We are a strong family and we care for our own." Traditional Chinese culture avoids direct verbal discussion of sensitive issues. This practice "saves face" so that the person is not embarrassed by emotions and can maintain her serenity. It is common for the family to withhold information from the patient and for the patient to pretend that she or he does not understand what is happening. The obligation that children will care for parents is termed "filial piety." Even with acculturated second generation Americans, hospice assistance must be discussed with great sensitivity so that the family members still feel they are fulfilling their duty (Kagawa-Singer & Glackhall, 2001).

Traditional Chinese healing includes herbs, amulets, acupuncture, bleeding, massage, moxibustion, and cupping (Spector, 2000). Moxibustion, for example, applies heated pulverized wormwood to the skin at certain points of the body. Cupping involves applying small hot glasses on the skin, often the back, to increase local circulation. Both moxibustion and cupping can create marks on the body, which can be misunderstood as manifestations of physical abuse. When applied by skilled practitioners, these healing methods often bring significant comfort to many people of Asian heritage.

A plan of care for Mrs. Chin involves initially addressing the first priority: relieving her severe dyspnea. The nurse would elevate the head of the bed, ensure that her home oxygen supply is effective, review palliative medications ordered to be sure they are effective and administered properly, call for a new order such as morphine by nebulizer, and arrange for sublingual morphine and benzodiazepine to be available for the family to administer in case of a respiratory crisis.

Now you turn your attention to cultural issues. You ask about the bruises on Mrs. Chin's back and learn that they are indeed from cups applied by a healer in the community. Had you not been culturally competent, you may have strongly suspected abuse by her caregivers. The patient denies that they hurt and says she always feels better when the healer comes. You ask about other practices the healer suggested, and the patient shyly reveals several paper amulets or charms that have been pinned on her clothing. You reassure her and the family that "anything that makes her comfortable is good." Since the family requests that they make the decisions and that there be no direct discussion of death-related subjects, you ask permission to ask one question that will then be documented in the hospice records, "Do you want to know about your disease and make all the decisions about your treatment, or do you want your family to do that?" Mrs. Chin clearly states that she wants the family to know and decide. Then, you assure the family that you will not bring up prognosis and treatment and will speak to the rest of the health-care team about how this will be essential to care for Mrs. Chin. After they agree to hospice services and Mrs. Chin signs, you focus the rest of the visit on teaching this family to care physically for Mrs. Chin at home until she dies. Thus, they will honor her last wish.

CONCEPTS IN ACTION

A Native American Man at the End of Life

The 350 Native American tribes in the United States vary greatly in customs and values. For example, the contrast between the Cherokees and the Crows is as great as the contrast between Chinese and English (Irish, Lundquist, and Nelsen, 1993). Thomas Running Bear is a 58-year-old veteran of the Vietnam War, currently living in a large Midwestern city. He grew up on a Lakota Sioux reservation where his sister and two cousins still live. Tom was diagnosed with insulin dependent diabetes mellitus when in the military. Over the years, he has suffered many cardiac and vascular complications. Currently he has a right side below-the-knee amputation and gangrene of his left foot. His heart is failing after two bypass surgeries. He has pulmonary edema that is not responding to diuretics. His breathing is loud and wet. His physician has signed a Do Not Resuscitate order. You learn from a change-of-shift report that "a bunch of drunken Indians have been making a lot of noise in his room. We think some of them are smoking dope." You enter the room to find three men chanting and a stick of dried grass burning. Two women are sitting silently and looking very sad. No one looks at you. You assess Thomas and find he has no palpable blood pressure. He is having long periods of apnea. One woman looks up and asks, "Would you please call Reverend Matthews?"

(continued)

CONCEPTS IN ACTION   (CONTINUED)

The Lakota Sioux are the second-largest American Indian nation (Irish, Lundquist, and Nelsen, 1993). As is true with most other Native American tribes, end-of-life rituals often include both tribal and Christian practices (Irish et al., 1993). Respect requires avoiding eye contact and maintaining a respectful distance. Native people are particularly vulnerable to the destructive effects of alcohol, which was not used until Europeans settled in North America. Because of the high incidence of alcoholism, health-care providers can easily stereotype them as alcoholics, which the nurses did during the change-of-shift report.

* How might you comfort Mr. Running Bear?
* How can you come to understand the family behavior?
* How would you approach the family? What words would you say to the family?
* How could you explain the family to the health-care team?
* How might you express your respect to the family?

References

Bateson, M. C. (2000). *Full circles, overlapping lives*. New York: Ballantine.

Bhungalia, S., & Kemp, C. (2002). (Asian) Indian health beliefs and practices related to the end of life. *Journal of Hospice and Palliative Nursing, 4*(1), 54–58.

Crawley, L., Marshall, P., Lo, B., & Koenig, B. (2002). Strategies for culturally effective end-of-life care. *Annals of Internal Medicine, 136*(9), 673–679.

Crawley, L., Payne, R., Bolden, J., Payne, T., Washington, P., & Williams, S. (2000). Palliative and end-of-life care in the African-American community. *Journal of the American Medical Association, 284*(19), 2518–2521.

Crow, K., Matheson, L., & Steed, A. (2000). Informed consent and truth telling: Cultural directions for health care providers. *Journal of Nursing Administration, 30*(3), 148–152.

ELNEC (End-of-Life Nursing Education Consortium). (2000). *Cultural considerations in end of life*. Washington, DC: American Association of Colleges of Nursing.

Henry, D., & Kemp, C. (2002). Culture and the end of life: Nigerians. *Journal of Hospice and Palliative Nursing, 4*(2), 111–115.

Hughes, A. (2001). The poor and underserved. In B. Ferrell & N. Coyle (Eds.), *Textbook of palliative nursing* (pp. 461–466). New York: Oxford University Press.

Irish, D., Lundquist, K., & Nelsen, V. (1993). *Ethnic variation in dying, death, and grief: Diversity in universality*. Washington, DC: Taylor and Francis.

Jackson, F., Schim, S. M., Seely, S., Grunow, K., & Baker, J. (2000). Barriers to hospice care for African Americans: Problems and solutions. *Journal of Hospice and Palliative Nursing, 2*(2), 65–72.

Kagawa-Singer, M., & Blackhall, L. (2001). Negotiating cross-cultural issues at the end of life: "You got to go where he lives." *The Journal of the American Medical Association, 286*(23), 2993–3001.

Kemp, C. (2001). Culture and the end-of-life: Hispanic culture (Mexican

American). *Journal of Hospice and Palliative Nursing, 3*(1), 29–33.

Kemp, C., & Rasbridge, L. (2001). Culture and the end of life: East African cultures: Part I, Somali. *Journal of Hospice and Palliative Nursing, 3*(2), 59–61.

Leininger, M., & McFarland, M. (2002). *Transcultural nursing: Concepts, theories, research and practice* (3rd ed.). New York: McGraw-Hill Companies.

Mazanec, P., & Tyler, M. K. (2003). Cultural considerations in end-of-life care. *American Journal of Nursing, 103*(3), 50–58.

McGee, C. (2001). When the golden rule does not apply: Starting nurses on the journey toward cultural competence. *Journal for Nurses in Staff Development, 17*(3), 105–112.

Mitty, E. (2001). Ethnicity and end-of-life decision-making. *Reflections on Nursing Leadership, 27*(1), 28–31, 46.

Spector, R. (2000). *Cultural diversity in health and illness.* Upper Saddle River, NJ: Prentice-Hall.

St. Marie, B. (2002). *Core curriculum for pain management nursing.* Philadelphia: WB Saunders.

Tripp-Reimer, T., Brink, P.I., & Pinkham, C. S. (1999). Cultural brokerage. In G. Bulechek & J. McCloskey (Eds.), *Nursing interventions: Effective nursing treatments* (pp. 637–649). Philadelphia: WB Saunders.

Wuzbach, M. E. (2002). *Community health education and promotion.* Gaithersburg, MD: Aspen.

Zerwekh, J. (2000). Caring on the ragged edge: Nursing persons who are disenfranchised. *Advances in Nursing Science, 22*(4), 47–61.

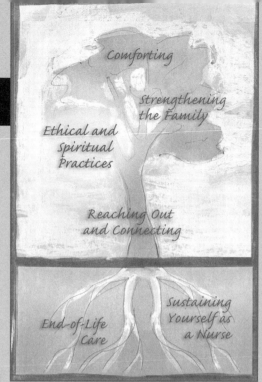

Comforting

Strengthening
the Family

Ethical and
Spiritual
Practices

Reaching Out
and Connecting

End-of-Life
Care

Sustaining
Yourself as
a Nurse

ETHICAL AND
SPIRITUAL
PRACTICES

CHAPTER 9

Ethical Issues at the End of Life

Philosophical Reflections

"It has become increasingly clear that the ability to prolong life has outpaced medical, philosophical, bioethical, and societal efforts to reach a value-based consensus on the goals of and criteria for care. . . . Ethical dilemmas on macro- and micro-levels emerge daily as the debate on extending life versus postponing death continues."

KAREN STANLEY AND LAURIE ZOLOTH-DORFMAN, 2000

Learning Objectives

1. Explain the importance of nurses questioning the ethical implications of interventions that they are expected to implement at the end of life.
2. Explain the relevance of compassion and courage in end-of-life ethical practice.
3. Define the end-of-life relevance of ethical duties, including beneficence, nonmaleficence, autonomy, veracity, fidelity, and justice.
4. Describe the impact of utilitarian ethics at the end of life.
5. When families are in conflict at the end of life, explain how a focus on care ethics fosters resolution.
6. Discuss the limits of advance directives and the advantages of the health-care power of attorney.
7. Explain the principles that a health-care surrogate is expected to use to make decisions when the patient has lost decisional capacity.
8. Describe the circumstances of social injustice at the end of life.
9. Define futility, proportionate good, and ordinary versus extraordinary treatments.
10. Contrast the ethical implications of withholding and withdrawing therapies.

11. Discuss the end-of-life benefits and burdens of antibiotics, food and water, turning, and positioning.

12. Contrast active euthanasia and assisted suicide, and explore associated ethical issues.

13. Discuss the ethical implications of withdrawing life-sustaining interventions for patients in persistent vegetative states.

Ethics is a process of reflecting on moral beliefs, and bioethics refers to the study and analysis of ethical issues that arise in the fields of health care and biological sciences. Nursing ethics comprises one dimension of bioethics. This chapter addresses the challenges of nursing ethics at the end of life. Ethical and Spiritual Caring represent one branch of the End-of-Life Caregiving Tree; both involve the search for meaning and acting in a manner that is consistent with the deepest human values. This chapter begins by acknowledging that nursing at the end of life often poses striking ethical challenges. The chapter explains the fundamentals of ethics based on virtue, duty, consequences, and relationships. It also discusses in depth end-of-life challenges regarding autonomy and avoidance of killing.

NURSING IN THE MIDDLE

To nurse at the end of life, you need to become conscious of how value-laden the choice of medical and nursing interventions can be. We practice in the middle of an ethical minefield. Even the most ordinary nursing measures, such as turning, feeding, and bathing, can elicit ethical conflicts. Physicians, families, patients, and a combination thereof make decisions. Nurses are often the ones asked to carry out their value-laden choices. Nurses remove the tubes and lines and administer the morphine. Sometimes, without discussion, physicians order us to intervene in ways that may end life or cause permanent unconsciousness (Schwarz, 1999). Nurses can become the "delegated providers" of assisted dying. These decisions—made by others—inflict on us significant moral turmoil. "Nurses experience moral distress when they are unable to translate their moral choices into moral action or when they feel that nursing virtues are undermined" (Volbrecht, 2002).

❝ *Naming and clarifying ethical issues is a prominent nursing role at the end of life.*

We can learn to manage and avoid moral distress by defining an issue as having ethical implications, analyzing conflicting moral obligations, and participating in meaningful collaborative dialogue to reach an ethical solution. Naming and clarifying ethical issues is a prominent nursing role at the end of life. Nurses witness patients' lives and hear their concerns. To mitigate our own moral distress and practice our caring role as nurses, we must continually guide the focus of the interdisciplinary team to emphasize what is good for the patient and those who love him. We must strengthen our voices and ask, "Is what we are doing good for this person and family? Is this what the person wants?" We cannot stay silent. Speaking out requires us to develop the virtue of moral courage. Often nurses feel morally uneasy about implementing specific therapies, but we are uncertain how to put our moral distress into words. This chapter will help the reader to identify the issues and articulate the questions specific to each patient's situation. It is helpful to be guided by ethical frameworks.

 We must strengthen our voice and ask, "Is what we are doing good for this person and family?"

ETHICAL FRAMEWORKS

Ethical decision-making is guided by a person's character or virtue, adherence to defined moral duties that respect human beings as persons, consideration of the consequences of decisions, and honoring relationships and the context of ethical decisions.

Virtue Ethics: Decisions Determined by Character

Aristotle described virtues as habitual patterns of perceiving, feeling, and behaving (Volbrecht, 2002). Virtues are strengths of character. For example, compassion and the courage to speak out are virtues that are central to effectively care for the dying. Compassion includes empathy, a deep sense of shared humanity, and a disposition to comfort and relieve suffering. Moral courage is necessary to question physician or institutional authority. The practice of virtue ethics integrates character and action. It posits that a person does the right thing because she cares deeply about it. Moral character is developed through mentoring by expert clinicians and peers. Ethical decisions are made based on critical reflection and ongoing dialogue about ethical issues as they are presented in the clinical setting. An important dynamic in critical reflection is the examination of ethical obligations as they have been defined by ethicists.

Moral Duties Based on Respect for Persons

Whereas a pure interpretation of virtue ethics emphasizes that a person will make a good decision because of her well-intentioned moral character, contemporary health-care ethics asserts that good decisions should be guided by fundamental ethical duties that require respect for persons. The obligation to respect each person emphasizes essential moral duties or principles: doing good, avoiding harm, respecting freedom of choice, speaking truthfully, being loyal, and promoting justice. Laying the groundwork for further discussion, each of these duties is briefly described here, including the name of the ethical principle identified. Consideration of these fundamental ethical duties should guide all ethical decisions.

Doing Good (Beneficence)

Beneficence involves simply doing good for others. At the end of life, beneficence is expressed through attentive listening, knowing the patient as a person, inquiring about well-being, and persistently trying to relieve suffering. Caring actions are a manifestation of beneficence. It is vital to patient well-being that nurses ask themselves whether their actions are truly doing good. So often fear actually prevents nurses from doing good. For instance, we might fear relieving suffering because stopping to listen carefully exposes our own vulnerability (Zerwekh, Riddell, and Richard, 2002). Or, we might fear comforting because we are afraid that medicating to relieve suffering will kill the patient. Or we might fear the anger of those in authority if we ask too many questions about how the medical regimen is benefiting the patient. Beneficent nursing practice at the end of life requires courage to confront our own fears. If a nurse is afraid to listen to a patient talk about how much he is hurting, the nurse will not be able to assess and relieve his pain. If a nurse is afraid to call the physician to request more pain medication, she will not be able to relieve pain. Such fears render us unable to practice beneficence.

66 | *Beneficent nursing practice requires courage to confront our own fears.*

Avoiding Harm (Nonmaleficence)

Nonmaleficence, the inverse of beneficence, is avoiding causing emotional and physical harm. It also involves an effort to foresee harms that might not at first be obvious. It includes the mandate to avoid killing and to prevent suffering. The moral requirement to do no harm has generated great controversy in end-of-life care because of the debate about medical decisions that may cause death. Alternatively, how do we fulfill our obligation of nonmaleficence when we are obligated to prolong life regardless of suffering? In the everyday world of nursing practice, nonmaleficence should play heavily into our decisions about whether to cause suffering at the end of life with common nursing actions like vigorous wound care, suctioning, turning, blood drawing, forcing fluids, forcing mobility, and performing frequent vital signs. Fear can lead nurses to cause harm because we feel powerless to question physicians' orders or the authority of an institution.

66 | *The moral requirement to do no harm has generated great controversy in end-of-life care because of the debate over medical decisions that may cause death.*

Respecting Freedom (Autonomy)

Individual liberty or self-determination is highly regarded in American society and in health care. The practice of requiring informed consent for medical intervention reflects this respect for autonomy. Autonomy was not emphasized in the United States until the latter half of the 20th century, however.

Before that, the Hippocratic tradition and oath, dating from around the fifth century B.C.E., emphasized paternalistic beneficence as the highest moral ground. Physicians believed they knew what was best, and patients were expected to comply without question (Veatch, 2003). This tradition still influences medical practice around the world. As a person dies, he loses the capacity to make his own decisions. This inevitable loss of autonomy presents significant end-of-life ethical challenges as clinicians and family members must take over decision-making for the patient. Traditional cultural perspectives on what is the right or wrong action at the end of life often diverge significantly from mainstream American bioethical emphasis on individual freedom. Chapter 8 examines dying from a cross-cultural perspective.

Speaking Truth (Veracity)

Veracity is fundamental to ethical relationships. Speaking truth involves avoiding lying, deception, and fraud. Multiple studies have revealed that most Americans want to know the truth about their illness and prognosis (Glass & Cluxton, 2004). Self-determination is not possible without knowing the truth. Patients from traditional cultures may choose not to be told the truth about their illness. In that case, they should be asked what they wish to know. If they refuse to hear information about illness and prognosis, they need to identify someone else to receive that information and make decisions.

Loyalty (Fidelity)

Fidelity involves establishment of a trusting nurse-patient relationship. Fidelity is usually achieved by persistence over time. But even brief nurse-patient encounters should be marked by trust. In a nurse-patient relationship, fidelity is the opposite of abandonment, neglect, and abuse. Fidelity at the end of life requires all clinicians to confront their own fears to develop and maintain trusting relationships with those near death.

Respecting Equality (Justice)

Respect for justice involves treating people fairly and without discrimination. Social or distributive justice requires fair distribution of community resources, a difficult ethical mandate in contemporary United States health care, which is characterized by a great contrast between health and health resources of the rich and poor. The poor die sooner and are less likely to receive hospice and palliative care (Williams, 2004).

Utilitarian Ethics: Focus on Consequences

Utilitarian thinking also influences contemporary American health-care ethics. Utilitarian thinking focuses on the consequences or outcomes of a decision. Social utilitarian thinking considers actions to be right in proportion to their ability to promote the greatest good for the greatest number of affected people. Utilitarian thinking applies to decisions about individual treatment when weighing the beneficial and burdensome consequences of treatment. This decision-making framework considers the beneficial consequences in determining whether or not an intervention should take place. Benefit/burden analysis is often used in end-of-life ethical decision-making to examine the anticipated consequences of a decision. One problem with this thinking framework is that individuals differ on what they believe to be a beneficial consequence.

Consider a social utilitarian perspective on extending the life of profoundly incapacitated individuals who cannot live without expensive medical regimens. A utilitarian perspective leads to questioning whether there are enough benefits for society to sustain their lives when the cost burdens are great. A growing number of facilities house children and adults who cannot swallow or breathe on their own. Inexpensive, fatal conditions have been turned into expensive, chronic conditions (Callahan, 1998).

Social utilitarian thinking asks us to weigh the benefits (more people are alive) and the burdens (cost of their care). Utilitarians look at the consequences to society. They assert that medical successes are turning into social hazards as medicine consumes ever more resources, which then are not available to fund other social needs, such as feeding and educating our children.

Care Ethics: Decisions Determined in Relationship

Beyond the language of conflicting duties and consequences, feminist and caring theorists have proposed a relational ethics of care to guide nursing practice (Volbrecht, 2002). Care ethics focuses on moral decision-making attentive to the context of relationships. Conflicts are resolved in ways that preserve community, family, and connection. Ethical decisions must always consider context of the decision and the well-being of caregivers as well as the patient. Care ethics emphasizes that patient and nurse are all part of one community. Such thinking stands in dramatic contrast to assumptions that human beings are intrinsically separate, and that autonomy is the highest moral imperative.

Family Good and Family Harm

Contemporary health-care ethics focuses primarily on what is good for the individual, and sometimes on what is good for society. The individual, however, lives in context of the family. A purely individualistic focus ignores the consequences of decisions made and gives little regard to family well-being. In fact, the family and other loved ones are intensely involved when a family member is dying. "The patient is in fact the patient-in-relation" (Ladd, Pasquerella, and Smith, 2000, p. 105). Respect for patient autonomy requires that the nurse ask the patient-in-relation to define what role he wants the family to have in decision-making. The needs of the family must be balanced with the needs of the suffering family members. It is vital that conflicts between patient and family needs be identified and carefully weighed, sometimes by the gathered health-care team and sometimes through ethical consultation. Consider conflict of needs in the following situations:

- A family's need to ensure food and shelter for themselves leads to neglect of a patient's comfort and safety.
- A family's desire that the patient remain alert as long as possible leads to failure to give sedating medication to relieve suffering.
- A family over-sedates the patient to avoid demands for care.
- A family desires to reduce its burden and accelerate dying by refusing all life-prolonging therapies for a family member.
- A family desires to prolong dying by insisting on all life-prolonging therapies.
- A family insists on a treatment that it believes will be helpful, although such treatment is known to be burdensome for the patient. Examples are oral suctioning and high volume hydration.
- Families are divided with some members wanting aggressive care to continue and others choosing palliation.

In the home environment, burden/benefit analysis must consider the impact of caregiving on all involved. Caregiver burden can involve lost schooling, lost income, lost relationships, and lost health. Ethical decisions should consider the limits of family obligation and how community resources can be mobilized to relieve caregiving burden. At the end of life, it is particularly important that the family and other loved ones be considered in all ethical decision-making. When there is conflict regarding life prolongation or palliation, the nurse, in close collaboration with social work and clergy, seeks to listen attentively, discover common ground to focus on the well-being of the dying person, and work out solutions where there is mutual agreement. Care ethics focuses on maintaining the delicate web of human relationships. When values collide, care ethics requires that nurses develop strong skills of mediation and conflict resolution to discover solutions that preserve human relationships. Family and loved ones must be refocused on considering the best interest of the patient. Help them listen to each other and look beyond opposed positions to discover shared and compatible values.

66 | *When values collide, care ethics requires that nurses develop strong skills of mediation and conflict resolution to discover solutions that preserve human relationships.*

CHALLENGES IN ETHICAL DECISION-MAKING

This section explores three types of ethical challenges commonly faced by nurses caring for patients at the end of life: respecting autonomy, fostering social justice, and avoiding killing while relieving suffering. It puts into practice the decision-making frameworks and principles discussed earlier.

Challenges to Respecting Autonomy at the End of Life

The liberty of the individual has dominated American health-care ethics since the 1970s (Veatch, 2003). Patients are expected to determine what is best for themselves. Authority lies in the individual's decision. For a person to act autonomously he must have truthful information, be free from controlling influences, and possess the capacity to make deliberate decisions (Ersek, 2004). There are many challenges to this ideal at the end of life, which pose ethical dilemmas for nurses and other health professionals. Challenges include uncertain and denied truth, informed consent, decisional capacity, noncompliance, advance planning, and surrogate decision-making. Despite these challenges, however, nurses should play an active role in promoting autonomy at the end of life.

Uncertain and Denied Truth

The truth about disease and prognosis always has an element of uncertainty. Contemporary treatment can significantly prolong life. Nevertheless, the reality of dying must be addressed with people with advanced life threatening illness. Denial of difficult truths is a common defense mechanism for patients, families, and professionals. In addition, family, physician, or other health team members may sometimes believe that being completely honest may cause more harm than good. Misinformation or actual deception is common (Glass & Cluxton, 2004). It is common for providers to disclose only incomplete information, while emphasizing the positive aspects. Providers may redirect questions to focus on encouraging information. Without complete information that includes their terminal condition, patients are unable to make decisions about their last days. Autonomy is denied. Consider the following example:

>An oncologist for a patient with prostate cancer metastasized to the brain, liver, and bone says to the patient:
>*Oncologist:* Your scans are looking good. There are no new lesions in your brain. Liver enzymes are coming down. We've got the pain in your pelvis under control. You're in good shape.
>*Patient:* I don't feel like I'm in good shape. You know, doc, I keep losing weight and I'm so tired.
>*Oncologist:* Well, there is a new clinical trial that looks promising.
>*Patient:* No, no doc. I want to die with my hair on! Do you think I'll make it to Christmas? I'm thinking of asking my whole family to come home one last time.
>*Oncologist:* Well, Dr. McNamara has a real promising clinical trial going on over at Memorial Medical Center. Let's call him.

Thus it happens that by hedging on the truth a physician encourages the patient to focus entirely on medical treatment and the patient loses the opportunity for self-determination in his last days.

Nurses support such deceit for many reasons, including concern about contradicting the physician's optimism, difficulty facing mortality, failing to overcome personal fears in order to have honest conversations, making assumptions that people really do not want to know the truth, believing that the only way to help is to focus on cure, and being unable to grieve their

---

Box 9-1 ■   TRUTH-TELLING STEPS

1. Ask difficult questions. Example: "What did your doctor tell you about how serious your illness is?"
2. Time your questions by watching for verbal and nonverbal cues that the patient desires discussion. When the patient turns away or changes the subject, respect that.
3. Balance what you know to be true with what the patient can accept.
4. Respect patient and family avoidance.
5. When patients desire open discussion, let go of encouraging words about prognosis. Follow the patient's lead.
6. Remember that some cultural and religious traditions require that terminal prognosis be withheld from the patient.

Source: From Zerwekh (1994).

Box 9-2 ■   STEPS IN ENCOURAGING CHOICE

1. Follow the steps of truth-telling.
2. Bring up the possibility of choice about treatment options and how they want to live the rest of their lives.
3. Encourage the patient to recognize his own needs.
4. Translate medical information into human terms.
5. Question the patient regularly to discover his or her desires and clarify options.
6. Propose a trial-run of choices about which the patient is unsure. The trial might include a living arrangement or a palliative treatment.
7. Help family communicate with one another. Listen and try to help members find common ground.
8. Respect the choice not to choose. Remember that cultural and religious traditions may require that family or medical authorities are the decision-makers.

Source: From Zerwekh (1994).

patients' dying (Glass & Cluxton, 2004). Perhaps the most prominent rational-ization for avoiding truth-telling is the fear of taking away hope. But hope can come in different shapes and sizes. At the end of life, realistic hope evolves beyond desire for a cure to hope for pain-free days and visits from friends. Ultimately, the hope shifts to the possibilities for reconciliation and meaning.

Nurses foster autonomous decision-making by telling the truth and encouraging choice (Zerwekh, 1994). Box 9-1 identifies the steps of truth-telling and Box 9-2 identifies the steps for encouraging choice. It is only through telling the truth that patients have enough information to make informed choices. A hospice nurse expert explains this ongoing process of encouraging choice with one patient:

> Everything became a decision. He couldn't swallow. Should he have TPN? We spent our time talking about what that meant. He decided to finish his PhD. We had to organize the bedroom so he could set up his computer. He thought about whether he wanted to kill himself, but he decided he had some more to do. He was hesitant to take pain meds. That was the way it went, trying to give him total control. When he needed several dressing changes, I gave him one dressing that he was in charge of and I was in charge of the other (Zerwekh, 1994, p. 33).

Noncompliance

It is important for nurses to understand that patients have many reasons for being noncompliant with beneficent medical and nursing recommendations. Their noncompliance often has nothing to do with impaired decisional capacity. They may alter their prescribed regimen because they cannot afford it, do not understand it, or find the side effects intolerable. Likewise, they may: find the regimen to be too intrusive or stigmatizing, seek to avoid chemical dependence, or desire that the illness not take control of their life. Respect for patient autonomy requires that nurses inquire deeply to under-stand patient decisions and to work with them to develop acceptable pallia-tive regimens.

Informed Consent

In order to make an autonomous decision, a patient must possess and under-stand the necessary information relevant to that decision. The doctrine of informed consent has two dimensions (Glannon, 2005). First, the physician is expected to truthfully disclose diagnosis, prognosis, treatment possibilities, risks, benefits, and consequences of accepting and refusing treatment. Second, the patient must have the mental capacity to understand this infor-mation and the consequences of accepting or refusing. Without extensive study of medicine, it is not possible for a patient to understand certain com-plexities of medical information; the patient can comprehend only a health professional's translation of that medical information into lay terms. Physicians often explain medical information incompletely and with an emphasis on the positive. Patients do not necessarily receive the objective information needed to make a truly autonomous decision. In addition, a severely ill patient's ability to comprehend life and death information is compromised by emotional stress and physiological impairments. The nurse frequently ends up asking the patient to sign papers indicating informed consent, and often is asked to witness this process. Sometimes she must question whether the patient comprehends the decision he is making and whether he possesses the mental capacity to decide.

Decisional Capacity

The ability to make reasoned decisions is called decisional capacity or competence. Patients with decisional capacity have the right to refuse all life-sustaining treatments, such as resuscitation, artificial ventilation, food, fluids, blood, dialysis, chemotherapy, surgery, or antibiotics. Such decisions may cause great distress on the part of family and caregivers, who may seek to deny that the person is in her "right mind." When the patient who is not cognitively impaired refuses life-saving intervention or chooses a physically harmful course of action, respect for patient liberty prevails. In such situations, the nurse listens with compassion to the patient and those who care for her. Some people have a strong drive to control their own destiny, and those who love and care for them must let them die without intervention.

Decisional capacity usually deteriorates at the end of life, due to both disease and medication. Evaluating decisional capacity entails asking the following (Dalinis, 2005):

1. Can the person understand and communicate information?
2. Is the person able to reason and deliberate about a decision?
3. Can the person identify personal values and goals?

When a patient's decisional capacity is impaired, family members or legally appointed surrogates make decisions in the patient's stead.

At some point, individuals, who have always been in charge of their own lives, and sometimes in charge of the family's life, can no longer be trusted to make good decisions. Families then need to be taught that the disease has advanced to the point where it has impaired their loved one's thinking. This can be a difficult transition in a family used to doing "whatever mother says." Strategize with the caregivers and other members of the health-care team about changing roles and responsibilities and about ways to preserve their family member from harm. When autonomous decision-making is no longer possible, patients must be protected from their own unsafe decisions as caregivers take over control. Nevertheless, a great effort should always be made to respect reasonable autonomous decisions while protecting the patient from harmful decisions.

Advance Planning

When a person makes and records a decision about limiting end-of-life treatment options when he still has decisional capacity (legally competent), he anticipates that health professionals will respect that decision when he becomes incapacitated (legally incompetent). Through the ethical principle of *autonomy extended,* an *advance directive,* often called a living will, can be written in which a patient defines his end-of-life wishes. In addition, a competent person can appoint a *proxy or surrogate decision-maker* to make a *substituted judgment* based on the patient's values (Veatch, 2003). Either way, the patient is seeking to safeguard his ability to make an autonomous decision. Box 9-3 contains a glossary of the complex language used in reference to advance planning.

Box 9-3 ■	THE LANGUAGE OF ADVANCE PLANNING

Advance care planning: Identifying wishes for specific treatment in anticipation of a time when the person will be unable to make decisions.

Advance directive: Statement made by a competent individual about preferences for future treatment.

Best interests: A health-care proxy or substitute is expected to make decisions for an incompetent person based on what that person would have wanted and what is believed would protect or benefit him.

Competency: Legal term implying capability of making rational decisions. Unless a court of law determines incompetence, people over 18 years old are assumed to be competent.

Decisional capacity and incapacity: Clinical determination of patient's ability to make rational decisions. A person with decisional capacity is not cognitively impaired.

Forgoing life-sustaining treatment: Also known as withholding treatment. Choosing not to have specific life-extending treatment. Examples of treatments include a ventilator, artificial food and fluids, antibiotics, and blood.

Health-care proxy: Another person appointed to make medical decisions when the patient is no longer competent.

Health-care surrogate: Same as health-care proxy.

Living will: An advance directive.

Patient Self Determination Act of 1990: Required that all hospitals inform patients of the right to complete advance directives.

Withdrawing life-sustaining treatment: Removing life-sustaining treatment once it has been initiated. Examples include the ventilator, vasopressors, parenteral fluids, and enteral nutrition.

ADVANCE DIRECTIVES

Advance directives address patient wishes when they no longer have the capacity to decide. In 1990, the Patient Self Determination Act stated that all patients admitted to a hospital receiving federal funds must be informed of their right to complete an advance directive. The law in every state provides for advance directives. Written advance directives need to identify patient wishes clearly; many wishes are too general and nonspecific to be useful. For instance, they may request no "extraordinary means" be used when the person is "imminently dying." These requests are too vague and subject to diverse interpretation. In contrast, advance directives should identify specific treatments refused and desired, when the directive should take effect, and who will be appointed as proxy decision-maker. Recommended specifics include (Preston, 2000):

- Clear definition of the circumstances covered, including terminal illness and/or permanent unconsciousness.
- Statement about whether or not to withhold or withdraw intervention that is artificially prolonging dying.
- Statement about whether or not to initiate resuscitation.
- Statement about administration of artificial food and fluids.
- Statement about administration of blood, antibiotics, or ventilator.
- Request to use analgesics in sufficient amount to relieve suffering.

There are different names for advance directives. They may be called Directives to Physicians, Health-Care Directives, or living wills.

WWW.   Internet Resource Box

Go to the Partnership for Caring Web site to find advance directive forms for your state: *www.partnershipforcaring.org/Advance/adconfirm.php.*

Unfortunately, creation of advance directives is difficult because of the problems with frankly discussing and making such difficult decisions in advance. Often, people do not know enough about illness and treatment to make decisions about a future time when they are sick and near death. They are asked to "conjure up preferences for an unspecifiable future confronted with unidentifiable maladies with unpredictable treatments. . . . The healthy may incautiously prefer death to disability. Once stricken, competent patients can test and reject that preference. They often do" (Fagerlin & Schneider, 2004, pp. 33–34). Only 18% of Americans have advance directives, and education does not seem to increase the number. The choice to avoid the topic of death prevents many older persons from filling out the forms (Winland-Brown, 1998). Most patients prefer to leave final resuscitation decisions to physician and family, rather than have their own prior uninformed (as to the specific situation) preferences prevail (Fagerlin & Schneider, 2004).

When advance directives have been written, a major problem is their reaching clinicians. Very few of these forms end up on the hospital or nursing home chart (Fagerlin & Schneider, 2004) and clinicians disregard past decisions if they believe they should act otherwise (Preston, 2000). In the absence of advance directives, and when patients lose decisional capacity, aggressive life-saving measures usually prevail unless surrogate decision-makers intervene.

SURROGATE DECISION-MAKING

A health-care proxy or surrogate is a person appointed by the individual while he still retains decisional capacity; the surrogate is expected to make medical decisions in the best interest for the patient when he loses decisional capacity. If the person never expressed his wishes or appointed a proxy, the next of kin is the presumed proxy decision-maker. The following have decision-making authority in descending order: spouse, adult children, parents, and siblings. This order can vary in different states. They are expected to use a *substituted judgment* standard by expressing the patient's previously stated preferences or inferring preferences from previous actions or statements (Jonsen, Siegler, and Winslade, 2002). They are expected to act in the patient's best interest. They should consider what the patient would want for himself and put aside their own wants. Quill (2005) proposes the following question to clarify the patient's wishes:

> If the patient could wake up for 15 minutes and understand his or her condition fully, and then had to return to it, what would he or she tell you to do? (p. 1632)

Nurses often are in a position to encourage discussion among friends and family members to clarify decisions that are in the patient's best interest. You can contribute to an understanding of what the cognitively impaired patient would have wanted by sharing your knowledge of what the patient told you. During the time before a patient loses decisional capacity, it is particularly helpful to document in writing in the medical record any statements about how he would have wanted to live or die.

Health-care surrogates or proxies are identified in a form called a health-care proxy or durable power of attorney for health-care decisions. This is different than a durable power of attorney for financial decisions. The health-care surrogate may also be called an attorney-in-fact, proxy, or agent. This person should be a close relative or friend and cannot be a physician or employee of the health-care organization providing care. In contrast to living wills, decisions of the durable power of attorney stand up strongly within the medical community and in court. There are several other advantages of the durable power of attorney (Fagerlin & Schneider, 2004):

- Requires a simple choice of a trusted person to make future decisions.
- Makes little change in the current practice of family decision-making.

- Improves quality of decision-making because surrogates know in the present time more than patients can know in advance.
- Inexpensive.

Appointing a health-care durable power of attorney ensures both the patient and health-care providers that the principle of autonomy will be respected in all ethical decisions.

Challenges to Social Justice

A commitment to social justice is a commitment to treat all people equally and to work toward ensuring that all people have access to food, water, shelter, and health care. While the privileged world worries about withholding or withdrawing life-sustaining artificial feeding and ventilation for dying people, millions of impoverished people throughout the world are brought closer to death for lack of food, clean water, clean air, and health care. They are denied the very means to sustain life. It is important for nurses to maintain this broad perspective whenever we are able to influence social and health policy in our agencies, communities, or nation. Given limited resources, how can we act to promote life? Nurses need to look at the big picture and promote social justice.

66 | *While the privileged world worries about withholding or withdrawing life-sustaining artificial feeding and ventilation for dying people, millions of impoverished people throughout the world are brought closer to death for lack of food, clean water, clean air, and health care. They are denied the very means to sustain life.*

In the United States, socially marginalized people continue to be disenfranchised from the health-care mainstream and to die young, posing ethical burdens on health professionals. For instance, among African Americans, who are disproportionately poor, 43% of deaths occur before the age of 65 as compared to just 22% for whites (Williams, 2004). Because minority and poor people have the highest rates of death from major types of disease, they are likely to have been exposed to dying family and friends. People living "on the ragged edge" (Zerwekh, 2000) fear and mistrust health-care providers, and in turn are themselves often feared and mistrusted by nurses and physicians. So it is that when the racially and economically disenfranchised are dying, they experience inadequate communication, broken continuity of care, no advance care planning, poor palliation of symptoms, and superficial response to their social and spiritual suffering (Moller, 2005). "At the intersection of poverty and minority status, the stigma of being poor, black, and dying young creates a state of being whose pain is intolerable at best and excruciating at worse. . . . Treating the total pain of the patient demands attending to social suffering in a systematic way" (Williams, 2004, pp. 35–36).

Poor African American patients are underserved by the hospice and palliative-care movement. Factors that challenge quality of care at the end of life include lack of stable housing, unavailable family members to assist and give care, and poor access to supportive care services (Kvale, Williams, Bolden, Padgett, and Bailey, 2004). Social justice at the end of life requires the development of comprehensive community programs for all who are dying, especially those facing financial or social barriers. This requires the willingness to go beyond traditional models of end-of-life care and mobilize broad-based financial support from community partnerships. This has been illustrated in the accomplishments of the Balm of Gilead Project that provides palliative and hospice care for the impoverished minority population of Birmingham, Alabama. Their name is based on the African American spiritual that includes the lyric: "There is a balm in Gilead, to make the wounded whole" (Kvale et al., 2004). Practicing with a commitment to social justice requires valuing and standing beside those most disadvantaged in our society, and drawing them into a supportive human community at the end of their lives.

WWW.　**Internet Resource Box**

Go to *www.promotingexcellence.org*, Web site of Promoting Excellence in End-of-Life Care and type in Balm of Gilead.

The Challenge of Avoiding Killing and Relieving Suffering

Contemporary technologies make it possible to extend organic lives. But with this technology, lives are often extended to the point of little quality, no evident benefit to the patient, and sometimes great suffering. This presents ethical dilemmas never before encountered in human history. Questions revolve around how to make decisions that result in good (beneficent decisions) and avoid harm (nonmaleficent decisions). More specifically, this section examines the dilemmas posed by: double effect; futility, including indications for withdrawing and withholding treatments; active euthanasia and assisted suicide; and defining death and vegetative states.

Double Effect

In clinical situations where a proposed intervention can result in both good and harm, the principle of double effect is commonly used to guide ethical reasoning. The principle of double effect asserts that a morally objectionable act is permitted if the intention is to produce a moral good. When the clinician intends a positive outcome—even if a negative outcome may result—it is morally acceptable to pursue the intervention.

66 | *The principle of double effect asserts that a morally objectionable act is permitted if the intention is to produce a moral good.*

Double-effect thinking was developed by St. Thomas Aquinas in the 13th century (Schwarz, 2004). His original formula identifies four conditions that must be met before an action with both good and bad results can be justified. These remain useful for consideration today:

1. The act must not be intrinsically wrong.
2. The intention must be to do good. The undesirable bad effect must not be the true goal of action.
3. The bad secondary effect must not be the means to achieve the good effect.
4. The good effect must outweigh the bad.

Consider the following examples. A nurse makes an independent decision to administer potassium chloride intravenously to end the life of an 85-year-old unconscious woman who is dying from a progressive neurological disorder. Applying condition No. 1, we can conclude that this action is intrinsically wrong. The killing of innocents is prohibited by all major religious systems and by medical and nursing codes of ethics. Applying condition No. 2, assume that the nurse's intention is good; she intends this to be a merciful end to a life she judges will be filled with suffering. The principle of double effect still cannot support her decision because the bad effect is the true goal of the action. Applying condition No. 3, killing is the means to achieve the good effect (relief of assumed suffering), so the action cannot be justified. Applying condition No. 4, the bad effect (death) outweighs the good effect, so No. 4 also does not justify the action.

The principle of double effect is commonly invoked to support administering high doses of sedatives and opioids to relieve suffering at the end of life. For example, a nurse may choose to administer high doses of morphine as ordered by the physician to relieve suffering. Certainly this act is not intrinsically wrong. The intention is to do good, to relieve pain. The feared secondary effect is respiratory suppression so severe as to cause death. However, death is not the means to relieve suffering. The morphine subduing the pain is the means to relieve suffering. According to the principle of double effect, the relief of suffering outweighs the risk of causing death. All conditions for the double effect are satisfied so that the nurse is morally justified. This example is commonly used to explain double effect. But use of that example has one terribly troubling consequence. It perpetuates the myth that there is a serious risk of killing patients by administering opioids at the end of life (Schwarz, 2004). This is simply not the case. The presence of pain is an antidote to respiratory depression caused by opioids and as the pain accelerates, tolerance of respiratory side effects develops. When a patient receiving high doses of opioids dies, it is because of disease progression. See Chapter 15 to understand opioid effects and side effects.

The principle of double effect can be applied to guide moral reasoning in many other end-of-life circumstances as well. Consider the experience of a nurse following a physician's order to administer palliative sedation, which involves inducing and maintaining a deep sleep to relieve agitated delirium when aggressive symptom-management efforts have failed. Administering a continuous infusion of barbiturates is not intrinsically wrong (condition No. 1). The intention is to do good, to promote restful sleep (condition No. 2). The barbiturate dose is titrated so that it does not directly cause respiratory suppression and death, so condition No. 3 is satisfied. Finally, condition No. 4 is satisfied because the good effect (elimination of uncontrolled agitation) is judged to outweigh the bad (total sedation). Some clinicians reject this argument because they point out that death is a predictable consequence of sedation therapy that renders a patient unconscious and immobile. The nurse has a responsibility in such circumstances to question the decision to sedate, embrace the principle of double effect, and/or conscientiously object.

Futile Interventions

From an ethical perspective, futile interventions should be withheld or withdrawn. An intervention is considered futile if it is incapable of achieving any positive result. For example, cardiopulmonary resuscitation (CPR) should not be initiated in a patient with crushed ribs. Blood would not be administered in a patient with arterial bleeding that cannot be repaired. Renal dialysis is futile for a patient whose heart failure cannot be controlled. The process of judging an intervention to be totally useless is usually controversial unless that patient has devastating disease that makes any desired physiological response impossible. Usually, however, a determination of futility is not 100% certain, so clinicians talk about futility in terms of probabilities or percentages. For instance, procedures might be considered futile if they have 10% or less chance of achieving a useful effect (Jonsen et al., 2002). Contemporary medicine sometimes disregards the futility of a measure. Futile heroic measures are sometimes initiated to signify commitment to life. Extreme life-saving efforts can symbolize an affirmation that the person is worth great effort (Benner, Hooper-Dyriakidis, and Stannard, 1999). For this reason, health professionals often do not even consider withholding what may be a futile measure.

When the usefulness of interventions is questionable, it may be helpful to weigh the benefits and the burdens imposed by initiating or continuing interventions. The concept of proportionate good justifies potentially harmful medical procedures. Proportionate good is determined using a benefit-to-burden ratio. Benefit/burden analysis should be used to decide on the proportionate good of resuscitation orders, withholding therapies, and withdrawing therapies, for instance. Ethicists also distinguish between the obligation to maintain life through "ordinary means" but not "extraordinary means." Extraordinary means are not ethically justifiable. Over time, extraordinary means have come to be defined as treatments that are considered useless and burdensome to the patient and others (Volbrecht, 2003).

RESUSCITATION
Basic CPR involves mouth-to-mouth breathing and chest compression. Advanced CPR includes chest compression, intubation with ventilatory

Box 9-4 ■	**THE DO NOT RESUSCITATE ORDER**

DNR orders should be written when (1) medical judgment indicates that the code would be futile, (2) the informed patient or surrogate consents, and (3) the quality of life that can be expected after resuscitation is poor (Jonsen, Siegler, and Winslade, 2002). DNR orders are written in the patient's chart with rationale identified in the progress notes. Recently, DNR orders have become "portable" in the form of bracelets, necklaces, wallet cards, or standardized forms that are legalized in most states.

assistance, defibrillation, cardioversion, vasopressors, and cardiotonic drugs. The Joint Commission on Accreditation of Healthcare Organizations (JCAHO) requires that CPR be performed on every patient who has a respiratory or cardiac arrest and does not have a Do Not Resuscitate (DNR) or "No Code" order. Following a judgment that a code would be futile, DNR orders are written by the physician. See Box 9-4, The Do Not Resuscitate Order. New "portable" DNR forms allow the orders to be honored outside the hospital, particularly by emergency medical providers. For instance, the state of Oregon uses the POLST (Physician Orders for Life-Sustaining Treatment) document, printed on a shocking pink card, and placed in the front of medical records in hospital and home, as well as encouraged to be prominently posted at home.

■
WWW. **Internet Resource Box**

The POLST is available through the Oregon Health and Sciences University Center for Ethics in Health Care at *www.ohsu.edu/ethics.*

Nurses working at the end of life need to understand that CPR seldom restores cardiac function for people with end-stage disease (Scanlon, 2003). One estimate is that fewer than 5% of terminally ill patients who are resuscitated survive to be discharged from the hospital. Consider the effects of coding a patient who has lost most bodily function and is suffering from emotional, physical, and spiritual distress. If the patient dies despite the code, his last minutes will have consisted of a team of strangers pushing the family aside, pounding on his chest, perhaps cracking his ribs, inserting needles, inserting tubes, and repeatedly shocking him. If the patient lives, he may survive only with artificial ventilation or with the effects of cerebral hypoxia that cause a persistent vegetative state. Therefore, nurses must be attentive to the need to speak to patients and/or their families about the futility of resuscitation efforts in those with advanced terminal disease, and therefore the need for a DNR order. Families need to understand that approving a DNR order does not mean abandoning their family member with no treatment; only cardiopulmonary resuscitation will be withheld.

WITHHOLDING OR FORGOING

Throughout the medical world, a critical ethical distinction is made between actively killing the patient and simply allowing the person to die by withholding or forgoing life-prolonging treatments that are believed to be futile. Natural Death Acts, passed in many states, grant patients the right to refuse life-saving therapies. Killing involves an affirmative act committed with the intention to end a person's life. On the other hand, withholding treatment involves never beginning an intervention believed to be futile. A treatment is not morally required if either there is no benefit to the patient or if it is burdensome to the patient and perhaps to the family. Benefit/burden analysis determines whether a proposed treatment should be withheld. Unfortunately, interpretations of benefit and burden are highly controversial. Some religious groups oppose withholding of life-prolonging therapies (see Box 9-5). It is extremely important that nurses, who work alongside the patient and know what they are experiencing, carefully consider benefit and burden and help the patient and family to make conscious decisions regarding withholding treatments. It is important to keep in mind that patients are dying from disease, not from withholding of a therapy. Withholding therapy allows the disease process to go forward without interruption.

A treatment is not morally required if either there is no benefit to the patient or if it is burdensome to the patient and perhaps to the family. Benefit/burden analysis determines whether a proposed treatment should be withheld.

Box 9-5 ■	ORTHODOX OPPOSITION TO WITHHOLDING THERAPIES

Some conservative Christians and Orthodox Jews do not support withholding life-sustaining treatments. Orthodox Jewish medical ethics places high value on preserving human life with few exceptions (Bleich, 1989). Life with suffering is regarded as preferable to death and cessation of suffering. There is no distinction between ordinary and extraordinary means. "The physician may withhold otherwise mandatory treatment only when the patient has reached the state of *gesisah*, i.e., the patient has become moribund and death is imminent" (p. 53). Only in the final hours of life when all treatment is futile, may therapies be withdrawn; at that time resuscitation is not required. In the moments before death, the patient should not be moved or manipulated lest these movements hasten death.

Consider the benefits and burden of withholding four routine interventions at the end of life: antibiotics, food and fluids, frequent turning, and daily baths.

What is the benefit of antibiotics at the end of life? If effective, they may be able to prolong meaningful life. Depending on the site of infection, an effective antibiotic may be able to reduce distressing symptoms, such as respiratory congestion or fever. The burden is that they may be able to extend a life that has been reduced to great suffering or to profound mental incapacity. Some will proclaim that burdensome life must always be chosen over death; others will say that extending a burdensome life is wrong. Nurses serve as moral agents when we are able to help patients and families weigh decisions about choosing or forgoing antibiotics. In the last days of life, decisions also need to be made about forgoing food and fluids.

The artificial administration of food and fluids in the end of life is a particularly controversial ethical issue. In order to promote benefit/burden analysis, it is particularly helpful that the nurse have a clear understanding of the arguments for and against administering food and fluids.

A variety of ethical arguments are used to support the position that it is always necessary to provide artificial food and fluids (Lynn & Childress, 1986). First of all, there is a common presupposition that food and fluids are essential to patient comfort and dignity. This argument holds that food and fluids are so basic and ordinary that they cannot ever be considered optional; they comprise a basic standard of care. The second line of argument holds that there is always a strong moral obligation to provide food and fluids to those who experience hunger and thirst. Without food and fluids, it is assumed that suffering will be great. Hydrating and nourishing have great symbolic value; denying these treatments is considered tantamount to starving a person to death, which elicits a deep-seated aversion for some observers. Artificial nourishment is assumed to be nurturing and caring. A third argument asserts that withholding food and fluids is the same as killing a patient prematurely.

But there are also a number of arguments supporting withholding artificial food and fluids, if they are unlikely to benefit the patient and are likely to be burdensome. In fact, administration of food and fluids often fails to bring comfort to the dying person (Ersek, 2003; Zerwekh, 2003). Those close to death are reported not to hunger or thirst. Dehydration does not cause suffering in the dying as it does for the living. The complications of enteral tube feedings and fluid infusions for those with end-stage organ failure are enumerated in Chapter 16, illustrating that artificial food and fluids can potentially increase suffering. Likewise, diminishing cognition requires that many patients be tied down so that they do not remove lines and tubes. Thus, the ideal of ensuring comfort and dignity with artificial food and fluids imposes literal restraints on dignity and comfort in practice. The idea of nurturing with food is legitimate, but when feeding takes place through needles, tubing, bags, and pumps, the nurturing aspects of it fall to the wayside. Clearly, technological feeding is not the same as nurturance. Finally, counter to the argument that withholding food and fluids may precipitate a premature death, in the event of end-stage organ failure, there is a surprising amount of evidence that artificial food and fluids do not extend life (Ersek, 2003). See Chapter 16. For patients who are not imminently terminal, clinical judgment may determine that artificial food and fluids are of clear benefit to prolong life and well-being. An ethical choice of artificial food and fluids at the end of life requires thoughtful burden/benefit analysis.

Sometimes dying patients choose on their own to stop eating and drinking. In a study of 307 Oregon hospice nurses, one third reported that they had cared for patients who chose to hasten death deliberately by voluntarily refusing fluids and food (Ganzini, Goy, Miller, Harvath, Jackson, and Delorit, 2003). The patients reasoned that they felt ready to die, no longer found meaning in living, and were experiencing poor quality of life. Most died comfortably within 2 weeks of beginning their fast. Such autonomous choices should be respected by nurses. Those opposed to such a choice by a patient with decisional capacity should remove themselves from the case after finding another nurse to take over patient care. Sometimes continuing common nursing practices can pose ethical dilemmas.

All routine nursing practices should be questioned in terms of benefit and burden at the end of life. The ethical issue is whether to cause suffering when little or no benefit of an action can be identified. For instance, soap and water baths are traditionally considered beneficial to remove sweat and microorganisms, to provide comfort, and to offer nurturing human contact. However, the skin of the elderly is dry and fragile, easily broken. Traditional bathing, long associated with comforting, actually can be harmful. Soap removes oil and can cause irritation and pruritus; friction from scrubbing and drying can cause skin tears. Conventional bathing actually causes serious distress in some demented patients who sometimes become combative during the process. At the end of life, standard bathing practice should be reconsidered (Lentz, 2003). One alternative is a bag bath in which multiple washcloths are soaked in an emollient solution. Ethical action involves choice of comfort instead of imposing burdensome routine that offers no benefit.

Frequent turning can also be burdensome at the end of life. When death is not near, turning reduces the likelihood of immobility complications, particularly skin breakdown. When pressure sores are already present, frequent turning and positioning are intended to prevent their worsening. However, turning and positioning at the very end of life cause serious incident pain in some patients and offer little chance of healing when circulation, oxygenation, and nutrition are extremely compromised. A palliative approach should seek to avoid hurt and respect patient choice. Ethical action involves choice of comfort instead of burden without benefit.

WITHDRAWING INTERVENTIONS
Ethicists have consistently proclaimed that stopping an intervention is considered morally comparable to withholding it initially. In other words,

.removing a feeding tube is morally the same as never inserting it. Withholding a life-sustaining intervention was once called passive euthanasia, but this terminology is no longer used because of the association with mercy killing. Withdrawing an intervention entails stopping an artificial measure so that the disease process comes to a natural end; no lethal act is committed to bring about death. Stopping an intervention is not considered by ethicists to be the same as killing. The criteria for withdrawing interventions are the same as the criteria for withholding them: the interventions are deemed futile and burdensome. The burdens of continuing the treatment outweigh any benefits.

Although ethicists argue that withholding and withdrawing are equivalent morally, removing an intervention usually causes greater moral distress for a nurse and family at the bedside. To feel that she is acting ethically, the nurse needs to be able to work through the decision and be clear about the futility and burdens of continuing therapy. Likewise, she should help the family with this reasoning.

In contrast to withholding or withdrawing life-sustaining treatment, assisted death involves deliberately committing a lethal act intending to bring about death. Ethically (and legally) such an act is more difficult to justify.

> 66 | *In contrast to withholding or withdrawing life-sustaining treatment, assisted death involves deliberately committing a lethal act intending to bring about death. Ethically (and legally) such an act is more difficult to justify.*

Assisted Death: Active Euthanasia and Assisted Suicide

Assisted death is also called "assistance in dying" or "aid in dying." Usually this includes both euthanasia and assisted suicide.

- Euthanasia is translated as "good death" and is often considered the same as "mercy killing" in which the patient is killed by another person with merciful intent.
- Assisted suicide involves the patient killing himself with the assistance of a physician prescribing lethal medication.
- Voluntary active euthanasia involves interventions administered with the intention to end a patient's life. "Voluntary" means that the patient has asked to have assistance to die.
- Nonvoluntary euthanasia is when the patient is incapable of making a decision, and involuntary euthanasia is when patients are killed against their expressed wishes.
- "Active" euthanasia involves commission of an act with intent to kill.

Nonvoluntary and involuntary active euthanasia are universally condemned by contemporary ethicists. The American Nurses Association also opposes nurse involvement in active euthanasia and assisted suicide.

Likewise, most ethicists and religious leaders oppose the deliberate taking of human life for any reason. However, organizations such as End of Life Choices support the choice and right of cognitively intact patients to hasten their own death.

■
WWW.   Internet Resource Box

The American Nurses Association end of life position statements can be found at *www.nursingworld.org/readroom/position.*
End of Life Choices Web site is at *www.endoflifechoices.org*

When a physician or nurse administers a lethal drug or procedure *that the patient has requested,* he or she is participating in voluntary active euthanasia, which is illegal everywhere in the United States. When a physician prescribes a lethal drug that the patient administers himself, it is called "physician assisted suicide," which is legal only in the state of Oregon. Box 9-6 clarifies the difference between active euthanasia and assisted suicide. The main difference between the two is that in the former, the health professional actually administers the lethal intervention, whereas in the latter, the patient self-administers it.

Voluntary active euthanasia can be defended morally based on the obligation to respect individual autonomy and promote beneficence by reducing suffering and eliminating loss of dignity. Advocates of voluntary active euthanasia and assisted suicide believe that legal safeguards can be developed to ensure safe ethical assisted death. The primary objection to voluntary euthanasia is that intentional killing profoundly disregards the sanctity of life and is thereby maleficent. Killing the patient is believed to be the same as abandoning him. It violates the very ethical foundations of the health professions. Other objections include concern that patients may choose death

---

Box 9-6 ■	THE LANGUAGE OF ASSISTED DEATH

ACTIVE EUTHANASIA	ASSISTED SUICIDE
Family member, friend, or health professional administers a lethal medication or intervention with a merciful intention to end life.	Family member, friend, or health professional makes a means of suicide available to a patient, who then administers it himself.

because their care is inadequate or because they would rather be dead than become a burden for their families. The "slippery slope" argument asserts that permitting clinicians to end life intentionally sets a dangerous precedent for society to slip into more widespread inappropriate killing by clinicians who traditionally have been sworn to protect life. For instance, clinicians may judge that the disabled or chemically dependent or mentally ill might be better off dead than continuing to burden society. In addition, those experienced in end-of-life care argue that the end of life can be time for growth and reconciliation, which would be lost by killing the patient. And of course, there is always the possibility of wrong diagnoses and new treatments that could have saved the life of the terminally ill patient seeking assistance in dying. Box 9-7 summarizes these arguments.

Nursing at the end of life frequently involves patients inquiring about euthanasia. Some patients may choose to stop eating and drinking, which some clinicians recommend as an alternative to physician-assisted suicide (Ganzini et al., 2003). Thirty percent of oncology nurses in one New England study reported that they had received requests for lethal drugs in the previous

---

Box 9-7 ■   ASSISTED DEATH ARGUMENTS

FOR ASSISTED DEATH	OPPOSED TO ASSISTED DEATH
Patients have a right to choose.	Honoring the sanctity of life overrides the right to choose one's own death.
Assisting a suffering patient to stay in control and end his suffering is beneficent.	Assisting a person to die is abandoning that person.
Refusing to assist someone to die destroys trust (fidelity) with the clinician.	Assisting a person to die destroys trust with the patient and obligation with society to protect life.
Safeguards can be written to ensure safe assisted death that avoids the "slippery slope."	When society permits assisted death, it creates a "slippery slope." The precedent may lead to vulnerable people being killed so that they are not burdensome to family or society.

Source: Adapted from Ersek (2004).

year; and 4.5% reported actually performing voluntary active euthanasia (Matzo & Emanual, 1997). Nurses become involved with requests to end life in the following ways:

- Patients want to talk about their desires and fears.
- Patients seek information about suicide, assisted suicide, or active euthanasia.
- Patients ask family members or friends to end their lives or supply the means to do so.
- Patients ask nurses or physicians to end their lives or supply the means to do so.
- Against the law, physicians write lethal orders, which nurses are asked to carry out, or which they witness being carried out.
- Nurses make home visits following unsuccessful or successful suicide attempts.

All of these circumstances cause nurses great moral distress. Nurses do have the right to conscientiously object to any involvement, but cannot abandon the patient until another nurse can be assigned. Therefore, you must become as clear as possible about your own beliefs and values.

Assisted Suicide in Oregon

Oregon is the only state that has legalized physician-assisted suicide (Oregon Department of Human Services, 2005). In 1994, the Oregon voters approved by 51% a Death with Dignity Act, permitting physicians to prescribe lethal medication for terminal patients to self-administer. It was immediately blocked by a restraining order, which a judge ruled unconstitutional. Again in 1997, Oregon voters decided by a 60:40 margin to oppose repeal of the act. In 1998, the first 24 patients died after self-administering lethal medication prescribed legally by physicians. Box 9-8 identifies requirements of the Oregon Death with Dignity Act. The federal government has repeatedly tried to block Oregon law and has threatened prosecution of participating physicians for violating federal drug laws by prescribing controlled substances to kill people. This move troubles even those who are adamantly opposed to physician-assisted suicide because it challenges state rights.

■

WWW. Internet Resource Box

Summaries, annual reports, and press releases for Oregon's Death with Dignity Act can be found at a Web site of the Oregon Department of Human Services: *egov.oregon.gov/DHS/ph/pas/.*

From 1998 through 2004, only 208 people ended their lives through physician-assisted suicide. Seventeen percent of dying Oregonians talk to

Box 9-8 ■	OREGON DEATH WITH DIGNITY ACT

Patient and Physician Requirements for Assisted Suicide

- The patient must be a mentally competent adult who is an Oregon resident.
- The patient must have a terminal illness with a prognosis of less than 6 months.
- The patient must voluntarily request a lethal prescription; the request must be oral and written with two witnesses who attest to the patient being of sound mind and voluntarily choosing to end his life.
- The physician must determine that the patient is terminally ill, competent to decide, and is making the request voluntarily; the physician must refer the patient to a consulting physician to confirm this.
- The physician must inform the patient of diagnosis and prognosis, result of taking lethal prescription, and palliative-care alternatives.
- The physician must refer the patient for counseling if he or the consultant conclude that the patient is suffering from a mental disorder.
- The physician must notify next of kin.
- The physician must thoroughly document in the medical record and report to the Oregon Health Services.

their families about the possibility, but only 2% formally request it (Tolle, Tilden, Drach, Fromme, Perrin, and Hedberg, 2004). The rate of assisted suicide is about 1 in 1000 deaths, much lower than had been feared. Numbers have not escalated. In fact, the rates of physician-assisted suicide are higher in states where it remains illegal (4 in 1000). Those requesting physician-assisted suicide in Oregon tend to be white, educated, and insured. The three most common end-of-life reasons for patients requesting lethal medication include loss of autonomy, decreasing enjoyment in life, and loss of dignity. Less than 1 in 4 said pain was their reason for requesting death. The three most common terminal conditions represented were amyotrophic lateral sclerosis (ALS), HIV/AIDS, and cancer. The patients must be able to administer their own medication and swallow it.

When patients are considering physician-assisted suicide, the nursing role is to listen compassionately and dialogue with patients and families about options, contribute to assessment of the patient's decisional capacity, and do everything possible to work with the hospice team to alleviate distress leading to requests for assistance to die. Some patients will request that nurses are present at their dying. The law does not protect a nurse who participates in the assisted suicide by delivering the medication to the home, awakening the patient to administer the drug, placing the medication in the mouth, emptying capsules into food, crushing tablets, or administering medication through a gastrostomy tube (Oregon Nurses Association, 1995). The patient must be able to follow through with these activities by himself. The Oregon Nurses Association supports conscientious objection for nurses who want no involvement in this process. They must continue to provide care until a replacement is found. Nurses who choose to be involved should continue to explore options to physician-assisted suicide with the patient, provide emotional and physical comforting for patient and family, and be present without assisting in administration.

WWW.   Internet Resource Box

See the Oregon Nurses Association guidelines on the nurse's role in assisted suicide at *www.oregonrn.org*.

Determination of Death and Vegetative States

Throughout human history, death has been defined as the irreversible cessation of heart and lung function, which either caused or was caused by the loss of brain function. Then, the ventilator was developed to permit breathing and oxygenate a beating heart, even when the brain stopped functioning. In the late 1960s, a Harvard University committee and a commission appointed by the federal government proclaimed that a person could be declared dead when all brain functions, including the cerebral cortex and the brain stem, ceased to function (Glannon, 2005). Patients whose entire brain has been destroyed can be declared dead and their organs harvested for transplant.

Some patients suffer from higher-brain death (Veatch, 2003). Those in a persistent vegetative state are permanently unconscious with most brain functions gone, including all functions of the cerebral cortex, but they have limited reflexes maintained by the brain stem. Persistent vegetative state should be diagnosed by neurologists; a flat electroencephalogram (EEG) characterizes partial brain death. The two most common causes of higher-brain death are external trauma to the brain and hypoxia. These patients are no longer able to think or interact. Although these patients can no longer think, they may randomly blink, grimace, smile, or move their limbs. These actions are not intentional, but are reflexes that continue because the brain-stem is intact. These patients can no longer swallow, but their bodies can survive for prolonged periods through artificial tube feeding. From an ethical perspective, it is important that friends and family understand that a person in a vegetative state is no longer conscious of either benefits or burdens of life-sustaining intervention. Persons in a vegetative state are unaware of themselves and their environment; they cannot experience hunger, thirst, or pain. Frequently, the family has difficulty believing the medical evidence and chooses to wait in hopes that cognition may return. Nevertheless, family members will eventually need to make a decision about withdrawing life-sustaining interventions based on the best interests of their loved one. How long should the body be sustained despite this lack of consciousness?

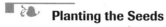 **Planting the Seeds**

Family and friends who are sitting vigil at the bedside of a patient in a persistent vegetative state need ongoing explanation to understand the meaning of involuntary movements. They may see every smile or hand grasp as an indication that their loved one is recovering. Explain to everyone at the bedside that only the primitive regions of the brain are functioning. Because of cerebral damage, patients are not able to comprehend or interact. Movements like grimacing, smiling, making sounds, and moving extremities are reflexes and are not purposeful. When uninstructed people who are involved with the patient observe this behavior, it can be over-interpreted as meaningful. They may develop groundless hopes for recovery.

Separating Personhood and Body

If human beings are defined in terms of their capacity for consciousness, then a person dies when the cerebral cortex, which makes consciousness possible, permanently stops functioning. However, some faith traditions believe that human beings are still persons even when they permanently lose capacity for consciousness. In April of 2004, John Paul II, then Pope of the Roman Catholic Church, declared that patients in a vegetative state are always human beings with moral standing (Kavanaugh, 2004). He asserted that personhood cannot be reduced to cognitive skills. The traditional Roman Catholic position had been that artificial feeding of a person in a persistent vegetative state is a medical treatment that can be halted using ethical benefit/burden analysis. But with his 2004 statement, the Pope proclaimed that in such circumstances, artificial food and nutrition are morally obligatory in order to preserve human life at any cost.

This position will certainly influence ethical decisions on behalf of people who are no longer capable of consciousness. It may increase tube feeding in Catholic hospitals, and more nursing home beds may fill with patients in vegetative states being artificially nourished. Is this care useful or useless as it preserves bodily life with no chance of restoring cognitive capacities? Is it beneficial to preserve bodies that are no longer capable of conscious benefit? Because the person is no longer capable of perceiving benefit, those who benefit from prolonged life would be family or community. All human societies have limited resources and make trade-offs in terms of where resources are expended. Should we feed the unconscious while mothers and children have no food on their table and no access to health care? The social justice issues cannot be ignored. We are severely challenged as a moral community by the power of life and death in our hands.

CONCEPTS IN ACTION

Events in the case of Ms. Terri Schiavo are summarized from Annas (2005), Dresser (2005), Quill (2005), and Tanner (2005). In 1990 Terri Schiavo, age 26, who had been married to Michael Schiavo for 5 years, experienced a cardiac arrest due to hypokalemia and was diagnosed with ischemic encephalopathy. EEGs were flat and computed tomography (CT) scans eventually showed severe cerebral atrophy (Quill, 2005). The consensus among neurologists was that she had lost all cognitive function and was in a persistent vegetative state. A feeding tube was inserted and sustained her life as various efforts at rehabilitation failed.

Conflict between Michael Schiavo and Terri's parents, Bob and Mary Schindler, began in 1993. The Schindlers began to seek court decisions to have Michael Schiavo removed as Terri's guardian. They questioned his motives, accusing him of abuse and neglect, and asserted that he was not acting in their daughter's best interests. In 1998, after 10 years of Terri living in a vegetative state, Michael Schiavo began to try to have his wife's feeding tube removed. He asserted that his wife would not want to live under these circumstances, whereas her parents believed that she would want to live. Terri had no written advance directive. A Florida circuit court approved Michael's request to have the tube removed, but Terri's parents appealed. In 2001, the tube was removed for the first time, but a judge soon ordered it replaced. Michael made another legal effort to withdraw the tube in 2002–2003. Three neurologists testified in court that Terri was in a vegetative state and could not improve, but a physician for the parents proclaimed that she could be helped with hyperbaric and vasodilation therapies, for which there is no research evidence. Her parents consistently asserted that they still believed Terri was interacting with them and could recover. The tube was removed for the second time in October 2003, but then an emergency appeal was made to the Florida State legislature. Highly edited videotapes of Terri, which captured pictures of Terri looking responsive and interacting, were shown to legislators and to television viewers. Many viewers concluded that Terri was "being killed." Governor Jeb Bush signed Terri's Law, mandating reinsertion of the feeding tube. In April of 2004, Pope John Paul II reversed the church's previous position on tube feeding vegetative patients, and declared that feeding tubes are morally mandated for all patients in vegetative states. The Schindlers are devout Roman Catholics. In September of 2004, the Florida Supreme Court declared "Terri's Law" to be unconstitutional.

In February 2005, the Florida circuit judge gave Michael permission to remove the tube. On March 18, 2005, the tube was removed for the third time. However, the appeal this time went all the way to Washington, D.C.

(continued)

CONCEPTS IN ACTION

The U.S. Congress viewed the videotape and rushed to pass a bill calling for a federal court to review the case. President Bush signed the bill but the U.S. district court judge reviewed the case and denied the parents' request for a restraining order. On March 31, 2005, the U.S. Supreme Court declined to intervene, just as they had on five previous occasions. Terri Schiavo died that day. The case drew international attention with great passion from right-to-life groups and dramatic response from those who feared that their own self-determination at the end of life could be prohibited by government intrusion.

1. Apply the duties of beneficence and nonmaleficence to this case.
2. What role does veracity play in the Schiavo tragedy? What would be the nurses' role in truth-telling?
3. How would events have been different if Terri Schiavo had completed a written advance directive or health-care power of attorney?
4. Apply the concepts of autonomy extended and substituted judgment. Read again the question Quill proposes to clarify best interest in terms of what a reasonable person in the same circumstances would want.
5. Assume a social utilitarian stance to consider the societal impact of unquestioned artificial nutrition for patients in the same condition as Terri Schiavo.
6. Apply Care Ethics to imagine a nursing role when conflict first developed between Michael Schiavo and the Schindlers.
7. Examine the concept of futility as applied to Terri Schiavo's circumstances.
8. Do a burden/benefit analysis for withdrawing artificial nutrition in Terri Schiavo's circumstances.
9. Right-to-life groups claimed that removing Ms. Schiavo's tube feeding was equivalent to killing her. Contrast withdrawal of life-sustaining therapy with "mercy killing."

References

Annas, G. (2005). "Culture of Life" politics at the bedside—The case of Terri Schiavo. *New England Journal of Medicine*. Retrieved from www.nejm.org.

Benner, P., Hooper-Dyriakidis, P., & Stannard, D. (1999). *Clinical wisdom and interventions in critical care*. Philadelphia: WB Saunders.

Bleich, J. (1989). The obligations to heal in the Judaic tradition. In R. Veatch (Ed.), *Cross cultural perspectives in medical ethics: Readings* (pp. 44–58). Boston: Jones and Bartlett.

Callahan, D. (1998). *False hopes: Overcoming the obstacles to a sustainable, affordable medicine*. New Brunswick, NJ: Rutgers University.

Dalinis, P. (2005). Informed consent and decisional capacity. *Journal of Hospice and Palliative Nursing, 7*(1), 52–57.

Dresser, R. (2004). Schiavo: A hard case makes questionable law. *Hastings Center Report, 34*(3), 8–9.

Ersek, M. (2003). Artificial nutrition and hydration: Clinical issues. *Journal of Hospice and Palliative Care*, 5(4), 221–230.

Ersek, M. (2004). The continuing challenge of assisted death. *Journal of Hospice and Palliative Nursing*, 6(1), 46–59.

Fagerlin, A., & Schneider, C. (2004). Enough: The failure of the living will. *Hastings Center Report*, 34(2), 30–42.

Ganzini, L., Goy, E., Miller, L., Harvath, T., Jackson, A., & Delorit, M. (2003). Nurses' experiences with hospice patients who refuse food and fluids to hasten death. *New England Journal of Medicine*, 349(4), 359–365.

Glannon, W. (2005). *Biomedical ethics*. New York: Oxford University Press.

Glass, E., & Cluxton, D. (2004). Truth-telling: Ethical issues in clinical practice. *Journal of Hospice and Palliative Nursing*, 6(4), 232–242.

Jonsen, A., Siegler, M., & Winslade, W. (2002). *Clinical ethics*, (5th ed.). New York: McGraw-Hill.

Kavanaugh, J. (2004, June 21–22). Another opinion: Artificial feeding. *America*, 7.

Kvale, E., Williams, B., Bolden, J., Padgett, C., & Bailey, F. (2004). The Balm of Gilead Project: A demonstration project on end-of-life care for safety-net populations. *Journal of Palliative Medicine*, 7(3), 486–493.

Ladd, R., Pasquerella, L., & Smith, S. (2000). What to do when the end is near: Ethical issues in home health care nursing. *Public Health Nursing*, 17(2), 103–110.

Lentz, J. (2003). Daily baths: Torment or comfort at end of life? *Journal of Hospice and Palliative Nursing*, 5(1), 34–39.

Lynn, J., & Childress, J. (1986). Must patients always be given food and water? In J. Lynn (Ed.), *By no extraordinary means* (pp. 48–60). Bloomington, IN: Indiana University Press.

Matzo, M., & Emanual, E. (1997). Oncology nurses' practice of assisted suicide and patient-requested euthanasia. *Oncology Nursing Forum*, 24, 1725–1732.

Moller, D. (2005). None left behind: Urban poverty, social experience, and rethinking palliative care. *Journal of Palliative Medicine*, 8(1), 17–19.

Oregon Department of Human Services (2005). Physician assisted suicide: summaries, annual reports, press releases. Retrieved from http://egov.oregon.gov/DHS/ph/pas/.

Oregon Nurses Association (1995). Assisted suicide: ONA provides guidance on nurses' dilemma. Retrieved from http://www.oregonrn.org.

Preston, T. (2000). Final victory. Roseville, CA: Prima Publishing.

Quill, T. (2005). Terri Schiavo—A tragedy compounded. *New England Journal of Medicine*, 352(16), 1630–1632.

Scanlon, C. (2003). Ethical concerns in end-of-life care. *American Journal of Nursing*, 103(1), 48–55.

Schwarz, J. (1999). The 'delegated providers of assisted dying.' *American Journal of Nursing*, 99(6), 9.

Schwarz, J. (2004). The rule of double effect and its role in facilitating good end-of-life palliative care. *Journal of Hospice and Palliative Nursing*, 6(2), 125–133.

Stanley, K., & Zoloth-Dorman, L. (2001). Ethical considerations. In B Ferrell & N. Coyle (Eds.), *Textbook of palliative nursing* (p. 663). New York: Oxford University.

Tanner, R. (2005, March 22). The Schiavo fight: The battle over the Florida woman's care has been raging for years. *The Oregonian*, A6

Tolle, S., Tilden, V., Drach, L., Fromme, E., Perrin, N., & Hedberg, K. (2004). Characteristics and proportion of dying Oregonians who personally consider physician-assisted suicide. *Journal of Clinical Ethics*, 15(2), 111–118.

Veatch, R. (2003). *The basics of bioethics* (2nd Ed.). Upper Saddle River, NJ: Prentice-Hall.

Volbrecht, R. (2002). *Nursing ethics: Communities in dialogue*. Upper Saddle River, NJ: Prentice-Hall.

Williams, B. (2004). Dying young, dying poor: A sociological examination of existential suffering among low-socioeconomic status patients. *Journal of Palliative Medicine, 7*(1), 27–37.

Winland-Brown, J. (1998). Death, denial, and defeat: Older patients and advance directives. *Advanced Practice Nursing Quarterly, 4*(2), 36–40.

Zerwekh, J. (2000). Caring on the ragged edge: Nursing persons who are disenfranchised. *Advances in Nursing Science, 22*(4), 47–61.

Zerwekh, J. (2003). End-of-life hydration—benefit or burden? *Nursing 2003, 33*(2), 32hn1–32hn3.

Zerwekh, J., Riddell, S., & Richard, J. (2002). Fearing to comfort: A grounded theory of constraints to opioid use in hospice care. *Journal of Hospice and Palliative Nursing, 4*(2), 83–90.

Zerwekh, J. (1994). The truth tellers: How hospice nurses help patients confront death. *American Journal of Nursing, 94*(2), 31–35.

CHAPTER 10

Spiritual Caring

THERIS TOUHY AND JOYCE ZERWEKH

Philosophical Reflections

"How strange this fear of death is! We are never frightened at a sunset."
GEORGE MACDONALD

Learning Objectives

1. Differentiate between spirituality and religion.
2. Demonstrate understanding of how spirituality is part of holistic nursing.
3. Appreciate the major world religions and the rituals and traditions important to people from different faith systems at the end of life.
4. Explain the elements of spiritual assessment.
5. Identify spiritual interventions.
6. Reflect on ways to develop one's own spirituality.

Spirituality is a primary concern for dying patients and their families and an essential component of end-of-life care. Spiritual caring is a vital branch of the End-of-Life Caregiving Tree. Nursing tradition, theory, codes of professional conduct, and professional organizations recognize spiritual care as an essential component of nursing care. Health-care organizations such as the Joint Commission on the Accreditation of Healthcare Organizations, the American Association of Colleges of Nursing, and the Association of American Medical Colleges have recognized the importance of addressing spiritual needs in health care. Yet, nurses and other health professionals often struggle with their role in providing spiritual care; and spiritual care at the end of life remains inadequate. This chapter will discuss spirituality as an essential dimension of holistic nursing, with a focus on end-of-life care. It will compare the similarities and differences between religion and spirituality, discuss nursing approaches for assessment and provision of both religious and spiritual care, and offer ways for nurses to develop and deepen their own spirituality and caring.

HOLISTIC NURSING AND SPIRITUALITY

The essence of being spiritual is being whole or holistic, and attention to the spiritual needs of patients is a critical dimension of holistic nursing care. Most nurses express a commitment to holistic care, recognizing that humans have biological, psychological, social, and spiritual needs that all affect health. Although a great deal of emphasis has been placed on the first three of these needs in nursing education, practice, and research, the area of spiritual care has received far less attention. We can observe the body, we can imagine the mind in operation and measure intelligence, but there is no computed tomography (CT) scan of the spirit (Bell & Troxel, 2001). Understanding spirituality is far more elusive than learning about the pathology associated with illness and disease. Surveys with practicing nurses suggest that most have had little, if any, education in spiritual care. Spiritual care entails assisting patients to find a sense of meaning and reconciliation with others and with a transcendent reality, encouraging patients to strengthen their spiritual life, as they choose.

An emphasis on spirituality in nursing is not new; nursing has encompassed the spiritual from its origin. In years past, nursing students were educated in care of the body, mind, and spirit, often in schools of nursing with religious affiliation. The science of nursing was not seen as separate from the art and spirit of the discipline. Florence Nightingale's view of nursing was derived from her spiritual philosophy, and she considered nursing a spiritual experience. She believed that "Nursing should be a search for truth, a discovery of God's laws of healing and their proper application" (Macrae, 1995, p. 9). Nightingale considered spirituality "intrinsic to human nature, our deepest and most potent resource for healing" (Macrae, 1995, p. 8). She saw spirituality as an awareness of our inner connection with a higher reality that creates, sustains, and organizes the universe. Many nursing theories address spirituality, including those of Neuman, Parse, and Watson (Martsolf & Mickley, 1998).

The secularization of the Western world, with its focus on that which is touchable, present, and material, has displaced concepts such as spirituality in favor of modern scientific thinking. Nursing theory, research, and practice, in attempts to establish the discipline as scientific and research-based, have followed these trends. Spirituality is abstract, cannot be measured, and is often associated with religion, an area considered off limits for scientific medicine. The de-emphasis on spiritual concerns and the contemporary lack of attention to spirituality in nursing education and practice have relegated spirituality to the clergy, leaving patients perceiving that nurses focus on the body and emotions but not the spirit.

These trends appear to be changing, however, and both nursing and medicine are beginning to reclaim some of the essential healing values from their roots. Spirituality is an intrinsic part of holism and overlooking a person's spiritual needs hinders a comprehensive understanding of the whole person.

 The essence of being spiritual is being whole or holistic, and attention to spiritual needs of patients is a critical dimension of holistic nursing care.

SPIRITUALITY CONTRASTED WITH RELIGION

Distinguishing between religion and spirituality is a concern for many health professionals. "Religion can be described as a social institution that unites people in a faith in God, a higher power, and in common rituals and worshipful acts. A god, divinity, and/or soul is always included in the concept" (Strang &, Strang, 2002, p. 858). Each *religion* involves a particular set of beliefs. *Spirituality* is a broader concept than religion and encompasses a person's search for meaning, relationships with a higher power, with nature, and with other people. Ultimately, spirituality involves a sense of unity with a reality more enduring than the individual self. Religion may be considered one path by which some people create a sense of the spiritual and support the personal sense of self. Everyone has a spirit or is spiritual whether or not they consider themselves religious or belong to an organized religion or faith community. The word spirit is derived from the Latin *"spirare"* meaning to breathe life. The spirit can be thought of as that which gives us the breath of our life, the meaning and purpose for our living. Religious systems and needs are not universal and are different for each individual. Spiritual needs, on the other hand, are essentially the same for everyone. The way people meet these needs will be different and may change over the course of a person's life, but the core spiritual needs are universal. The concept of spirituality is found is all cultures and societies (Bell & Troxel, 2001). See Box 10-1, The Five Rs of Spirituality.

Box 10-1 ■ **THE FIVE R'S OF SPIRITUALITY**

Reason and Reflection—Search for meaning and purpose in one's life. Finding the will and reason to live. Reflection and meditation on one's existence (may be enhanced through art, music, or literature).
Religion—Means of expressing spirituality through a framework of values and beliefs, often actively pursued in rituals, religious practices, and reading of sacred texts. Religion might be institutionalized or informal.
Relationships—Longing to relate to oneself, others, and a deity/higher being (may be expressed via service, love, relationships, trust, hope, and/or creativity). Appreciation of the natural environment.
Restoration—Ability of the spiritual dimension to influence health and well-being positively.

Source: Adapted from Covier (2000).

The definition of spirituality proposed by the 1971 White House Conference on Aging endorsed this view:

> The term spiritual pertains to one's inner resources, especially one's ultimate concerns; the basic values around which all other values are focused; the central philosophy of life—religious, non-religious or anti-religious—which guides conduct, and the non-material and/or supernatural dimensions of human nature (Moberg, 1984).

A hospice nurse describes her relationship with a patient who lived a deep spiritual life outside of organized religion:

> He had terrible things to say about television evangelists and the organized church. At various times I asked him questions like, "What has life meant to you?" and "What has brought harmony to your life?" He described his connection with nature. He was so attuned to nature, like what I've read about Native American spirituality. His belief was that when he died he was going to be the blossoms in the spring, or the clouds in the sky. That was under a crusty gruff exterior.

With few exceptions, research on spirituality, and even instruments used to measure and assess spirituality, have had a Christian focus. There is a need to broaden the research to focus on the various ways spirituality may be expressed, both within and outside the context of different religious beliefs. Outside organized religion, many contemporary people have developed individualistic spiritual convictions. For instance, they may practice meditation while adhering to no specific religion. They may find experiences of the transcendent in music or nature without adhering to a specific creed. This is especially important in contemporary America where a multicultural population with diverse faith systems and views of the spiritual is increasing. Nurses of today reflect this growing diversity and must be knowledgeable about how concepts of faith and spirituality influence not only their lives and practice, but also the lives and health of their patients. The increasing diversity of the nursing profession will add insight and richness to our understanding of the concepts of spirituality, religion, and faith, and their importance to the health of our patients.

Nurses often view spirituality and spiritual care in religious terms and as the responsibility of chaplains or other religious leaders. They worry about the ethics of health professionals entering into discussions that may be construed as religious in nature, or the implied risk of imposing their own beliefs on patients. Conflicts may occur when nurses are faced with caring for a patient whose beliefs differ from their own. One hospice nurse told the author that she chose hospice nursing because she felt she could bring her deep Christian-based faith to help patients accept her God at the end of their life. After a short time in practice, she realized that her role with care of the dying was not one of imposing her own beliefs, but rather supporting the patient in finding his or her own meaning and purpose in life. Her own beliefs gave her the strength to perform her work, guided her care, and strengthened her own spirit. However, she learned to respect and support her patients' beliefs and values rather than impose her own. Many nurses struggle with these same issues and this has been identified as one of the reasons they may be hesitant or uncomfortable with spiritual care.

> *Spirituality is a broader concept than religion and encompasses a person's search for meaning, relationships with a higher power, with nature, and with other people . . . Ultimately, spirituality involves a sense of unity with a reality more enduring than the individual self.*

ORGANIZED RELIGIOUS TRADITIONS

For many people, spirituality is rooted in organized religious traditions. For the faithful, religious practices such as prayer and worship services help develop their sense of meaning and purpose in life and nurture their spiritual needs.

Judeo-Christian Religions

The most ancient of the major contemporary world religions began approximately 3500 years ago with Judaism in North Africa and Hinduism in India (Kemp & Bhungalia, 2002; Levey & Greenhall, 1983). Out of Judaism emerged Christianity about 2000 years ago and Islam about 1400 years ago. These have become the religions of North Africa, Europe, the Americas, Australia, and New Zealand. All religions emerging out of Judaism believe in worship of and prayer to one God. Prayer includes giving thanks, asking for forgiveness, and asking for help. The forms of worship and prayer and rules for behavior vary dramatically between subgroups and sects. Prayer, readings from sacred texts, and centuries-old rituals are comforting at the end of life. Psalm 23 has comforted people of Judeo-Christian heritage for generations. It follows in an American Bible Society (1976) contemporary translation:

> The Lord is my Shepherd.
> I have everything I need.
> He lets me rest in fields of green grass
> and leads me to quiet pools of fresh water.
> He gives me new strength.
> He guides me in the right paths,
> as he has promised.
> Even if I go through the deepest darkness,
> I will not be afraid, Lord,
> for you are with me.
> Your shepherd's rod and staff protect me.
>
> You prepare a banquet for me,
> where all my enemies can see me;
> You welcome me as an honored guest
> and fill my cup to the brim.
> I know that your goodness and
> love will be with me all my life;
> and your house will be my home as long as I live.

Eastern Religions

Out of Hinduism emerged Buddhism about 2600 years ago (Kemp & Bhungalia, 2002; Levey & Greenhall, 1983). These Eastern traditions are widespread throughout Asia in various divisions and sects. Both Hinduism and Buddhism believe in the cycle of death and rebirth. Freedom from that endless cycle of reincarnation and suffering is brought about by meditation and right actions. Buddhism teaches that suffering ends when a person is able to let go of attachment to life and its desires. Followers of Eastern traditions do not usually conceive of spiritual reality in terms of a single god; some pray to multiple gods. At the end of life, they seek comfort through ancient rituals, chanting, and meditation.

Box 10-2 presents an overview of major religious belief systems with traditions and practices that may be associated with end-of-life care. Each religious group has many divisions with unique beliefs and practices. Likewise, each individual may interpret the tenets of faith in his or her unique way. Keep in mind that many patients derive their spirituality outside the context of organized religion. The nurse and the patient may not be religious, but can still be spiritual. Everyone has spiritual needs and everyone meets them in their own unique way.

Note that within tradition, there is a wide divergence in beliefs and practices. Below are generalizations about the most commonly held beliefs and practices

CHRISTIANITY

Beliefs

Jesus Christ was born about 2000 years ago. He taught compassion and forgiveness, was tortured and hung on a cross (Crucifixion) for his teachings, and rose from the dead (The Resurrection). Jesus was the Messiah or Savior. All who believe in him can have their sins forgiven and go to Heaven after they die. Each group of Christians believes they have the truth. There are three major divisions: Roman Catholic, Protestant, and Orthodox. For all, the groups, the sacred text is the Bible, including the Old Testament (Hebrew Bible) and the New Testament, which describes the life and teachings of Jesus.

Practices Including Those at the End of Life

Roman Catholic Christians

Participation in sacred rites called sacraments is important throughout life.
Baptism involving sprinkling of water as a symbol of washing away sin. In infancy or at the time conversion, baptism admits the person to the church. A dying person must be baptized to enter the afterlife.
Anointing the Sick by a priest for those near death. Formerly called Last Rites.
Sacrament of Reconciliation (Confession) in which a priest grants forgiveness from God.
Eucharist (Holy Communion) in which the participant receives bread consecrated by the priest and believed to be the Body of Christ. Deacons and eucharistic ministers, who are not clergy, may administer Communion. The foundation of the Catholic worship service or Mass is the celebration of Communion. Prayer and sacraments are comforting at the bedside of the dying.

(continued)

Box 10-2 ■ RELIGIOUS BELIEFS, TRADITIONS, AND PRACTICES AT THE END OF LIFE (CONTINUED)

Protestant Christians

Sacred rites or sacraments are less important in many branches of the Protestant Church. Most believe that baptism is essential to life after death. Frequent reception of Communion is comforting to members of some denominations, particularly Lutheran and Episcopalian. Prayer, Bible readings, and hymns are comforting at the end of life. Pentecostal and charismatic churches believe in faith healing. Christian Scientists rely on spiritual healing rather than medicine.

Orthodox (Greek and Russian) Christians

Confession and Communion are important sacred rites as death approaches. Last anointing may occur before or after death.

Practices Including Those at the End of Life

Orthodox strictly observe Jewish law. Conservatives follow that Law but believe it can be altered within the context of contemporary culture. Reform do not believe that the Torah was written by God and interpret Jewish law liberally. The Sabbath or Shabbat begins just before sunset on Friday and ends just after sunset on Saturday. On Shabbat, certain rituals and prohibitions are followed.

JUDAISM

Beliefs

Jewish faith dates from approximately 1500 to 1000 B.C. The central belief is in one God. Practicing Judaism involves following the Law, practicing rituals, and supporting the people chosen by God. Sacred texts are the Hebrew Bible (Includes the Torah) and the Talmud (legal code for living). There are three main divisions: Orthodox, Conservative, and Reform.

ISLAM

Beliefs

Islam is defined as submission, and a Muslim is one who submits to Allah, the Arabic word for God. Muslims, Jews, and Christians worship the same God. Mohammad founded Islam. During a vision, the Koran (Qur'an) was revealed to him. Another sacred text is the Tradition or Hadith. Islam recognizes the prophets of the Hebrew

The dying person can be comforted with readings from the Torah and Psalms, which is acceptable to be read by those who are not Jewish. Prolongation of life is usually emphasized. The dying person is not left alone. After death, the body is straightened and covered.

Among the Orthodox and observant Conservative Jews, cremation, embalming, and ornate coffins are forbidden. Burial occurs within 24 hours of death. In the first week after death, the mourners sit "shivah," which includes many restrictions. Kaddish, an ancient Jewish prayer which exalts God, is recited by groups of 10 men throughout the mourning period lasting 30 days.

Practices Including Those at the End of Life

There are Five Pillars of Islamic Practice:

1. Daily confession of faith
2. Prayer five times daily preceded by ritual cleaning
3. Fasting during Ramadan, except for those who are ill
4. Giving to the needy
5. Pilgrimage to Mecca, if possible

At the end of life, discussions about death are often not wanted. Cousins or uncles may be the contact people who will decide whether to tell the patient and family about diagnosis and prognosis.

(continued)

Bible, as well as Jesus. Mohammad is considered to be God's final Prophet.

Patients may choose to face toward Mecca, which is West or Southwest in the U.S.

Prolongation of life is usually emphasized. Only same sex caregivers should touch the person's body. After death, non-Muslims should not touch the body. They can wear gloves if necessary.

It is usually not comforting or acceptable for non-Muslims to read aloud from the Qur'an.

HINDUISM

Beliefs

Hinduism began in India about 1000 to 1500 B.C.E., about the time of Moses. The goal of Hinduism is freedom from suffering and repeated reincarnation, caused by actions in this life and past lives. Karma is the law that determines consequences of past actions. Enlightenment occurs through meditation. Some believe in one God (Brahman the Creator) and others believe in multiple Gods. Major scriptures are the Vedas, the Upanishads, and the Bhagavad-Gita.

Practices Including Those at the End of Life

Believing in the cycle of death and rebirth, a devout Hindu is likely to be accepting of death.

Choice of consciousness as death nears may limit acceptance of symptom management.

Chanting, prayer, incense, and rituals accompany dying.

Family members should be the only ones touching the body. Preference is for cremation.

White is the color of mourning.

BUDDHISM

Beliefs

Buddhism began as a reform of Hinduism. Siddhartha, born in the 6th century B.C., became enlightened while sitting under a banyan tree, and was then known as the Buddha. He taught that freedom from being reincarnated repeatedly can be attained through absence of desire. There are two major branches: Theravada and Mahayana. Buddhism teaches Four Noble Truths:

1. All sentient beings suffer.
2. The cause of suffering is attachment to life and other people.
3. Suffering ends when we stop desiring.
4. Suffering will cease if you follow the Eightfold Path of right beliefs and right actions.

Practices Including Those at the End of Life

Consciousness in dying is highly valued. Death is accepted. Expect chanting, prayer, incense, and rituals at the deathbed. White is the color of mourning. Cremation is common. A new incarnation occurs right after death. There are no specific regulations about handling the body.

Source: From ELNEC (2003); and Kemp (2003).

> **Box 10-3 ■   FOUR CENTRAL SPIRITUAL DOMAINS AT THE END OF LIFE**
>
> Hope: Expectation of achieving a future good
>
> Meaning: Sense that one's life has purpose or significance
>
> Reconciliation: Reunion with other people or with God; bringing life into harmony after estrangement.
>
> Transcendence: Going beyond the bounds of human experience

CORE SPIRITUAL NEEDS AT THE END OF LIFE

Death confronts dying people with issues related to hope, meaning, reconciliation, and transcendence. Therefore, nursing goals at the end of life should foster hopefulness, meaningfulness, reconciliation, and transcendence. We do not undertake this alone, but in collaboration with the entire health-care team, particularly the spiritual counselor or chaplain if accepted by the patient. See Box 10-3, Four Central Spiritual Domains at the End of Life.

Meaning

For many, living in the face of death compels examination of their purpose on earth and whether they will live after death. They search for meaning. Meaning refers to a sense of one's individual life having had a purpose or significance. Puchalski (2002, p. 290), a physician expert in spiritual care, says:

> Dying should be as natural an experience as birth. It should be a meaningful experience for dying persons, a time when they find meaning in their suffering and have various dimensions of their experience addressed by their caregiver. These dimensions are: the physical (pain and symptom control); the psychological (anxiety and depression); the social (feelings of isolation from friends and family); the spiritual. It is our responsibility to listen to people as they struggle with their dying. We need to be willing to listen to their anxieties, their fears, their unresolved conflicts, their hopes, and their despairs. If people are stuck in despair, they will suffer deeply. It is through their spirituality that people become liberated from despair. As people are faced with serious illness or the prospect of dying, questions of meaning often arise.

- Why did this happen to me?
- What will happen to me after I die?
- Why would God allow me to suffer this way?

- Will I be remembered?
- Will I be missed?

Spiritual meaning is central to the dying person and should receive greater emphasis by health professionals. In one survey, patients ranked coming to peace with God and praying nearly identical in importance to pain control (Steinhauser, Christakis, Clipp, McNeilly, McIntyre, and Tulsky, 2000). Patients are comforted by believing that death is a normal part of life and that they will be remembered and live on, either through their relationships, their accomplishments, or their good work. Dying patients want to believe that they have done their best in life, have a purpose for living, and will be in the presence of a loving God or Higher Power after death (Puchalski, 2002).

> *Dying patients want to believe that they have done their best in life, have a purpose for living, and will be in the presence of a loving God or Higher Power after death.*

Stephenson, Draucker, and Martsolf (2003) asked hospice patients to describe the experience of spirituality in their lives and how their experience with spirituality had changed since they became ill. They were also asked to describe a spiritual experience in their life, reflect on their spiritual needs, and discuss how nurses can help them meet those needs. Few participants used the terms spiritual or spirituality, and none reported newly found religion or life-altering spiritual experiences in the face of impending death. Rather, they shared life stories that illustrated how they found meaning in their lives, their values, and their relationship with others, God, and the environment. One author remembers reflecting with Mother Essie Law, leader of her Pentecostal church, while she was on her deathbed. For 2 hours she talked about all the people she had come to love. Spirituality involves a search for purpose and connectedness with others and God or a Higher Power. According to the Stephenson study, dying patients do not expect theological epiphanies, but rather they want us to be supportive listeners who help them explore meaning. To do this, a nurse asks questions and encourages life review:

- Tell me more about your life.
- What has been most meaningful in your life?
- How have you found strength throughout your life?

A hospice nurse explained the possibility of finding a deepened sense of meaning with a dying patient:

> We talked about terminal illness as a real paradox. There are some positive things that can happen that never would have happened otherwise: a new point of view, a new spirituality, renewed family relationships, or just appreciation. At the same time you are losing that great joy and experiencing great pain.

Hope

Palliative interventions should be offered in the context of hope rather than as a response to a hopeless situation. Hope can be described as confident expectation of achieving a future good that is personally significant. At the end of life, there are two kinds of hope: hope to live more fully and deeply in the time remaining and hope to live beyond death (Kemp, 2001). Unless caregivers understand the nature of hope and the many ways it can be expressed, our care can impede rather than promote hope. Factors identified by patients as impediments to hope include hopelessness in others, depleted energy, uncontrollable pain and suffering, negative hospital experiences, dehumanizing messages, feeling that no one cares, lack of information, and physical and emotional distancing of caregivers (Herth, 1993; Miller, 1989). For example, providing emotional and physical comfort to minimize suffering and maximize the patient's energy to invest in hope is an important nursing response at the end of life. Carrying out an intervention such as relieving a symptom, or creating a peaceful and beautiful environment, suggests that you are hopeful and that you care.

❝ | *Palliative interventions should be offered in the context of hope rather than as a response to a hopeless situation.*

Hope is a powerful force against despair and helps patients and families journey through the difficult times leading up to death. At the end of life, hope is not just associated with cure but extends beyond a physical nature to that of a social, psychological, and spiritual nature. "Because we have declared limits on treatment or cure does not mean that we have pronounced the limits of human potential. Patients are invited to open themselves to new targets of hope, to draw on strengths not yet experienced" (Jevne, 1993, p. 126).

Central to the instillation of hope is the caring relationship between nurses and patients. Nurses can inspire hope by helping patients and families focus on living the moment as fully as possible. A patient's hope for a cure may change to his or her hope for freedom from pain, day to day experiences to enjoy precious moments of life, time to accomplish life goals before life is over, sharing love with family and friends, relief of suffering, death with dignity, and eternal life (Matzo, 2001).

Nursing responses that instill hope can foster harmony, healing, and wholeness (Watson, 1988). Caring relationships characterized by unconditional positive regard, encouragement, and competence help patients feel loved and cared about, thus inspiring hope. Nurses may need to help family focus on goal directed interventions that emphasize what the patients still wants to accomplish. Nursing interventions that foster hope (Ersek, 2001) are as follows:

- Control symptoms
- Encourage patient and family to become involved in positive experiences that transcend their current situation
- Foster spiritual processes and finding meaning

Box 10-4 ■	**HOPE-PROMOTING EXPERIENCES**

Feel the warmth of a sunbeam
Share experiences children are having
Note the crystal blue of the sky
Savor the richness of black coffee at breakfast
Feel the tartness of grapefruit to wake up the taste buds
Watch the activities of an animal in a tree outside the window
Benefit from each encounter with another person
Write messages to grandchildren, nieces, or nephews
Study a favorite painting
Listen to a symphony
Build highlights into each day such as meals, visits, Bible reading
Keep a journal
Write letters
Make a tape recording of your life story
Have hope objects or symbols nearby
Share hope stories
Focus on abilities, strengths, and past accomplishments
Encourage decision-making about daily activities; foster a sense of
    control
Extend caring and love to others
Appreciate expressions of caring concern
Renew loving relationships

Source: Adapted from Miller (1983); and Jevne (1993).

- Promote connection and reconciliation
- Help in the development of realistic goals
- Focus attention on the short-term future

Box 10-4 offers suggestions for experiences that foster hope for patients at the end of life.

Consider how nurses foster hope for Ms. Harriet Truman, age 87, who lived at home until last year, when her husband died suddenly from a heart attack. For the last 7 months, Harriet has lived in a skilled nursing facility with excellent nurses and an active group of volunteers. Her emphysema has worsened, with repeated respiratory infections necessitating hospitalization. Now Harriet has signed a living will, requesting not to be re-hospitalized or resuscitated. The nurses and aides are fostering hope by controlling her growing breathlessness and chronic osteoarthritis pain, encouraging visits from daughters and grandson, and taking her into the garden every day. She wants to complete a legacy of her childhood stories on audiotape; a volunteer comes twice a week to help her with recording. Nieces have brought her tapes of her classical and folk music favorites. She looks forward to a reunion with her eldest son, who has been living out of the country for the last 14 years. Every week, a Eucharistic minister from her Roman Catholic church brings Communion and prayer to her bedside.

For patients whose religious life is a source of hope, providing opportunities for prayer, reading hope-filled Scripture, and creating an environment in which the patient feels comfortable expressing hope in God or a Higher Power are hope-promoting interventions. Hope is promoted by having a clear sense of meaning.

Connectedness and Reconciliation

The sense of connectedness through relationship is a spiritual need that contrasts with the sense that many people have of being alone and isolated from others and from God. Terminal illness brings that loneliness and need for connectedness into sharp focus. Related to the need for connectedness, there is opportunity for reconciliation at the end of life. Reconciliation involves healing past estrangements from other people and from God. In America, many people have lived lives cut off from close friends and family. They have been committed to self-help and individualism. Even for those who live in tight-knit family and social circles, there may be those who have been lost to past quarrels and disagreements. At the end of life, some choose reconciliation. Nurses encourage reconnecting with cut-off relatives and friends. Sometimes we can even serve as go-betweens to bring people together.

Likewise, for many individuals, dying is an opportunity for reconnection with God and their faith. Patients should be offered religious counsel and ritual that brings them opportunity for reunion with the transcendent. One facet of reconciliation is the need for forgiveness or acceptance. Sin, regret, and guilt are common to the human experience, and dying brings opportunity to forgive and be forgiven. This is the last chance to find reunion and peace. Sadly, some are never able to let go of their anger and resentment; they cannot find their way beyond broken relationships and estrangement.

Nurses helped brothers Craig and Joe to reconcile, for example. When their mother died, they had fought bitterly over the provisions of her will and never spoken again. Over the years, they completely lost touch. Nine years later, when Craig was dying of multiple myeloma, the palliative unit nurse asked if there was anyone he should be talking to or seeing. At first he thought he would write a letter to Joe, but then he asked his wife to see if she could find him. When Joe walked into the room, they both started weeping. Craig died 2 days later.

Transcendence

Transcendence is defined by philosophers and theologians as going beyond the limits of lived human experience. Transcendence involves detachment and separation from life as it has been lived to experience a reality beyond oneself and beyond what can be seen and felt. Dying people often experience such transcendence in one form or another. Nurses cannot make transcendence happen, but should have open minds and listen carefully when we hear stories of transcendence or witness the unexplainable.

Two hospice nurses, Callahan and Kelley (1992), describe their repeated experiences with the "nearing death awareness" of patients on the verge of death. They assert that "the experience of dying frequently includes glimpses of another world and those waiting in it. Although they provide few details, dying people speak with awe and wonder of the peace and beauty they see in this other place. They tell of talking with, or sensing the presence of, people whom we cannot see—perhaps people they have known and loved" (pp. 22–23). Their messages often include preparing for a change or travel. They may talk about traveling, packing, or finding a map. Some will describe the place where they are going. One patient described his upcoming journey:

> He was frustrated at the boat he saw across the river. It was carrying both his wife and his sister, who were dead. . . . The boat wouldn't come across the river. Finally, at 4:30 in the morning, he told me the boat was coming across the river, closer and closer. He died at 4:47 AM (Zerwekh, 1993, p. 29).

Nurses at the deathbed sometimes share their own mystical experiences that are outside explanations of everyday reality. One nurse described seeing a luminescent angel at a dying patient's bedside when she was still a nursing student. For fear of being considered crazy, she told no one for many years. Other nurses describe once-in-a-lifetime experiences of witnessing a spirit leave the body at the moment of death. One nurse recalls:

> He began to have periods of apnea. I turned to look out of the window. . . . I remember hearing some birds singing. Then I looked back at the patient and watched his spirit come up out of his head (Zerwekh, 1993, p. 29).

Another nurse asserts:

> When the patient is edging out of this world, I want to be there. It's a spiritual experience beyond words.

Nurses can help families understand and accept transcendent experiences that they are witnessing. One nurse tried to comfort a dying patient's family by describing her patient's transcendent experience:

> Three days before she died she talked about a comforting person who would take her across. She would tell me that she believed the person was coming to lead her. It was so meaningful to her, so comforting. She wasn't frightened at all. She thought it might be an angel, but she wasn't sure. She would talk with the angel

while I was there. It was kind of eerie to be with her. I explained that her experience wasn't unusual for people near death, and tried to convey to the family the comfort she was receiving from the experience.

The nurse's response to the spiritual need for transcendence is to recognize and be open to it, and to be willing to explain experiences of the transcendent to patient and family if they choose.

RECOGNIZING SPIRITUAL DISTRESS

Spiritual distress at the end of life is an impaired ability to experience meaning, hope, connectedness, and transcendence. Spiritual distress at the end of life commonly involves an intensification of alienation and disconnection, while dying forces a progressive series of separations and detachment from life itself. Manifestations of spiritual distress include anger, guilt, blame, hatred, expressed absence of meaning, expressions of alienation and turning away from friends and family, inability to enjoy, and inability to participate in religious activities that have previously provided comfort (Doenges, Moorhouse, and Geissler-Murr, 2004). A hospice nurse expert gives an example:

> I felt there was a lot of spiritual stuff going on with him. A lot of unrest in his soul. He was in constant motion. I got Trilicate for his bone pain and called in the chaplain. It turned out he was very angry at God because he had given his life to the church and now he was dying so soon.

Another nurse gives an example of suspected spiritual distress:

> She was suffering at some level and I didn't know where. I wanted to spend some time with her to try to find out. Somewhere, I really felt that she had some past secret, something that she felt was totally unforgivable.

Building on a fundamental understanding of the core spiritual needs and spiritual distress occurring when these needs are not met, the next section examines how a nurse can complete individualized spiritual assessments to identify spiritual distress and respond to meet spiritual needs.

SPIRITUAL ASSESSMENT AT THE END OF LIFE

Patients welcome a discussion of spiritual matters and want health professionals to consider their spiritual needs (O'Brien, 1999; Post, Puchalski, and Larson, 2000). For instance, three fourths of patients in a rehabilitation center considered their religious and spiritual beliefs to be important, but three fourths said that no one from the health-care staff ever spoke to them about their spiritual and religious concerns (Anderson, Anderson, and Felsenthal,

1993). A spiritual history opens the door to a conversation about the role of spirituality and religion in a person's life. People often need permission to talk about these issues. Without some signal from the nurse, patients may feel that such topics are not welcome or appropriate. The role of the nurse is to listen and encourage people as they search for their own answers.

Obtaining a spiritual history involves simply listening to patients as they express their fears, hopes, and beliefs. A spiritual assessment is intended to elicit information about the core spiritual needs and how the nurse and other members of the health-care team can respond to them. Just as a medical history is completed using a systematic review of physiological systems, hospices and palliative-care programs incorporate spiritual assessment instruments into their medical records; these are used to steer conversations about spirituality. They are not intended to be used as checklists or routine paperwork, but rather as guides to begin a spiritual history and to focus listening as patients talk about their beliefs and what gives their lives meaning (Puchalski & Romer, 2000). Listening and responding to spiritual needs and concerns are best conducted within the context of a relationship. An assessment form may offer some ideas regarding spiritual-care needs but does not replace relationship as the context for the delivery of spiritual nursing care. Checklists are merely starting points to begin in-depth dialogues about faith and meaning.

WWW. Internet Reference Box

Examine the spiritual assessment tool available through Last Acts:

http://www2.edc.org/lastacts/assess.asp.

Open-ended questions within the context of the nurse-patient/family relationship can be used to begin dialogue about spiritual concerns. Samples of the types of questions that you might try out in your practice follow (Blues & Zerwekh, 1984):

Concept of God or Spiritual Reality

- Is spiritual peace important to you? What would help you achieve it?
- Is your religion or God significant for you? Can you describe how?
- Is prayer or meditation helpful?

Sources of Hope or Strength

- What matters most to you in your life?
- What is your source of strength and hope?
- To whom do you turn when you need help?
- What brings you joy and comfort?
- What are you afraid of right now?
- What are your worries?

Religious Practices

* What spiritual or religious practices bring your comfort?
* Are there religious books or materials that you want nearby?

ᘔ Planting the Seeds

Nurses who are so busy with medical and nursing tasks should examine their priorities. What really matters for your patients who will soon not be among the living? They are facing the loss of self, all they love, and the only reality they have known. Take time to discover their stories and their struggles. Ask them, "What really matters to you now?" At the same time, respect patients' privacy on matters of spirituality and religion. Avoid imposing your own beliefs.

Throughout life and around the world, human beings cry out:

* To be known
* To feel connected
* To feel appreciated
* To feel useful
* To love and be loved
* To be compassionate
* To give and share
* To have hope
* To experience meaning and purpose

At the end of life, these spiritual needs intensify in the final search for hope, meaning, reconciliation, and transcendence. The person must let go of life and go beyond the limits of lived human experience. Through a continual process of spiritual assessment, we seek to be attuned to their struggle.

SPIRITUAL CARING INTERVENTIONS

Cassidy (1998) proposes that the most powerful caring intervention is to be a companion to the dying:

> The spirituality of those who care for the dying must be the spirituality of the companion, of the friend who walks alongside, helping, sharing, and sometimes just sitting empty-handed, when we would rather run away. It is the spirituality of presence, of being alongside, watchful, available, being there. . . . We who would be a companion to the dying therefore must enter into their darkness, go with them at least part of the way, along their lonely and frightening road . . . enter into the suffering and share in some small way their pain, confusion and desolation (Cassidy, 1998).

There are some specific approaches that foster the practice of this "spirituality of the companion." Keep in mind the overall goals of fostering meaning, hope, connection, and recognizing transcendence. Interventions identified as particularly important to accomplish these goals include (Emblen & Halstead, 1993; Goldberg, 1998; Nagai-Jacobson & Burkhardt, 1989; Stiles, 1990; Touhy, 2001a; Touhy 2001b; Zerwekh, 1993):

- Relief of physical discomfort, which permits refocus on the spiritual
- Comforting touch, which fosters nurse-patient connecting
- Authentic presence and being there
- Attentive listening
- Knowing the patient as a person
- Listening to life stories
- Sharing caring words
- Fostering reconciliation
- Fostering connections with that which is held sacred by the person
- Respecting religious traditions and rituals
- Referring the person to a spiritual counselor

WWW.   Internet Reference Box

Discover Manning's three Hs of empathic presence and active listening by visiting the Hospice Foundation Web site:

http://www.hospicefoundation.org/caregiving/conclusion.htm.

Fostering Reconciliation

As nurses, we often have opportunity to suggest that people review their past and make needed reconnections with those they have lost and faith traditions they have neglected. The goal is to come to some resolution of the past. We can encourage them to tell the story of their lives, and to examine past pains that need healing. A hospice nurse proclaims simply, "The work of the people is to review their life." Where there are estrangements, we encourage giving and receiving forgiveness. A nurse might say, "You haven't seen your son in 11 years. Why not call him? Is now the time?" We do not push or preach. We offer to help heal the brokenness. Patients make their own choices.

Authentic Presence

Authentic presence, for example, becomes possible when nurses deliberately choose to keep their minds uncluttered by distracting thoughts and preoccupations so that they are able to pay full attention in caring relationships with their patients. The practice of presence is described in Chapter 6.

It takes courage and a deep sense of one's own spirituality to be able to have a healing presence with the person nursed. Presence at the end of life involves "talking soul to soul." A hospice nurse describes this as "The essence of me is sharing with the essence of them beyond the words we're talking about" (Zerwekh, 1993, p. 27).

> 66 | *Authentic presence becomes possible when nurses deliberately choose to keep their minds uncluttered by distracting thoughts and preoccupations so that they are able to develop caring relationships with their patients.*

There are a number of spiritual-caring interventions in the following story told by a nurse in a nursing home:

> She wasn't real sure that she had lived a good life, nor was she real sure she was going to have a place in heaven. She was very afraid of pain of dying, of being alone, and being that way eternally. She shared some of her life's experiences. I tried to point out to her that if she had not been in this world that there would have been many lives that would have been affected differently. I tried to help her see some of the positive impact she had on other people in her life. We cried together, hugged, and she thanked me very much and just asked if I would be there when the time came. I told the staff that if she looks like she is getting close to death, call me. And they did, and I was able to be with her and hold her hand as she passed on.

This nurse listened to the patient's life story and came to know her as a person. She was present and listening with her whole being to the fears and doubts expressed as she and the patient talked soul to soul. In an attempt to share how important this person's life was, she was fostering connections and sharing love and caring words. The nurse and patient touched, hugged and cried, and when the time of death came, the nurse was able to comfort and be there, holding her hand.

The nurse cannot prevent death from occurring but can accompany the patient some of the way just by staying, watching, and being there. By helping patients express their beliefs and by staying with them during the events of their illness, nurses are providing spiritual care. A patient dying in a hospital once described to a nurse the two kinds of people who came into the room (Levine, 2003, p. 47):

> One kind could hardly sit still in their chairs, could hardly touch her, or be present and there was very little eye contact. The other kind could merely sit with her without having something to say, having even to reassure her. Their presence, their acceptance of her situation was reassurance enough. Their fingers might just toy gently with her forearm, they didn't have to grasp her, they could touch her with love.

A lovely example of this type of comforting and quiet presence was shared by Wright (2001, p. 22) in a reference to A.A. Milne's *Winnie the Pooh*:

> Piglet sidled up to Pooh from behind.
>
> 'Pooh,' he whispered.
>
> 'Yes Piglet?'
>
> 'Nothing,' said Piglet, taking Pooh's paw.
>
> 'I just wanted to be sure of you.'

Referral to a Spiritual Counselor

Spiritual care should not be provided by the nurse or any other member of the caregiving team in isolation. Instead, it is always enhanced by a strong spiritual counselor or chaplain. Spiritual counselors are essential members of hospice teams and are often included in palliative-care teams. The best spiritual counselors are prepared by clinical pastoral education (CPE) programs to understand psychosocial and spiritual needs at the end of life. They must be able to provide spiritual support to people from a variety of faith traditions and from no identified tradition. The best spiritual counselors are able to listen and offer unconditional love, without focusing on evangelism. They offer religious teaching for those individuals from traditions similar to their own.

An effective spiritual counselor will sit with dying persons to help them discover their own spiritual end-of-life journey. A hospice nurse describes one case needing referral:

> He began to talk about the Trinity and what it meant and was it real. I felt like it was important for me to have the answers and to make sure that I wasn't telling him something that would send him in the wrong direction after he died. So I had his minister come to the house. He helped me reflect on my thinking that I had the power to control whether a person goes to heaven or hell by what I say. So there was some mutual learning and we laughed.

66 | *An effective spiritual counselor will sit with dying persons to help them discover their own spiritual end-of-life journey.*

The nurse should offer to call church, synagogue, temple, or mosque for all patients who identify with a specific faith community. Clergy and designated laypersons should be available to offer the traditional end-of-life ministries of their religion. However, they may be ill-prepared to confront the profound questions of hope and meaning that overwhelm some dying individuals. In such cases, patients may choose to explore these issues with hospital or hospice spiritual counselors as well as receiving comfort from the sacred traditions of their religion.

NURTURING THE SPIRIT OF THE NURSE

"Because spiritual care occurs over time and within the context of relationship, probably the most effective tool at the nurse's disposal is the use of self" (Soeken & Carson, 1987, p. 607).

Thinking about what gives your own life meaning and value helps in developing your spirituality and assists you in being able to support patients. Giving your patient the best spiritual care stems from taking care of your own spiritual needs first (Bell & Troxel, 2001). Following are ways to take care of your own spiritual needs:

- Finding quiet time for meditation and reflection
- Keeping your own faith traditions
- Being with nature
- Appreciating the arts
- Spending time with those you love
- Journaling

Find at least three ways to nourish your own spirit. Nurses often do not take the time to do so and become dispirited. This is especially true for nurses who work with dying patients and experience grief and loss repeatedly. Having someone to talk to about your feelings is important. Chapter 3 explores strategies for self-care. Practicing compassion for oneself is essential to authentic practice of compassion for others. Box 10-5 lists some personal spirituality questions for reflection.

66 | *Giving your patient the best spiritual care stems from taking care of your own spiritual needs first.*

Box 10-5 ■ PERSONAL SPIRITUALITY QUESTIONS FOR REFLECTION FOR NURSES

What do I believe in?
What gives my life meaning?
What do I hope for?
Who do I love and who loves me?
How am I with others?
What would I change about my relationships?
Am I willing to heal the relationships that trouble me?

Source: Adapted from Newshan (1988).

CONCEPTS IN ACTION

As you read the following passage think about these questions:

Are you a glassy-eyed or clear-eyed nurse?
Have you met nurses who are glassy-eyed? Clear-eyed?
How is their nursing care different?
What can you do to become more a more clear-eyed nurse?

Stephen Wright (2001, p. 3) describes the observations of a desperately ill hospitalized friend who said that there are only two types of nurses—the glassy-eyed and the clear-eyed.

> Glassy-eyed ones came into the room, did all the nursing as good as any other, but you could tell by the look in their eyes, no matter what they were saying to you or you to them, that they weren't really with you. They were already thinking of what they want to tell you or have already moved on in their minds to something else. Clear-eyed nurses are absolutely present for you. You can tell by the look in their eyes—clear, attentive, nothing else was going on with them. They weren't thinking about the next job or patient or what they did the night before. They were just right there for you. Clear-eyed nurses were just as busy as the others but the grace of their presence made the difference. The work of the expert nurse is not just built on professional knowledge and skills, it is also dependent on understanding the immense healing power of our uncluttered selves—and that is a spiritual path requiring spiritual practices . . . Illness and dying are attacks upon the soul and the suffering that emerges from such an assault upon the core of our being can be relieved in the respite we find in a clear-eyed nurse. No matter how brief the contact, our presence can be a form of sanctuary as well.

References

American Bible Society. (1976). *Good News Bible*. Nashville, TN: Thomas Nelson Publishers.

Anderson, J., Anderson, L., & Felsenthal, G. (1993). Pastoral needs for support within an inpatient rehabilitation unit. *Archives of Physical Medicine Rehabilitation, 74*, 574–578.

Bell, V., & Troxel, D. (2001). Spirituality and the person with dementia: A view from the field. *Alzheimer's Care Quarterly, 2*(2), 31–45.

Blues, A., & Zerwekh, J. (1984). *Hospice and palliative nursing care*. Orlando, FL: Grune and Stratton.

Callahan, M., & Kelley, P. (1992). *Final gifts*. New York: Simon and Schuster.

Cassidy, S. (1988). *Sharing the darkness*. London: Darron, Longman and Todd.

Covier, I. (2000). Spiritual care in nursing: A systematic approach. *Nursing Standard, 14*(1), 32–36.

Doenges, M., Moorhouse, M., & Geissler-Murr, A. (2004). *Nurse's pocket guide: Diagnoses, interventions, and rationales*. Philadelphia: F. A. Davis.

Emblen, J., & Halstead, L. (1993). Spiritual needs and interventions: Comparing the views of patients, nurses and chaplains. *Clinical Nurse Specialist, 7*(4), 176–182.

ELNEC (End of Life Nursing Education Curriculum). (2003). AACN and COH.

Ersek, M. (2001). The meaning of hope in the dying. In B. Ferrell and N. Coyle (Eds.), *Textbook of palliative nursing* (pp. 339–351). New York: Oxford University Press.

Goldberg, B. (1998). Connection: An exploration of spirituality in nursing care. *Journal of Advanced Nursing, 27*(4), 836–842.

Herth, K. A. (1993). Hope in older adults in community and institutional settings. *Issues in Mental Health Nursing, 14*, 139–156.

Jevne, R. (1993). Enhancing hope in the chronically ill. *Humane Medicine, 9*(2), 121–130.

Kemp, C., & Bhungalia, S. (2002). Culture and the end of life: A review of major world religions. *Journal of Hospice and Palliative Nursing, 4*(4), 235–242.

Kemp, C. (2001). Spiritual care interventions. In B. Ferrell & N. Coyle (Eds.), *Textbook of palliative nursing*. New York: Oxford University Press.

Levine, S. (2003). Mercy in the room. *American Journal of Nursing, 103*(9), 47–48.

Levey, J., & Greenhall, A.(1983). *The concise Columbia encyclopedia.* New York: Columbia University Press.

Macrae, J. (1995). Nightingale's spiritual philosophy and its significance for modern nursing. *Image: Journal of Nursing Scholarship, 27*(1), 8–10.

Martsolf, D., & Mickley, J. (1998). The concept of spirituality in nursing theories: Differing world views and extent of focus. *Journal of Advanced Nursing, 27*, 294–303.

Matzo, M. (2001). End-of-life care: Nurses should help patients to live fully, inspire hope. *American Nurse, September-October*, 1–4.

Miller, J. F. (1989). Hope-inspiring strategies of the critically ill. *Applied Nursing Research, 2*, 23–29.

Miller, J. (1983). *Coping with chronic illness: Overcoming powerlessness.* Philadelphia: F.A. Davis.

Moberg, D. (1984). *Subjective measures of spiritual well being: Review of religious research.* New York: Religious Research Association.

Nagai-Jacobson, M., & Burkhardt, M. (1989). Spirituality: Cornerstone of holistic nursing practice. *Holistic Nursing Practice, 3*, 18–26.

Newshan, G. (1998). Transcending the physical: Spiritual aspects of pain in patients with HIV and/or cancer. *Journal of Advanced Nursing, 28*(6), 1236–1241.

O'Brien, M. E. (1999). Sacred covenants: Exploring spirituality in nursing. *AWHONN Lifelines, 3*(2), 69–72.

Puchalski, C. (2002). Spirituality and end-of-life care: A time for listening and caring. *Journal of Palliative Medicine, 5*(2), 289–294.

Puchalski, C. Retrieved February 2, 2004 from http://www2.edc.org/lastacts/assess.asp.

Puchalski, C. & Romer, A. (2000). Taking a spiritual history allows clinicians to understand patients more fully. *Journal of Palliative Medicine, 3*(4), 129–137.

Post, S., Puchalski, C., & Larson, D. (2000). Physicians and patient spirituality: Professional boundaries, competency, and ethics. *Annals of Internal Medicine, 132*(7), 578–583.

Soeken, K., & Carson, V. (1987). Responding to the spiritual needs of the chronically ill. *Nursing Clinics of North America, 22*, 604–611.

Steinhauser, K., Christakis, N., Clipp, E., McNeilly, M., McIntyre, L., & Tulsky, J. (2000). Factors considered important at the end of life by patients, family, physicians, and other care providers. *Journal of the American Medical Association, 284*(19), 2476–2482.

Stephenson, P., Draucker, C., & Martsolf, D. (2003). The experience of spirituality in the lives of hospice patients. *Journal of Hospice and Palliative Medicine, 5*(1), 51–58.

Stiles, M. (1990). The shining stranger. *Cancer Nursing, 13*(4), 235–245.

Strang, S., & Strang, P. (2002). Questions posed to hospital chaplains by palliative care patients. *Journal of Palliative Medicine, 5*(6), 857–864.

Touhy, T. (2001a). Nurturing hope and spirituality in the nursing home. *Holistic Nursing Practice, 15*(4), 45–56.

Touhy, T. (2001b). Touching the spirit of elders in nursing homes: Ordinary yet extraordinary care. *International Journal for Human Caring, 6*(1), 12–17.

Wright, S. (2001). Presence of mind. *Nursing Standard, 15*(4), 22–23.

Zerwekh, J. (1993). Transcending life: The practice wisdom of nursing hospice experts. *The American Journal of Hospice and Palliative Care, 20*(3), 40–45.

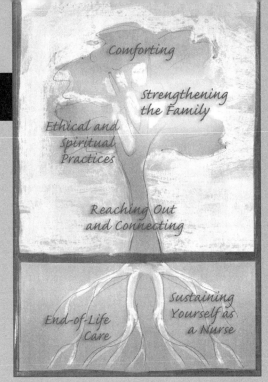

Comforting

Strengthening
the Family

Ethical and
Spiritual
Practices

Reaching Out
and Connecting

End-of-Life
Care

Sustaining
Yourself as
a Nurse

STRENGTHENING
THE FAMILY

CHAPTER 11

Understanding and Strengthening Families

Philosophical Reflections

He cannot bring up her fear.
She is afraid of being alone.
He cannot see that she is not angry at him.
They chase one another in ordinary circles.
They love each other.

LH IN LARSEN, 2002

Learning Objectives

1. Explain the impact of illness on the entire family.
2. Draw a genogram and ecomap to depict family structure and relationships outside the family.
3. Explain common family relationship patterns that will impact family coping with a dying member.
4. Identify the transition processes involved as a family adapts to the dying of a family member.
5. Describe the burdens of providing physical and emotional care to a dying family member.
6. Explain how nurses can guide families through the transition and redefinition that occurs when someone in the family is dying.
7. Identify strategies to teach stressed family caregivers how to care for their dying family member.
8. Describe how nurses can promote communication between family members.
9. Explain the nurse's limitations in being able to strengthen the family.

Understanding and strengthening families is a major branch of the End-of-Life Caregiving Model. This branch of the tree joins the trunk, which visually represents caring and connecting, with the leaves, which represent comforting. This chapter describes how to understand and work with contemporary American families when someone they love is dying. After defining family and family systems, the chapter covers the structure and function of families and networks, the family's experience of transition when someone is dying, the burden of caregiving for family members, and the ways nurses can strengthen families so that they can care for and comfort the dying person.

FAMILIES AND FAMILY SYSTEMS

The term family has come to mean many things in contemporary society. We are all familiar with the traditional understanding of a family as a group of individuals who are related through genetic ties, marriage, and adoption. We visualize mother and father, daughters and sons, perhaps grandparents, all living in the same household. However, families today include unmarried couples with or without children, single parent households, same gender families, and previously married parents who come together to create a blended family. For purposes of this chapter, we will look at "family" in its broadest sense, as a group of individuals who depend on one another for emotional, physical, and possibly economic support (Hanson & Boyd, 1996). Beyond this immediate network is a broader social support system that is essential to understand and strengthen.

  Planting the Seeds

Nurses should consider family to be whoever the patient tells us is family. This includes a wide variety of people whom we might also label as "friends" or "loved ones."

To understand the impact of serious illness on a family, it is helpful to understand the whole family as a system. Illness in one member affects the lives and relationships of everyone else. A metaphor is helpful to understand how family members are intertwined. First of all, imagine the family as a large flowerpot with a variety of flowers blooming individually but all rooted in the same soil. Now pull out one of the flowers and notice how it is tangled in the roots of the others. All will suffer some damage as one flower's roots are torn up; they will struggle to flourish again. "The family as a whole dies along with one of its members—the family will never be the same again" (Davies, 2000, p. 148).

FAMILY STRUCTURE AND FUNCTION

Who exactly comprises the family and how is the family functioning? To understand the human body, you must learn both anatomy and physiology. Likewise, to understand the family, you must learn how it is structured and how it functions.

Structure

It sometimes can take many visits or meetings with a patient to straighten out who are the household members, relatives, and influential friends. The "family" members will, in large part, determine the quality of living and dying for their dying family member. At the same time, these family members will suffer the loss of someone vital to their lives.

Many frameworks are useful to depict family structure. Genograms or family trees can be used to diagram relationships between relatives. Drawing a genogram is much easier than writing several narrative pages to explain family relationships. Detailed instructions for drawing a genogram are contained in most community health nursing and family nursing texts. In the most common way of drawing a genogram, males are symbolically represented as boxes and females as circles. When a couple is married, a box is connected to a circle with a horizontal line. When they are living together but unmarried, the line is dotted. Children are then identified as boxes or circles hung in birth order from the horizontal marriage line. The marriage line is slashed once for separation and twice for divorce. The household is represented with a dotted line encircling it. See Figure 11-1, Basic Genogram Rules.

Figure 11-1 Basic Genogram Rules.

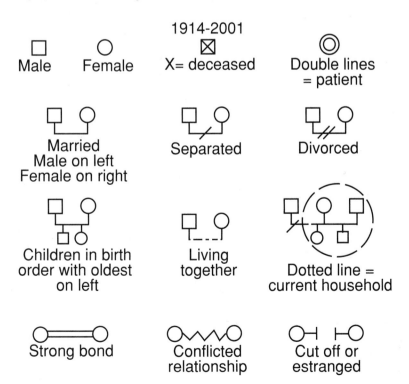

It is also important to understand the broader support network for individuals and families. In many cases, American preoccupation with mobility and self-reliance has left many people with minimal community support. Ecomaps are diagrams that are drawn to depict family connections to the community. A circle is drawn around a genogram of the nuclear family, and then lines are drawn like spokes extending outward to people and organizations with which the individual and family relate. Isolation, conflict, and relationships outside the family can be readily seen in a detailed ecomap. Figure 11-2, Genogram and Ecomap Illustrated, diagrams one family's genogram and ecomap.

Function

Knowing the usual ways that a family functions helps you to understand its present state and to assess whether it will be able to organize itself at the end

Figure 11-2 Genogram and Ecomap Illustrated.

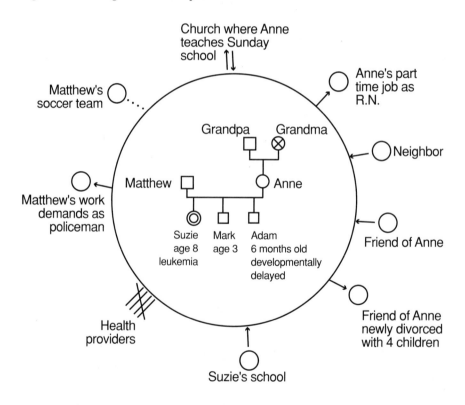

of life. Your nursing goal is not to provide family therapy, but to strengthen the family and enable its members to provide care. To do this, you need to discover the ways the family has functioned over time. Is there unspoken pain under the surface? Is this a family that does not talk about trouble? Are there long-kept secrets? Is there a history of drug abuse or alcoholism? Is there a history of mental illness? Have members of the family been physically or emotionally abusive to one another for years? Have there been suicides? Are they cut off from one another due to past hurts?

Nurses study family dynamics. You can become familiar with family patterns by watching body language and behavior as well as words. Some individuals may change the subject and walk out of the room when difficult subjects arise. Some may become agitated or blaming. Some may be persistently quiet and apologetic. To understand dynamics, it is useful to recognize some common family interaction patterns.

Communication Styles

Virginia Satir (1988) described four habitual unhealthy styles of communication when families come under stress: placating, blaming, distracting, and being super-reasonable. Individuals in families adopt habitual ways of coping that avoid directly addressing and solving distressing problems. Placating is the most common unhealthy communication habit. The placater avoids stressful realities by trying to smooth over conflict. When circumstances are stressful, the placater seeks to please others and continually apologizes and puts himself down. The placater assumes the blame when things go wrong. For the placater, self-esteem comes from winning external approval.

Blaming or fault-finding is the second most common unhealthy family communication pattern. When stressed, the blamer points at another person and puts him down. Blamers and placaters often come in matching pairs. A blamer can continue his pattern only if there is another family member who continues to accept the blame. The blamer avoids stressful realities by faulting someone for them.

The irrelevant or distracting style involves clowning or acting out rather than facing difficulties. In a family with constant stress, such as one experiencing an abusive alcoholic parent, the distracting style develops as a way of avoiding the frightening realities of the situation. For example, a child who has developed a distracting style might try to make everyone laugh in order to interrupt family conflict.

Finally, the super-reasonable style involves avoiding feelings, intellectualizing, and staying aloof rather than facing emotional realities. The super-reasonable family member tries to avoid confronting emotion by focusing on facts. For example, a super-reasonable husband might focus all of his discussion with the home visiting hospice nurse on the mechanics of the infusion pump or the pharmacology of morphine. Meanwhile, his wife is close to death and he avoids talking about that.

One nurse described walking into a home where all four habitual styles were being used at once, so that no one was actually addressing the problem at hand—poorly managed pain. The wife was standing over her husband, yelling at him for "overdosing on narcotics" to relieve his severe pancreatic cancer pain. She kept proclaiming, "You're gonna be an addict just like your brother." The husband was curled up on the sofa, apologizing repeatedly for complaining. One daughter was sitting next to the television, coiling and uncoiling her father's oxygen tubing and giggling on the cell phone. Another daughter began to ask the nurse about the pathophysiology of the cancer. They had fallen into unhealthy patterns of communication to avoid the harsh reality they were facing. The intervention for this family involved getting them to name their worries about dad's suffering and how it was affecting everyone. Once family members named the truth, the family could problem-solve together.

Family Interaction

In addition to recognizing unhealthy communication styles between family members, it is helpful to identify how the entire family interacts. A healthy American family has strong ties that unite members, but also encourages the development of individual identities. Healthy families are also characterized by having relationships with the community outside themselves. Salvador Minuchin and H.C. Fishman (1981) characterized two kinds of unhealthy families: enmeshed or disengaged. Enmeshed families are very dependent on each other and have a low sense of individual autonomy. Enmeshment is perceived as unhealthy from the viewpoint of mainstream American values because individuals, particularly women, are not given a chance to develop independently. From the perspective of providing health care, enmeshment can become a problem when the family cannot accept desperately needed external help. Women caregivers may be particularly burdened because they feel simultaneously obligated to care for their loved one and to reject outside assistance.

Enmeshed families are often described as having rigid boundaries with the outside world. They rarely interact with people or organizations outside the family. In enmeshed families, individual dying members may not be permitted to make end-of-life decisions. Depending on cultural tradition, decisions are often made by designated family members, such as the eldest son or the oldest matriarch in an extended family. Death of family members in those positions of authority can be devastating to the enmeshed family until it reorganizes itself.

Disengaged families are at the other end of the spectrum in terms of involvement with each other. Individual members have a low sense of belonging; everyone goes his own way. This may appeal to the American ideal of individualism and liberty, but the family functions poorly when someone in the family needs help. Members are not able to rally around one another to provide support and they cannot rely on each other as caretakers. They are difficult to organize for practical assistance in terminal illness.

To assess family functioning and relationship patterns, determine the following as you interact with a family over time. These are not questions to be asked directly. Rather, an observant nurse working with members of the interdisciplinary team begins to recognize patterns in the ways family members are interacting in the nurse's presence and in the way they describe family reaction to past events.

- Do family members trust each other?
- Can family members rely on each other for help?
- Do family members trust outsiders? Will they accept help?
- Is this family tied to a wider network/community?
- Does the family communicate feelings directly?
- Is expression of feelings avoided in this family?
- Are anger, blame, and fear the dominant feelings expressed?
- Does the family have a history of problem-solving or do members live from crisis to crisis?
- Does this family have a history of being open to change and new ideas?
- Is there a history of physical, sexual, or emotional violence in this family?

See Box 11-1, Unhealthy Family Coping Patterns.

Planting the Seeds

A practical way to get a snapshot view of how a family interacts is to ask several family members, "How did your family work things out last time there was a family crisis? Tell me about it."

Box 11-1 ■ UNHEALTHY FAMILY COPING PATTERNS

Unhealthy across all cultures:

- Low trust of each other
- Anger, fear, and blame frequently expressed
- Living from crisis to crisis
- History of past and present violence within the family

Unhealthy in American mainstream culture but may reflect healthy patterns in traditional families:

- Low trust of outsiders
- Indirect communication with unspoken rules
- Avoidance of emotional expression or persistent dramatic emotional expression
- Resistance to change and new ideas
- Rigid roles for family members

Keep in mind when assessing family interactions that culture also plays a role in family dynamics. For instance, ethnic families living outside the American mainstream culture may have cultural values and patterns that have worked for them for generations and should be respected. They may have indirect communication styles, avoid overt expression of feeling, resist change, and maintain rigid roles within the family. If they are recent immigrants to America, they may have strong boundaries that dictate against help from outsiders.

THE FAMILY TRANSITION PROCESS

Davies (2000 & 2001) describes how families adapt to a family member dying. As they realize that death has become inevitable, research reveals that most families disengage from their formerly held understanding of life, redefine the situation, and adopt a new understanding of life. Davies has described seven dimensions of the transition process; these dimensions begin when the family recognizes that the family member is not going to recover: redefining, burdening, struggling with paradox, contending with change, searching for meaning, living day-to-day, and preparing for death. See Box 11-2, The Process of Family Transition. If we understand these processes, we can better understand each family's experience. Note that the seven dimensions can be identified in most families, but not every family necessarily goes through each of these in stepwise fashion.

Redefining is the central process that influences all of the other dimensions. Families seek to maintain normal life as long as possible. However, illness will at some point force them to redefine and shift their roles and responsibilities to accommodate to the new situation. The patient's acknowledgment of serious illness makes that possible. If patient and/or family try to maintain "business as usual," while the patient's incapacities make normal routine impossible, anger and frustration at the failure to function will surface. If the dying family member's inability to maintain his role in the

---

Box 11-2 ■ THE PROCESS OF FAMILY TRANSITION

1. Redefining
2. Burdening
3. Struggling with paradox
4. Contending with change
5. Searching for meaning
6. Living day-to-day
7. Preparing for death

Source: From Davies (2001).

family is acknowledged and understood, other family members can begin to take on new responsibilities to fulfill the role the dying family member has left.

As patients redefine their roles, *burdening* becomes an issue for the family. As their conditions deteriorate, patients see themselves as burdens and family members try to bear the burden. If patients and family clearly redefine their roles, it becomes possible to discuss openly how to relieve and manage burdens. Burdens of caregiving are discussed further in the next section.

End-of-life care is filled with paradox, both for the families and for the dying family members. *Struggling with paradox* involves the reality that the patient is both living and dying. Family members hang on to hope for extended life, and yet face the reality that death is approaching. Each person struggles with that paradox differently. Some hold onto hope for life until the moment of death; some readily acknowledge the approach of death; and many live with both possibilities in mind until death occurs. Another dimension of the paradox is that caregivers want at the same time to care for their loved one and to return to "normal" life. Dying family members desire care from their family but do not want to pose a burden. This dimension of family transition is a difficult one to experience because the only resolution to the struggle is the one result that all family members are struggling against—death of the family member.

Contending with change describes coping with the dramatic changes in family life: relationships, roles, social relationships, and employment. All of these shift dramatically as the illness progresses. Caregivers are forced to break new responsibilities into manageable tasks and to maintain as much normalcy as possible. Even non-caregiving family members feel the push to change when roles are redefined.

Searching for meaning involves the search by many families for philosophical and spiritual answers. Coming face-to-face with death, they reflect on life and its meaning. For instance, the husband of a dying wife may come to realize that his most important purpose is family life, not making more money. The patient's sister may decide to return to her traditional Jewish roots to understand living and suffering better.

Some families develop an attitude of *living day-to-day*, which involves making the most of each day. When each moment may be the last conscious moment in a life, some families deliberately choose to appreciate it. They find satisfaction in making the most of everyday moments, like a shared meal or the fragrance of flowers.

Finally, the transition involves *preparing for death* itself by completing financial and legal tasks, and final arrangements. If awareness is open and redefinition has proceeded, family members are involved in responding to the person's final wishes. They will be involved in legal practicalities so that their family member prepares a living will, a regular will, and medical power of attorney documents. *Preparing for death* involves decisions regarding the future of the household, particularly children and spouses. Many families discuss funeral or memorial arrangements with their family member. When awareness is open, dying family members deliberately may choose to create family memories, such as journals, photo albums, audiotapes, or videotapes.

THE BURDEN OF CAREGIVING

Often, family members take care of their dying loved one in the last weeks, months, and even years of life. See Box 11-3, The Process and Consequences of Taking Care, which outlines caregiving responsibilities, interactions, and consequences. Although gratifying for many, such care provision also frequently takes a toll physically and mentally on those individuals providing care. Caregiver burden can be described as "the oppressive or worrisome load borne by people providing direct care for the chronically ill" (Hunt, 2003, p. 28). See Box 11-4, Assessment of Family Caregiver Coping, to identify questions for you to consider as you evaluate family coping with the illness itself. The stresses of family caregiving have been demonstrated to result in high levels of depression and impaired physical health while providing care (Haley, LaMonde, Han, Narramore, and Schonwetter, 2001). Caregiving burden with inadequate family support is also associated with poor physical and mental health during bereavement (Brazil, Bedard, and Willison, 2002). Nevertheless, a majority of chronically ill patients have family members and other lay providers as their primary caregivers. Much of the work of caregiving occurs during a process that Stetz and Brown (1997) have called "taking care," which can be understood as strategies, interactions, and consequences of caregiving.

Box 11-3 ■ THE PROCESS AND CONSEQUENCES OF TAKING CARE

RESPONSIBILITIES

1. Managing the illness and responding to suffering
2. Managing the environment
3. Facing and preparing for dying

INTERACTIONS

1. Responding to issues in family relationships
2. Struggling with the health-care system

CONSEQUENCES

1. Personal suffering
2. Coming to know one's own strengths

Source: From Stetz & Brown (1997).

Box 11-4 ■	ASSESSMENT OF FAMILY CAREGIVER COPING

- Who are the caregivers?
- Are the caregivers overwhelmed?
- How could the caregivers be relieved?
- Is there a way to simplify caregiving?
- Who in the family is suffering and needs help?
- Are there physical needs not being addressed?
- Are there emotional needs not being addressed?
- Are there family conflicts that prevent provision of care?
- What is this family's capability?
- Can this family make long-range plans?
- Would social work intervention strengthen this family?

≥ Planting the Seeds

Whenever you are caring for a patient who lives at home with life-threatening illness, never forget to consider the burdens of family caregivers. Keep the questions from Box 11-4 clearly in mind as you assess caregiver well-being. As nurses, we are responsible for promoting the health of those who will survive after our patient has died.

Caregiving Responsibilities

Caregiving responsibilities include managing the illness and responding to suffering, facing and preparing for dying, and managing the environment (Stetz & Brown, 1997). *Managing the illness and responding to suffering* involves physical care, such as assistance with eating, mobility, and therapies. It involves all of the practical assistance needed for daily living, recreation, and visits to health-care providers. It involves symptom management, including measures to provide physical and emotional comfort. Likewise, managing the illness requires monitoring and reporting symptoms. The physical demands of managing the illness accelerate as the patient's condition deteriorates. For instance, the physical demands involved in ensuring proper medication administration are minimal compared with those involved in helping a wheelchair-bound patient get in and out of bed.

Managing the environment involves seeking and obtaining information about the illness and helping resources. This endeavor may require extensive time on the telephone and the Internet. For example, caregivers may find themselves on the phone trying to find answers about insurance reimbursement or coverage. Information must be sorted and prioritized. Visitors and phone calls often need to be limited as the person's condition worsens.

Personal and family resources must be organized to provide care. Arranging physical space for the dying person in the home is challenging. Where will the bed be placed? Will the rest of the family's personal space be invaded because the patient needs to be downstairs and close to a bathroom?

Facing and preparing for dying is a third "taking care" strategy. Every caregiver becomes aware of death drawing near in his or her own way. The realization may be gradual or sudden. If death can be acknowledged, then the caregiver assists with arrangements for wills, financial and legal planning, and funerals or memorials. Caregivers may even facilitate personal visits and good-byes by friends and family.

Caregiving Interactions

Taking care involves the challenge of interactions with family members and health-care providers (Stetz & Brown, 1997). Caregivers must respond *to family relationship issues* as described earlier. Frequently, family dynamics require them to face conflict. Family members have different opinions about what is "best" for their loved one. For instance, one person insists on pushing the dying person to eat. Another family member is distressed about "drugging" the person at the end of life. Potential conflicts about goals of care are endless at this time of intense emotions. Likewise, caregivers often *struggle with the health-care system.* They must negotiate persistently with providers and agencies to secure needed support for their caregiving activities. For instance, in a single day, a family caregiver might need to keep calling the physician's office for advice when her husband's nausea is uncontrolled, face conflict with an oxygen supply company that delivers the wrong equipment, and speak to the manager of a pharmacy that has informed her that insurance will no longer cover one of her husband's medications.

Caregiving Consequences

Stetz and Brown (1997) describe two major consequences of "taking care": personal suffering and coming to know one's own strength. *Personal suffering* involves the sense of being alone, putting one's life on hold, experiencing mental and physical symptoms of stress, and anticipatory grieving. Caregiving is an isolated task in our busy society where most people are working outside the home and evenings are filled with activities outside the home. Discomfort with illness and dying leads many people away from visiting. The caregiver suspends his or her personal or professional life for periods of weeks to years. Stress and grief take their toll on physical and emotional well-being.

There are also positive consequences of taking care, which include *coming to know one's own strength.* Knowing one's own strength involves learning to live day-to-day, becoming a patient advocate, learning to care for oneself, gaining caregiving competence, and ultimately feeling stronger as a person. For instance, a 19-year-old daughter who had been estranged from her gruff father since she left home at age 16, moved back home to care for him physically during his last weeks of life. The hospice team actively supported her. After his death, she told the hospice nurse, "I never knew I could do anything this hard. My grandparents can't stop telling me what I good job I did. Now I'm going to go back to school to actually do something with my life!"

WWW.   Internet Reference Box

For more information on caregiving, access the American Medical Association's caregiving assessment questionnaire and the National Alliance for Caregiving at: *http://www.ama-assn.org/ama/pub/category/5037.html http://www.caregiving.org.*

NURSING INTERVENTIONS: STRENGTHENING THE FAMILY

Nurses can guide families by assisting with their transition and redefinition, developing their capacity as caregivers, making connections between family members, and recognizing limitations. Having gained these new abilities, skills, and connections, families become stronger and better able to deal with crises.

Guiding Families through the Transition

Although redefinition is an essential dimension in the transition process described by Davies, each family member is likely to redefine the patient, relationships, and responsibilities at a different pace. You need to listen repeatedly and recognize that they must let go of old orientations and hopes at a pace each can handle. You need to let go of your agenda about what would be best for them. Each family member needs individual attention, which may require referral to other disciplines and resources. Practical guidelines to counsel families through the transition include:

- Explaining normal grief, normalizing the difficult feelings of grief
- Listening to expressions of grief
- Focusing on intact abilities and ways the family can sustain normalcy
- Helping the family with prioritizing and role changes
- Helping the family with coordination of resources
- Helping family members to continue with their own lives
- Mobilizing resources so that each family member gets attention
- Encouraging expression of choices and preferences
- Encouraging life review, reminiscing about meaningful past events

For instance, a nurse *helping a family with prioritizing* might sit down with Marianne, an exhausted single mother who has taken her dying sister Judith into her home to provide care. Together they rank Marianne's daily responsibilities in importance and determine which activities she can discontinue and which she can delegate. She decides to give up remodeling projects and handmade Christmas presents. She will stop cleaning her teenaged children's rooms and will accept their offers to make dinner. She decides to ask for help from church members, who have offered to sit at Judith's bedside so that Marianne can get out to exercise and go to the store. *Helping family members to continue with their own lives,* the nurse encourages Marianne to ask for volunteers to drive so that her children can continue with after-school sports. Together they consider whether Marianne should ask a retired aunt to care for Judith 3 days a week so that she can return to work part-time. Finally, for example, the nurse discusses ideas for *life review* with Marianne. Marianne decides to ask Judith whether she would enjoy putting together a photo album with journal entries about their childhood in rural New England.

Developing Family Capacity as Caregivers

Nurses working in home health and hospice work directly with families at home, so their role in training family caregivers is critical. Nurses in hospitals and medical offices also can help strengthen family members' abilities as caregivers because there is limited access to community-based nursing and many patients are returning home to struggle with severe end-stage illness.

All teaching must be adapted to readiness to learn. Emotions are so overwhelming at the end of life that the learning process can be severely limited. Many times the family simply cannot hear what is said. Approach teaching with patience; use a lot of repetition and take steps slowly. Learning takes time. One nurse explains her approach to a family caregiver frightened of technology, "I couldn't just run in with the pump. First we got her to touch it and hold it and know it wasn't going to explode." Other families may be anxious for as much information as possible:

> In that family conference I discovered very organized controlled sons who wanted to know everything and have it written down. They taped our conversation to replay so that everyone would get the same information. They were very hungry for information about what to do to keep Mom comfortable.

Teaching caregiving requires multiple methods and flexible approaches. Some of the strategies you can use include translation, drawing pictures, systematic instruction, convincing argument, demonstration, modeling, and trial and regrouping. See Box 11-5, Teaching Strategies at the End of Life. Learn to *translate* medical knowledge to human terms. You can explain the disease process in simple language. Describe end-of-life symptoms as normal and predictable. Likewise, explain the range of feelings associated with grief and loss in human terms. Translation skills also involve considering how to modify medical procedures for the home. For instance, what

> ## Box 11-5 ■ TEACHING STRATEGIES AT THE END OF LIFE
>
> * Translating medical knowledge to human terms
> * Drawing pictures
> * Systematic instruction
> * Convincing argument
> * Demonstration and role-modeling
> * Trial and regrouping

compromises can be made regarding asepsis or wound dressings? What compromises pose risk for complications? All experienced visiting nurses have stories about how patients and families "push the envelope" regarding what we would consider acceptable in the hospital or nursing home! Nurses translate medical knowledge to human terms that help families cope.

Sometimes words are not enough. Consider finding pictures or *drawing pictures* to illustrate essential ideas and train caregivers in providing technological care.

Picture Challenges

She was one of my picture challenges. She had absolutely terrible circulation. Her hands and feet were always dusky. She started getting pedal edema and some breakdown on her feet. She just didn't understand what was happening. I did a lot of picture drawing to explain. She was afraid of taking narcotics. I drew a picture of how the tumor was pressing on her nerves. I find drawing pictures can be really effective. I have a catheter picture down pat. I show where it goes, how it works, and what the catheter balloon does to keep it in so you don't have to worry about losing it or having urine all over your floor.

Question and answer, in contrast to simply proffering information, is essential to teaching home caregiving. You explain, search for understanding, and they repeat and question. The teaching process should feature an ongoing dialogue instead of a lecture by the nurse authority. Always leave time for clarification and further clarification. Follow the family lead. Avoid asking them questions that can be answered simply with "yes" or "no." For instance, after reviewing a medication regimen, don't ask, "Do you understand?" Instead, teach one medication at a time and then inquire, "Now let's go over what this is good for and how to use it. How would you summarize what I just said?" Validate that they have grasped the essentials and repeat as needed.

Family caregivers often need extensive *systematic instruction* to provide home nursing:

I did a lot of teaching. Mark learned to manage the pump. We taught him to do the dressings around the epidural. He knew how to watch for redness and inflammation. We trained him in bowel management, to get plenty of p.o. medications or give her a suppository or enema. We taught him how to position her, what to do for skin care. He learned to do personal care for the Foley catheter.

Sometimes families need *convincing* about some aspect of palliative care:

Every time I went there I felt like I was on the hot seat. I went through Double Jeopardy. Did I win or lose? I never knew if the answers I gave were the ones they wanted. They were trying to make sense out of what happened and whether they believed in hospice. They wanted information. I felt like I was proving myself to them. I start early to plant seeds about morphine as our friend. You really have to confront people's mindset about addiction. I emphasize that it will prevent their family member from struggling and suffering.

Demonstration and role-modeling are powerful tools as well. You are demonstrating when you invite family members to watch you providing care, and then to practice what they have learned as you watch and coach them. You turn and position the patient, and then you invite the family members to do the same. Then you give them feedback. You role-model gentle touch to calm the patient, and then ask the husband to try it and see that his wife becomes quiet and relaxed. You role-model touching and speaking to the unresponsive patient as you bring the family to the bedside to do the same.

To enable the family to provide care at home when death is imminent, you prepare them by explaining normal processes at the end of life and how to manage any disturbing symptoms that develop. As alertness diminishes, the patient will become bedridden and is likely to need around-the-clock care. You might prepare the family for the final course of events by saying, "At the very end, people stop eating and drinking when the body can no longer handle food and fluids. We don't need to force fluids on him. He can't swallow. We'll keep his lips moist. His breath and circulation are going to slow down. There might be a rattle from mucus in his chest. We have medicine to keep him comfortable. I'll show you how to use it."

Often sustaining family capacity involves *trial and regrouping.* For example, you might encourage the family to try caring for their loved one at home for a 1-week trial period during which the hospice team and concerned family members are all mobilized to help. After that week, the plan is reexamined, resulting in alterations to the home care plan or a move to a skilled nursing facility where the hospice team visits. An expert nurse explains how she proposes a trial intervention using a convincing argument:

You don't know if it will work if you don't try it. You know, I had a patient in a similar situation and it helped a lot. If it

---

Box 11-6 ■   MAKING FAMILY CONNECTIONS

- Encouraging open communication
- Being present so family members can discuss difficult issues
- Interpreting family members to each other
- Getting family members together
- Acting as an intermediary between family members who are not communicating

---

doesn't work, we'll think of something else. How do you feel about that?

Making Connections Between Family Members

Expert end-of-life nurses are often able to help family members communicate with each other. We can do this by encouraging individuals to communicate, being present so family members can discuss difficult subjects, interpreting family members to each other, gathering family members together, and acting as an intermediary between family members who cannot speak to each other. Box 11-6 outlines Making Family Connections.

Encouraging Individuals to Communicate

You should encourage family members to say what they need to say to each other. We do not tell them what to say, but instead encourage them to talk about difficulties, express emotion as culturally appropriate, and plan together. People who love each other are often so engaged in protecting each other's feelings that they avoid talking about anything difficult. We advise them to speak the difficult words that they long to say.

> 66 | *You should encourage family members to say what they need to say to each other. We do not tell them what to say, but instead encourage them to talk about difficulties, express emotion as culturally appropriate, and plan together.*

Being Present So Family Members Can Talk

Often the words are too painful, and so the very presence of nurses or other team members can facilitate talking. When someone else is there encouraging expression, it can feel safe for those who don't know how to speak troubling words:

> Nobody was communicating until I got there. I got them all together and helped everybody to start talking. It's a victory to see

something not working at all, and then to pull it together so that the family starts working together.

I asked him to tell his partner what he was afraid about. I asked his partner to tell him what he was afraid of. They were so protective of each other. They just hadn't been able to talk about it. I facilitated their conversation.

Interpreting Family Members to Each Other

The nurse can often be helpful by interpreting one family member to another. Because of an understanding of illness and human responses, the nurse can offer explanations for troubling feelings and behavior. In particular, you can help each person understand the normalcy of feelings like anger, depression, and avoidance. For instance, you could explain normal adolescent grieving behavior to a mother caring for her dying husband. Her adolescent son has been escaping frequently to his friends' houses, which she thought meant that he "doesn't care about his Dad." Likewise, you can help family members understand the effects of disease on the mind and behavior of those they love.

I met the mother on the porch and explained the dementia and the fact that he was no longer capable of making decisions for himself.

You can help them understand that the behaviors and communication patterns of a lifetime are unlikely to change at the end of life. A nurse explains this to a young woman dying of breast cancer who is disappointed with her father:

"Maybe your father just can't do it. You want him to be at your bedside holding your hand and saying it's okay honey and I love you. He's got all that grief locked inside him since your mother died. He's never talked about feelings and he just can't do it." She got my point and after that, she accepted her father's limitations.

Gathering Family Members Together

Often, we are able to bring family members together to talk to each other when there are difficult decisions to be made or when death is close. They might meet by themselves at our urging, or we can facilitate a family meeting in the kitchen, living room, or bedroom. Frequently, family meetings are organized in close collaboration with social workers:

Marlene, the social worker, and I organized a family conference with the patient, all his kids, and one of the grandsons. They told him it was okay if he wanted to quit his tube feedings. We talked about children and grief and about having young kids in the house where someone is going to die. They felt pretty good about that. I taught them what symptoms to expect at the end of life and how hospice would help. They used this as an opportunity to state that it was not all right for him to shoot himself. He agreed they could take the gun.

Acting as Intermediaries

Finally, expert nurses describe their role as intermediaries when family members are unable to speak to each other. This role usually arises when there is a need for care and/or decisions but the family members who need to provide the care and make the decisions have been estranged. Following is a particularly vivid example:

> I had to go up and take care of Dan and then downstairs to talk to Marge. I felt like I was a go-between for these two, trying to get them to talk. They both loved each other. I was listening to each one and then trying to get them to talk about the issues and concerns with each other. Dan wanted hospice and she wanted a full code and to keep him alive as long as possible. I tried to get them to finally be able to talk directly to each other again.

Recognizing Limitations

Families are unique and each responds to dying in a unique way that is consistent with its own history and beliefs. Sometimes that way is not consistent with our own hopes for them. In this example, a nurse learned from facing obstacles with a complicated alcoholic family:

> I kept trying to get them to do things the way I thought it should be done. I could never relax and finally had to give the case to someone else. Since then, I've learned that when families do unhealthy things, I'm able to point it out to them, but it doesn't make me crazy when they don't change. I give them a lot of leeway in how they do things, and I don't feel like I have to fix them.

Some families may not be able to organize themselves, to listen to each other, to forgive, or to open themselves to outsiders. When someone is dying, their difficult history rears up and the nurse finds herself or himself caught in the middle. We witness their suffering; we offer what we can to help. We make suggestions. Then it is up to the family to choose. When they reject most of our help and advice, we must set clear limited goals and realize what we can and cannot accomplish. Often we need other health team members to help draw boundaries.

CONCEPTS IN ACTION

Ron Trader

Consider Ron Trader's situation. Ron, age 43, was diagnosed with a particularly dangerous kind of brain tumor, a glioblastoma, that has not responded to two surgeries, chemotherapy, or alternative therapies. He and his first wife, Luanne, divorced 3 years ago. She left him and their two children, Sarah and Jason, to pursue a romance that has now turned into a marriage. For 2 years, Ron managed as a single father until Luanne returned to town and began to share some responsibility for parenting. Ron is newly married to Marge, who also has two children, Hannah and Lucy. Now they are living as a newly blended family of husband and wife and four children, two of whom come and go to spend time with their mother. Ron's parents live nearby and are in their 70s; his mother Helen is caring for his father George, who has Alzheimer's. She is also coming over daily to help with Ron's care. Marge is trying to hold onto her job as schoolteacher, but Ron's physical and mental status is rapidly declining. The four children are fighting constantly. A couple of them are falling behind in school; one has been caught stealing. Ron's mother is exhausted and his father has now developed cardiac arrhythmias. Sometimes she snaps at Ron when he forgets what he is doing. Ron's close friends are coming over to provide some caregiving relief, but this is challenging their abilities since he can no longer walk and is incontinent. There is great strain every time his first wife comes into the house. She tends to find fault with everything from Marge's housekeeping to her failure to discipline the out-of-control children. Marge keeps apologizing and proclaims, "I'm just no good to anybody right now. I can't think straight."

- Draw a genogram for Ron Trader's extended family.
- What coping style do Luanne and Marge use when stressed?
- Consider the impact of Ron's dying on each family member. What are the needs of each?
- Ron's wife and his mother are his primary caregivers. How can you respond to their needs?
- Both caregivers are having trouble providing physical care as Ron's level of consciousness has plummeted. What would you recommend to them? What teaching strategies would be particularly important?
- How might the nurse promote connections between family members?

References

Brazil, K., Bedarde, M., & Wilson, K. (2002). Correlates of health status for family caregivers in bereavement. *Journal of Palliative Medicine, 5*(6), 849–855.

Davies, B. (2001). Supporting families in palliative care. In B. Ferrell & N. Coyle (Eds.), *Textbook of palliative nursing* (pp. 363–373). New York: Oxford University Press.

Davies, B. (2000). Anticipatory mourning and the transition of fading away. In T. Rando (Ed.), *Clinical dimensions of anticipatory mourning* (pp. 135–153). Champaign, IL: Research Press.

Haley, W., LaMonde, L. A., Han, B., Narramore, S., & Schonwetter, R. (2001). Family caregiving in hospice: Effects on psychological and health functioning among spousal caregivers of hospice patients with lung cancer or dementia. *The Hospice Journal, 15*(4), 1–18.

Hanson, S. M. H., & Boyd, S. T. (1996). *Family health care nursing: Theory,* *practice, and research*. Philadelphia: F.A. Davis.

Hunt, C. K. (2003). Concepts in caregiver research. *Journal of Nursing Scholarship, 35*(1), 27–32.

Larsen, L. (2002). *Facing the final mystery* (p. 84). First Books Library.

Minuchin, S., & Fishman, H. C. (1981). *Family therapy techniques*. Cambridge, MA: Harvard University Press.

Satir, V. (1988). *The new peoplemaking*. Palo Alto, CA: Science and Behavior Books.

Stetz, K., & Brown, M. (1997). Taking care: Caregiving to persons with cancer and AIDS. *Cancer Nursing, 20*(1), 12–22.

CHAPTER 12

Children Facing Death

Philosophical Reflections

"Freddie found himself losing his color, becoming brittle. It was constantly cold and the snow weighed heavily upon him. At dawn the wind came that took Freddie from his branch. It didn't hurt at all. He felt himself float quietly, gently and softly downward."

Buscaglia, 1982, "The Fall of Freddie the Leaf"

Learning Objectives

1. Identify children's normal grieving behaviors from toddler to adolescent.
2. Explain helping strategies for grieving children of each age group.
3. Describe unique ways of helping grieving children that include play, creative arts, literature, and ritual.
4. Identify common dying pathways for children.
5. List essential features of palliative care for children and barriers to its implementation.
6. Explain palliative psychosocial care for children and their families.
7. Discuss unique aspects of providing physical comfort for dying children.
8. Develop a palliative care plan.

Strengthening the family while a family member is dying is a branch of family caregiving at the end of life. This chapter discusses the unique dimensions of strengthening families when children face their own death or the death of a loved one. Children today seldom experience another person's death, especially that of a parent or sibling. Likewise, only a small number of children die in contemporary America. The death of a child challenges our understanding of the natural order. This chapter examines children's perceptions of death, grief, and coping in children and adolescents, and ways of helping grieving children. The chapter then shifts to look at children and death from a different perspective. It discusses contemporary causes and circumstances of children dying, palliative programs for children, and the psychosocial and physical needs of dying children and their families.

CHILDREN'S PERCEPTION OF DEATH

In the past, children died frequently. Before the middle of the 20th century, only a small number of children from large families survived into adulthood. Death was swift from infectious disease and accidents. As a result, traditional children's stories, games, prayers, and rhymes are filled with death. Consider this circle game played since the plague years of the 15th century when one by one people fell down and turned to ash. Their only defense was to hold onto one another (Kastenbaum, 2000):

> Ring-around-the rosey.
> Pockets full of posies.
> Ashes, ashes.
> We all fall down.

Or consider the words of the traditional American lullaby, another reminder of frequent child mortality:

> Rock-a-by baby in the treetop.
> When the wind blows, the cradle will rock.
> When the bough breaks, the cradle will fall.
> And down will come baby, cradle and all.

However, in contemporary America, children are often unprepared to face death. The child mortality rate is much lower and children commonly experience deaths of loved ones when they are older themselves. Death is seldom discussed. The death of the family pet or seeing a dead animal is usually the first experience. Children generally can recognize death by the time they are 3 years old (Faulkner, 2001). They first recognize what death looks like. Then, they begin to consider the effects of death on ability to function. Preschool children do not understand that death is final, however. As school-age children develop cognitively and emotionally, they grow to realize the impact of death, and finally they consider their own death and that of family members and other people in society. They gradually realize

Box 12-1 ■	CONCEPTIONS OF DEATH FROM EARLY CHILDHOOD TO ADOLESCENCE
AGE	UNDERSTANDING AND FEELINGS
Birth to Age 2 to 4	Cannot differentiate between death and separation
	Believe death is reversible
	Experience separation anxiety
	Concerns expressed by crying
Age 4 to 6	Come to understand that death is irreversible and final
	For younger child, death appears equivalent to sleep or going on a trip
	May believe they can cause death
	May have anxiety about separation and sleep
Age 7 to 1 1	Understand that death is irreversible and universal
	Developing logical thought, realistic understanding of causes of death
	May perceive human death as punishment
	Continuing concerns with separation
Age 12 and adolescent	Now have abstract understanding
	Death may be perceived as heroic or tragic
	Death associated with old age
	Commonly dislike showing emotion
	May choose escapism, denial, acting out

Source: From Faulkner (2001); and Oltjenbruns (2001).

that death is permanent, universal, and inevitable for everyone, including themselves. See Box 12-1, Conceptions of Death from Early Childhood to Adolescence.

CHILDREN'S GRIEVING

Signs of grief are initially apparent around the age of 2 years, when the child has observable responses to separation from a parent. Normal children's grief is manifested as somatic, psychological, and behavioral (Oltjenbruns, 2001). Somatic symptoms include difficulty sleeping and eating, wetting the bed, sleep disturbances, headaches, and stomachaches. Psychological symptoms include separation anxiety, loneliness, guilt, fear that others will die, fantasizing about death, learning difficulties, and school problems. Behavioral symptoms include crying, emotional outbursts, temper tantrums, extreme shyness, disinterest in playing, demand for attention, overdependence, and acting out. Acting out, for example, is a result of the anger the child feels because the parent or sibling cannot be brought back, and life is dramatically changed. Behaviors include arguing, disobedience, demands for attention, stubbornness, and aggressive anti-social behaviors, particularly in adolescents. These reactions are common right after death; however, some symptoms may not appear until as long as 2 years later, as the child comes to recognize the loss.

Children's grief is influenced by the kind of pre-death relationship the person had with the child, the nature of the death, the health and reaction of surviving parent(s), and the child's preexisting psychological difficulties. Emotional health of the family predicts a child's healthy adaptation to loss because a healthy family is able to provide a stable, loving environment that minimizes fear and promotes child growth. Recent studies do not reveal an increased risk of future depression for those who experienced a parent dying while they were children (Oltjenbruns, 2001).

As children who experienced death at very young ages move into more mature developmental stages, they may examine the death from a different perspective than was possible earlier. They may revisit grief periodically as they develop. This is called the "re-grief phenomenon." A preschooler misses a father as caregiver and provider. Then, later in adolescence he may wonder how his life would be different if his father was there to play baseball and take him hiking. Grief surges again as he misses his father as role model, "a man to tell me what to do."

Children's grief is often misunderstood. See Box 12-2, Myths about Grief in Children and Adolescents. Children grieve at any age, but it is manifested very differently depending on developmental stage. Children should not be shielded from death. They cannot be protected from inevitable loss without deception, which they can detect quickly. It is better to support and include

---

Box 12-2 ■ MYTHS ABOUT GRIEF IN CHILDREN AND ADOLESCENTS

1. Children do not grieve.
2. It is better to shield children from loss.
3. Children should not go to funerals.
4. Children should always attend funerals.
5. Children recover from loss quickly.
6. Children are permanently scarred by early loss.
7. Talking with children is the most therapeutic way to help them cope.
8. Helping children and adolescents cope with loss is the sole responsibility of the family.

Source: From Doka (2000).

them in age-appropriate ways. Children's ways of coping are determined by their developmental stage and the tasks needed to be accomplished at each stage (Oltjenbruns, 2001). For example, children should neither be forced to attend funerals nor prevented from attending them. When they are old enough to do so, children should be able to choose their role in such rituals after death. Although children do not recover quickly, death of a loved one does not scar children permanently. Grief from significant loss resolves slowly and frequently recurs. Yet children are remarkably resilient when given strong support. Talking may not be the most effective way of supporting them. Play, creative activities, and ritual have a vital role in fostering expression. Childhood grief is a great family burden, which should not be borne alone without support of the community at large, including schools and faith communities.

66 | *Children's ways of coping are determined by their developmental stage and the tasks needed to be accomplished at each stage (Oltjenbruns, 2001).*

It is important to understand and recognize symptoms of grief at the different levels of child development. The following section, which summarizes a study of childhood bereavement by Grace Hyslop Christ (2000), sheds some understanding on death and grief behavior in children of different ages. She identifies helpful interventions for each age group as well.

Ages 3 to 5 Years

Preschoolers cannot understand the significance of a terminal illness. They react strongly to separation from the sick parent and can become overwhelmed by their parents' intense emotions and loss of control. They have great difficulty understanding that death is irreversible. For months afterward, they may ask when the loved one is returning. They need repeated concrete explanations of what has happened. They may develop symptoms like intense separation anxiety, stomachaches, bed-wetting, whining, temper tantrums, and fretful sleeping.

Helpful interventions for preschoolers include:

- Strengthening the parent's ability to provide support for the child by realizing the child's need to stay close to the parent
- Using simple explanations and providing opportunities to ask questions
- Recognizing that expression of strong feelings can frighten the child
- Using play and drawing to express feeling
- Preparing for regressive symptoms after death and expecting the child to need to talk frequently
- Referring for counseling those children with persistent difficulty playing; persistent fears; aggressiveness; difficulty separating from the parent; preoccupation with dying; and regression in toilet training, eating, or sleeping

When Dinosaurs Die, written for preschoolers and young readers, describes feelings about death and illustrates children's reactions with various quotes from dinosaur children (Brown & Brown, 1996, pp. 12, 14–15):

> "It's not true. Grandma isn't dead."
> "She is too."
> "I'm not hungry. My tummy hurts."
> "Will I get sick and die like Cousin Boris?"

Preschoolers need triggers to help them talk. In addition to reading children's books about death, many activities may help them to remember and talk. For instance, taking them to visit the grave, giving them keepsakes to treasure, looking at photograph albums, or planting a tree or bush in honor of the person may bring back memories and encourage children to talk.

Planting the Seeds

In early childhood, grieving children need to be kept close to their parents and other family members. They have trouble understanding that death is permanent. Encourage family to maintain familiar routines and promote expression through play. Help families understand normal grieving for this age, such as regressive behavior and development of physical symptoms.

Ages 6 to 8 Years

Young school-age children are usually aware of serious illness and react intensely with anger, anxiety, fear, and sadness. They may become demanding, stubborn, and clingy. They understand that death is permanent, but they may reach the illogical and guilt-inducing conclusion that they are responsible. When told of a parent's death, their reactions may cover the gamut, from screaming to no response at all. Usually they are quite direct in expressing feeling, but they express intense feelings only briefly and then may want to return to school and playful activities. Helpful interventions for young school-age children include:

- Remembering that parental support is central
- Joining with the parents to inform them of the parent's illness and when death is imminent
- Sharing controlled expression of emotion so that they are not overwhelmed
- Encouraging continuation of developmentally appropriate activities
- Encouraging participation in traditional rituals
- Not being surprised by a child's brief episodes of mourning alternated with desire to return to normal activities
- Communicating with school personnel

- Referring for counseling those children living with persistent anxiety, depression, low self-esteem, or thoughts of suicide

Tommie was 8 years old when his father was killed in an automobile crash. Tommie's initial reaction was to scream and throw a tantrum. Then he turned back to his videogame. His mourning seemed to come in waves. He wore his dad's Red Sox cap everywhere, even in bed. In the first few weeks, he resisted going to school every morning and resisted going to bed at night. Sometimes he wet his bed. In the evening, he never let his mother out of his sight. His uncle started taking him to Little League practices, which he loved.

 Planting the Seeds

Young school-age children need truthful information with concrete details. They need to stay close to family. Encourage play dates and normal activities. Help family to understand normal grieving behavior for this age group, including intermittent periods of grief and forgetting.

Ages 9 to 11 Years

Preadolescents are rapidly developing their capacity for logical thinking. They are conceptually able to understand the implications of terminal illness. Their world is expanding outside the home, so that they have chances to distract themselves from parental dying and death. They are now able to control expression of feeling, so that they can restrain their reactions to the point of appearing callous and indifferent. They fear being overwhelmed by grief and so may not talk about it and choose to escape into activities. When they do grieve, they express a range of feelings similar to adults, including anger and sadness. For months following the death, many have difficulty paying attention at school. Helpful interventions for preadolescents include:

- Giving them information as soon as it is known about diagnosis and prognosis
- Encouraging participation in care of the patient
- Involving teachers
- Encouraging involvement in after-school activities
- Encouraging participation in rituals after death and activities that remember parent
- Structuring family activities and returning to predictable routines
- Referring for counseling those children who do not return to previous levels of functioning in school, activities, and peer relationships

Jeanine was 10 when her single mother was diagnosed with an inoperable brain tumor. She threw herself into basketball and swimming, but her grades deteriorated. Her grandmother called the school when her mother died, but Jeanine insisted on staying until the end of the school day. Several friends went with her to the funeral home to view her mom's open coffin, but she refused to get too close. For several months afterward, she argued frequently with her grandparents, who adopted her. Sometimes they heard her crying softly in her bedroom, but she never mourned in public. She gradually immersed herself in after-school sports and her grades bounced back.

Planting the Seeds

Preadolescents should be involved with decisions and encouraged to ask questions. Family needs to understand that these young people should have as much control as possible within boundaries that include clear expectations. Teach the family to understand normal coping behaviors of preadolescents, including apparent indifference, intense peer involvement, and oppositional behavior.

Adolescents 12 to 14 Years

Young adolescents are conflicted by their own need to develop independence from their parents and the intensified family needs for help and emotional closeness. They are quite self-centered. They may withdraw emotionally and have exaggerated needs for privacy. They may go to great lengths to avoid feelings and to express indifference. They withdraw into themselves and escape with peers. This apparent callousness can be extremely troubling to family members. It is not unusual for the grieving young adolescent to test limits by acting rebellious. Helpful interventions for young adolescents include:

- Providing detailed information
- Understanding their emotional withdrawal as developmentally related
- Allowing them to help but limiting caregiving tasks that may be excessively burdensome to a child so young
- Helping them express grief
- Letting them choose their role in rituals after death
- Supporting their desire to return to normal activities
- Setting limits on destructive behavior
- Referring for counseling those teens with clinical depression, suicidal thoughts, fears and phobias, refusal to attend school, withdrawal, use of alcohol and drugs, aggressive behavior causing injury, regression to childish behavior, and somatic symptoms that do not disappear

Andy was 14 when his 6-year-old sister died quickly from acute leukemia. He walked out of the room when his mother told him his sister was dying, but not before challenging her by yelling, "You don't know what you're talking about!" Following her death a week later, he agreed to carry her coffin into the church and to participate in the church service, but then he disappeared to a friend's house immediately afterward saying, "Our band's got to practice." In the weeks afterward, his mother smelled alcohol and marijuana on his breath and clothing. She sought counseling to learn how to set limits and found a counselor for him to express his grief through music therapy.

Adolescents 15 to 17 Years

Middle adolescents have become capable of abstract thinking that allows them to comprehend the realities of death and its impact. They are also growing in empathy and capable of deepening personal relationships. Therefore, they find it difficult to distract themselves with activities and friends. During the illness and in bereavement, they can be expected to function poorly in school and activities. Their mourning behavior is similar to that of an adult. However, they can also externalize their grief by episodes of anger, argument, drinking, and escape from the home. Helpful interventions for middle adolescents include:

- Informing them fully about illness and prognosis
- Anticipating some withdrawal from normal functioning
- Discussing ways they can be helpful
- Involving them in rituals after death, in roles they choose
- Anticipating intense mourning and helping them understand the process
- Communicating with the school
- Anticipating conflict around responsibilities and the need for independence
- Helping them identify a positive legacy of the deceased person
- Referring for counseling those teens with severe symptoms including severe withdrawal, depression, destructive acting out, severe aggression, problems in school, and eating problems

Planting the Seeds

Adolescents need clear, honest communication. Recognize that they have strong needs for independence and control. Teach family about normal grieving behavior including emotional withdrawal and the need to identify with peers.

WAYS OF HELPING GRIEVING CHILDREN AND ADOLESCENTS

Children and teens have a limited ability to explain their feelings with words and are often able to express those feelings through play, creative arts, ritual, and reading together.

Using Play with Grieving Children

Play is a natural medium for children to express their feelings. Play is the way that children work through their experiences, express themselves, cope with anxiety, and develop skills (Brown, 2001). Play allows children to feel some control over their world. Whether it is facilitated by adults or not, children will express their grief through play activities. Play offers a diversion from fear and anxiety, and can help children release pent-up feelings. Play can be used by parents, nurses, other health professionals, and play therapists to support grieving children. Play materials might include:

- Dolls, action figures, puppets
- Toys that re-create life, such as doll houses, telephones, doctor kits
- Aggression release activities like beating drums, punching bags, kicking balls, running, and hammering
- Construction toys
- Games

Jay is 5 years old. Last year, Jay's dad committed suicide. Since then, his preschool behavior has become unmanageable and aggressive. Jay and his mother have been visiting a family therapist who does play therapy. Jay chooses male and female action figures who take trips along highways or in space. The male action figures repeatedly have crashes and Jay throws them on the floor. Whenever they crash, he and the therapist talk about how "the boys always get killed. Daddy got killed."

> Play is a natural medium for children to express their feelings. Play is the way that children work through their experiences, express themselves, cope with anxiety, and develop skills (Brown, 2001).

Using Creative Arts with Grieving Children and Adolescents

The arts provide a medium for children and teens to identify and express their feelings (Webb, 2000). Artwork can be used by parents, nurses, other health professionals, and art therapists with special expertise. Many hospital pediatric units offer art and music therapy for seriously ill children. Hospices sometimes offer creative art programs for children with dying siblings or parents, and for bereaved children. A growing group of counselors offer art and music therapy for children in the community living with grief. In encouraging children's creative expression, it is important not to correct artwork or expect it to be beautiful. The adult should show interest, refrain from interpretation, and ask to learn more about what is created. Some creative arts examples include:

- Drawing and painting
- Drama
- Making up songs and changing the lyrics in songs
- Playing musical instruments like drums or triangles
- Writing poetry and stories
- Pounding and sculpting clay
- Making collages

These and other creative activities help children understand the loss, express feelings, commemorate the death, and discover ways to go on with their lives.

Using Ritual with Grieving Children and Adolescents

Rituals are solemn acts or ceremonies. Death rituals include memorials and funerals, as well as private acts that give meaning to the death and offer the comfort of people drawing together in mutual support. Funerals and public memorials directly confront the loss and give the death meaning within the community. Once children are able to understand and sit through a funeral ceremony, they should be given the choice to be present and to participate (Doka, 2000). They can select music and readings. They can write letters and draw pictures. For example, after the funeral of an environmentalist from the Pacific Northwest, his school-age children distributed fir seedlings to all guests present. Private rituals might be as simple as looking at picture albums every Saturday, remembering Daddy before every dinner, or lighting a candle in his memory at each family gathering.

Planting the Seeds

If a parent asks you whether children should attend the funeral, first explore what that parent is thinking. In deciding how to respond, respect the person's values. Parents may wonder if children need to be protected from mourning expressed during the service. Remind them that the children are experiencing their own grief and should not be isolated at this time. Reinforce the value of involving children in traditional ritual and community support to relieve their own suffering. They should not be left out. If possible, they should be given the choice to participate in services.

Using Children's Literature

The literature for grieving children and adolescents is growing. Many books are available for each developmental level. Consider the following in assessing books for the purpose of helping a grieving child (Doka, 2000):

- Evaluate the book for its fit with the particular child and select titles that fit individual needs.
- Examine the limitations of the book's explanations. Are they helpful and consistent with the family's values?
- Match the book to the concerns of the individual child.
- Read and discuss together.

WWW. **Internet Resource Box**

Books for and about children and grief are identified in *www. compassionbooks.com*.

Books and activities for children 12 or younger and 13 or older are found at *www.dougy.org*. This is the Web site for the Dougy Center, the National Center for Grieving Children and Families. Also included is advice for parents of grieving children.

DYING CHILDREN

Death rates in children have dropped dramatically so that children now constitute only 2% of all deaths reported annually, approximately 55,000 children (Institute of Medicine, 2003). Causes of death differ for different age groups:

- Infants from birth to age 1 year are at greatest risk of mortality. Leading causes are congenital abnormalities, low birth weight and immature body organs, sudden infant death syndrome, complications of pregnancy, and respiratory distress syndrome.
- For children 1 to 9 years, leading causes of death include unintentional injuries such as drowning and motor vehicle injury, congenital abnormalities, cancer, and intentional injuries (murder and suicide).
- For youth age 10 to 19, dominant causes of death are unintentional and intentional injuries, cancer, and heart disease.

Because of medical advances, there is a significant group of children living with complex chronic illness who can be expected to need care for years before they die in childhood. The rates of childhood death from causes such as injury and low birth weight are higher among people living in poverty. African American children have a higher mortality rate at all ages (IOM, 2003).

Pathways and Prognoses

The course of death in children varies dramatically and can be explained by identifying four different pathways: sudden death, death from a potentially curable disease, death from a congenital abnormality that is lethal, and death from a progressive condition (IOM, 2003).

Sudden unexpected death occurs with sudden infant death syndrome or a fatal injury. For example, a child's lifeless body is found in her crib or a child is struck by a car or killed by a bullet. The survivors have no chance to say good-bye. Their grief is often intense and complicated.

Death from a potentially curable disease often involves an initial positive response to treatment, followed by the return of the disease and eventual failure of all curative therapies. Often, preoccupation with therapies overshadows any discussion about death as a possible consequence. Comfort may be forgotten in the increasingly desperate rush to cure.

Some infants are born with problems that are incompatible with survival; they live only briefly. This includes infants with severe congenital anomalies and extremely premature babies. Comfort for parents and infant should be the predominant concern.

Finally, there is the extended pathway of children suffering from progressive conditions, such as degenerative neuromuscular disorders. The child repeatedly survives one crisis after another, often growing into adolescence and young adulthood, until a resuscitative effort fails or is rejected as too burdensome. The long-term emotional, physical, and economic burdens on families are immense. Caregiving systems that have focused on long-term illness may not be ready to provide end-of-life care. The team that may have worked with the child for years is trained and organized to maintain physiological functions aggressively, despite the futility of such activities.

Palliative Care for Children

Children often suffer needlessly at the end of life. In a study of parents' perceptions of their children's deaths from cancer, 89% described their children as suffering "a lot" or "a great deal" from at least one symptom (Wolfe et al., 2000). Medical professionals focused on aggressive treatment, including ventilatory support, and did not address suffering adequately.

Essential Features of Palliative Care for Children

Pediatric palliative nursing focuses on the child and family at the center of the care plan (Feeg, Miller-Thiel, and Will, 2001). The nurse recognizes emotional suffering throughout the course of a life-limiting illness, translates medical information to parents and children, collaborates closely with other members of the health-care team, and advocates for family and child wishes. She recognizes the uncertainty and fear that the family experiences from diagnosis through aggressive therapies. She advocates for compassionate comfort care throughout the course of treatment, not just when the child is finally identified as terminally ill.

The American Academy of Pediatrics proposes an integrated model of palliative care for children, with a focus on comfort and psychosocial support, from diagnosis of life-threatening illness throughout all the efforts aimed at cure (AAP, 2000). Children should have simultaneous palliative and curative care, according to this model. This integrated model seeks to relieve emotional and physical distress from the very beginning. The minimum standards proposed by this group of pediatricians include the following:

- Continuity of care by a consistent physician
- Availability of support 24 hours a day, 7 days a week
- Interdisciplinary care from a physician, nurse, social worker, spiritual counselor, and child-life therapist
- Care coordination from tertiary care medical center into the local community
- Home nursing
- Respite for families to take breaks from intensive bedside care

Chronically ill dying children can be treated effectively for many years, but treatment often requires multiple technologies and intensive bedside care. As they grow into school age and adolescence, these children need attention to developmental needs. They need to play. They need to achieve in school and in activities outside of school. In adolescence, they need to have a sense of independence and control. Thus, caregivers are involved in the paradoxical task of promoting growth while preparing for death.

WWW.   Internet References Box

See the Texas Children's Cancer Center End-of-Life Care for Children Web site at *www.childendoflifecare.org.*

See the Initiative for Pediatric Palliative Care at *www.ippcweb.org/initiative*

See the Children's Hospice International Web site at *www.chionline.org.*

Barriers to Palliative Care for Children

Barriers to palliative care for children include the compulsion to save life, parents' lack of information, lack of insurance to cover needed services, and inadequacy of the hospice model for children. The belief that children should not die is a persistent barrier to preparing for the death of a child. Parents usually desire every medical option to save or lengthen their child's life. Professionals likewise are committed to saving children's lives. Thus, parents and professionals commonly focus on survival at all costs. "Acceptance that cure or meaningfully prolonged life is not possible is painful and difficult—so difficult that some clinicians and parents may not recognize that they are pursuing treatments that bring suffering without benefit" (Institute of Medicine, 2003,

p. 31). Clinicians fail to assess and relieve suffering, and may even withdraw from the child and family during the final phase of a child's fatal illness, rather than face their own powerlessness and fear. By contrast, the pediatric palliative-care movement actively seeks to relieve suffering throughout the course of illness. Compassionate communication and relief of physical distress can be incorporated into the aggressive fight for survival, instead of limited to the last days or weeks when mortality is finally admitted.

Parents' lack of information is also a significant barrier to palliative care for children. Too often, physicians spend limited time discussing diagnosis, prognosis, and options. In the urgency to treat, parents may not be told of the limitations of and suffering imposed by treatments. Informed consent forms do list every possible side effect, but that information is often too alarming or too technical for authorizing parents to comprehend intellectually and emotionally. These parents often simply sign where they are told in hopes of receiving the treatment benefit the physician describes. Some do not have the literacy level to comprehend the complex information given. Frequently, parents are not brought in on decisions of the caregiving team, and they become outsiders in the care of their own children. Fear and anxiety complicate their ability to raise questions with professionals.

Because parents often feel that they are not given adequate information, and because they frequently do not know what to expect or what questions to be asking, nurses must ask parents what information they want, and guide them to ask the questions they want answered. Do they want to talk about the symptoms, the treatment, the impending death, funeral plans, or bereavement issues? What do they need to know?

Finally, many children and families have limited access to health care. Many are not insured through private or public health insurance. Even if they are covered, their insurance may limit reimbursement to physician and hospital care only, and may even include coinsurance and deductible payments that become increasingly burdensome for families. Multidisciplinary services such as social work, counseling, physical therapy, home nursing, and medical equipment are limited or absent in many insurance policies. Although a multidisciplinary team is essential to provide adequate palliative care for child and family, the U.S. health-care system is not organized to reimburse such services.

> 66 | *The belief that children should not die is a persistent barrier to preparing for the death of a child. Parents and professionals focus on survival at all costs.*

Because of these barriers, the switch to hospice care generally does not take place until the very end of life. In fact, most children die before receiving it. Even when a child does enter hospice, the current hospice model of care itself presents many barriers (AAP, 2000). The federal Medicare model for chronically ill adults and those over 65 has been used as a blueprint for private insurance and Medicaid benefits. This limits hospice admission to those people with a prognosis of 6 months or less to live. The course of children's illness is particularly difficult to predict, and it is hard emotionally to proclaim that only 6 months remain. Likewise, many hospice programs limit costly life-prolonging therapies, such as transfusions and parenteral nutrition, which physicians and families may be unwilling to give up. Even if a child is referred to hospice, most hospice professionals need additional pediatric training to care for dying children. To compound issues even further, some state Medicaid programs do not pay for hospice at all.

Children's Hospice International, with assistance from the federal government, has established a Program for All-Inclusive Care for Children (PACC) as a model to provide care for all children with life-threatening conditions and their families (Armstrong-Dailey & Zarbock, 2001). Model programs offer integrated care that includes home, outpatient, respite for family caregivers, and inpatient acute care. The goal is to avoid fragmented care, relieve psychosocial and spiritual distress, ensure access to needed services, and avoid crisis-driven costly hospitalizations. Family support services include medicine, nursing, social work, chaplains, therapists, home-health aides, day care, family support, care for siblings, and community services to prevent unnecessary institutionalization of the child. Interdisciplinary coordination of services saves money.

Moreover, the Pediatric Palliative Care Consulting Service of Children's Hospital in Seattle, Washington, has developed an innovative program for children who are not expected to survive childhood (A New Language, 2002). The hospital has forged an agreement with private insurance and the state's Department of Social and Health Services to provide care at home. Expert palliative services reduce the cost of repeated hospitalizations and emergency room trips. Palliative-care coordination is believed to be saving the state $3,000 a month for each child served. Working in close partnership with local hospices, the health-care team includes a care coordinator, insurance case manager, and health-care professionals working closely together to meet the goals of dying children and their families.

Managing Symptoms at the End of a Child's Life

For younger children, assessments by family members determine the degree of distress and are the roots of an effective plan of care. Parents must be consulted as experts on their child's comfort (IOM, 2003). Parents vary in the degree to which they recognize the extent of their child's suffering, but they report that physicians and nurses frequently do not notice or relieve many of the symptoms that they, as parents, recognize (Wolfe et al. 2000).

Managing Pain

Children at the end of life often suffer pain that is not recognized and not treated (Wolfe et al., 2000). Children respond to pain with growing fear and anxiety, and eventually withdrawal. Myths about children and pain contribute to (1) physicians not adequately prescribing pain medication, and

Box 12-3 ■	MYTHS AND REALITIES ABOUT CHILDREN'S PAIN

MYTH	REALITY
Infants and children do not experience pain.	Even the youngest infants experience pain. Children will tell you they are in pain. Children may believe adults will know they are in pain and so they do not report it. They may not report pain because they are fearful of taking medicine or going to the hospital again.
Children cannot tell you where they hurt.	Preschool children as young as 3 or 4 years can use visual pain rating scales.
Opioids are dangerous in children.	There is no evidence that opioids used with care are unsafe for children.
Children will become addicted to opioids.	Addiction is defined as a compulsive craving for drugs to get high. There is no evidence that children taking opioids to relieve pain will turn into addicts.

Source: From Huff & Joshi (2001).

(2) nurses not questioning children about pain and giving even less medication than prescribed. See Box 12-3, Myths and Realities about Children's Pain.

A pain evaluation tool especially developed for nurses working with children is called QUESTT (Huff & Joshi, 2001).

- *Q* stands for Questioning the child or parent to get full description of the location, quality, intensity, and pattern of the pain. Verbal questioning may be ineffective if the child is preverbal, does not speak English, or is cognitively impaired.
- *U* stands for Using pain rating scales. The Oucher scale with six photographs of a child's face, depicting "no hurt" and "biggest hurt," and the FACES scale with six cartoon faces, are the most common scales used from ages 3 to 13. See Box 12-4, The FACES Scale.
- *E* stands for Evaluating behavior and physiological clues. Documentation of behavioral changes reinforces the child's report on a pain rating scale. The child's normal behavior needs to be understood. Behavioral indicators of pain in children include irritability, restlessness, changes in sleep, changes in feeding patterns, head banging or rocking, changes in crying, including long periods

---

Box 12-4 ■   THE FACES SCALE

0 1	2 3	4 5 6	7 8	9 10
No Pain	Mild	Moderate	Severe	Worst

---

when the child cannot be comforted, immobility, and passivity. Of course these behaviors can indicate other distress besides pain, but they are clues that need to be looked at together.

- *S* stands for Securing parental involvement. Parents should be actively involved in recognizing signs and behaviors indicating pain. Some may already recognize these signs for their children and some may need coaching.
- *T* stands for Taking the cause of the pain into account. It is important to evaluate whether the pain is due to a scrape, a headache, or a metastatic lesion.
- *T* stands for Taking action. Nonpharmacological and pharmacological interventions for pain are discussed in Unit Six: Comforting.

Managing Pediatric Symptoms

Unit Six details symptom management for all ages. However, comforting dying children is different from comforting adults in many ways. Most obvious, medication doses for children must be adjusted according to weight. Furthermore, medication administration to a resistant child or adolescent may require the expertise of an experienced pediatric nurse. The patient cannot be separated from the family, which should be in control and actively participate in all aspects of care. Comforting interventions may involve familiar blankets and stuffed toys, beloved music and videos, a homelike environment, and physical care that includes cuddling and bathing by family members. At the very end of life, turn off monitors and infusions and eliminate discomforting assessments like blood draws. If the child is at home, the family will need extensive guidance to control the signs of imminent dying and to witness distressing breath sounds without calling for emergency medical assistance. If at all possible, a nurse should be at their side during the last hours.

Psychosocial Dimensions of Caring for Dying Children and Their Families

Children with life-threatening illness come to an understanding of death and their own death much earlier than healthy children. Although the children often have intuitive knowledge of their life ending, the adults around them often assume that they are too young to understand. Given adults' hesitance, inability, or lack of awareness of the need to listen, children often become reluctant to talk (Faulkner, 2001).

Talking to Parents Facing Children's Death

"To offer humane care to the dying and their families is to take time to listen, to respect their wishes for what they want to know and do, to support them in their grief, and to share with them that the professional is also affected by the situation" (Davies & Connaughty, 2002, p. 6). Physicians find it difficult to inform parents that their child's condition is not improving. Once the physician has explained the terminal prognosis, the nursing role is to support the parents in understanding the implications. Parents commonly report that hospital staff members do not understand how to provide emotional support (Davies & Connaughty, 2002). Attentive listening to feelings is always the first step. Often, after being heard, family members will say they feel better and more able to function. Following are Guidelines for Interactions with Families of children with Life-Threatening Illness (IOM, 2003):

- Listen carefully. Pay attention to questions.
- Reassure the family that intense reactions are normal. Remember the physical, mental, emotional, and behavioral aspects of grieving.
- Respect family need for hope.
- Get an early idea of what the family knows and how family members express themselves.
- Use everyday language instead of clinical language.
- Consider using drawings to explain diagnosis and prognosis.
- Seek guidance from families about amount and kind of information desired.
- Realize that the family needs time to process the information.
- Check understanding of what the family has heard.
- Provide written information to family if appropriate.
- Encourage family to write down questions.
- Offer to help family prepare to talk to the child.
- Respect family decisions to withhold information from the child, but inform them that this will block honest communication and isolate the child. Cultural or religious preferences may prohibit open communication about dying.
- Involve the family in developing and revising palliative goals.

Consider the example of Martin McAllister, who worked for an agency providing pediatric home care. His conversation with one family followed the

Guidelines for Interaction with Families. During his initial home visit to see 3-year-old Danny, who is dying of a rare malignancy, he spent the early part of the visit listening to the anger and sorrow the family was feeling. They kept apologizing for expressing their strong emotions, and he reassured them that these were normal grief reactions and acknowledged, "This is a sad time for everyone." His primary goal was to explain Danny's condition and palliative care to Eileen and Clara, his mother and aunt who were the primary caregivers. But when he handed them written literature from the agency, they didn't glance at it. Initially they couldn't think of any questions to ask about Danny's care. That was when Martin sat down at the kitchen table with Eileen and Clara to draw some pictures illustrating the tumor in Danny's lungs and liver. Then he drew arrows targeting where each palliative drug prescribed would make Danny more comfortable. He explained, they nodded, and they finally asked a few questions. He urged the family to write down more questions for the next visit, when he told them they would develop some goals for Danny's care together. This pleased Eileen, who said she would ask her husband to be part of the visit.

> To offer humane care to the dying and their families is to take time to listen, to respect their wishes for what they want to know and do, to support them in their grief, and to share with them that the professional is also affected by the situation (Davies & Connaughty, 2002, p. 6).

Talking to Children Facing Their Own Death

Parents usually decide when and how much to tell their children. Palliative psychosocial interventions foster communication between parents and their children. The child's questions guide the conversation, and art, music, play, and stories facilitate expression. Even when parents decide to "protect" the child from the news, children are often aware that they will not live to grow up. Over time, they pick up emotional cues from the adults who are trying to hide their feelings. For example, when one 5-year-old boy was asked what he was going to be when he grew up, he answered, "a ghost" (IOM, 2003). There is growing agreement that dying children should be informed in language appropriate to their developmental level and their wishes. However, you should respect contrary family and cultural values. Following are guidelines for nurses' conversations with terminally ill children when the parents decide to be open in communication:

- Listen to the child's questions
- Beware giving too much or too little information
- Remember that some children seek to protect their parents and other adults from distressing conversation
- Offer to talk but accept the child's silence or change of subject
- Use dolls, stuffed animals, and puppets to aid children's expression
- With parental permission, involve the child in identifying goals and making decisions about care.

The Life of Dying Children and Their Families

Children should continue familiar activities as long as they can. They should learn, spend time with other children, be expected to act responsibly, and be disciplined when they do not (Gibbons, 2001). If they are infants, they need visual and auditory stimulation, toys to manipulate, and to be touched and held. If they are toddlers or preschoolers, they need to play, draw and use other arts to express feeling, have consistent limits, and be held and comforted. Preschoolers need to understand that the illness and treatments are not punishment. They need to express their fears. Story-telling and books may help. School-aged children need to play, to go to school, to have contact with friends, and to express their fears. Adolescents are seeking greater independence while the illness is making them more dependent. It is essential that they keep in contact with friends and go to school as long as possible. School provides normal structure in their lives and connections with peers. Older teens need to challenge authority and question parental values at the very time that curative treatment requires them to comply with authority. It is essential to understand and respect their needs for autonomy and control. If they are actively part of decision-making, they will feel more secure and be less resistant. Younger teens may feel immortal, but older teens can see clearly that they may not live to adulthood. An adolescent's future orientation makes acceptance of death particularly difficult. Their strong will to live often coexists with an awareness that death is likely (Gibbons, 2001).

66   *Children should continue familiar activities as long as they can. They should learn, spend time with other children, be expected to act responsibly, and be disciplined when they do not (Gibbons, 2001).*

The everyday life of a terminally ill child presents many practical challenges for the family. See Box 12-5, Challenges to Family Life When a Child is Dying. The family needs the assistance of the multidisciplinary team in order to plan for health care at home and to normalize the child's life by continuing schooling and play activities, and welcoming the child's friends. The needs of siblings must not be forgotten. Caregiving responsibilities will challenge parental finances and employment. Finally, plans must be made for emergent symptoms and management of impending death. Everyone in the household will live in unrelenting uncertainty until the child dies.

Mothers, Fathers, and Siblings of Dying Children

Mothers are usually the primary caregivers for their children and provide most physical care when the child is at home. Caregiver burdens are discussed in Chapter 11. Mothers often give their jobs up to provide needed care. Fathers tend to function as wage earners, caregivers of siblings, advocates in the health-care system, and problem-solvers when there is trouble with medical technology (Lehna, 2001). Siblings should be informed and

> **Box 12-5** ■ **CHALLENGES TO FAMILY LIFE WHEN A CHILD IS DYING**
>
> - Adapting space in the home to the child's comfort and safety
> - Arranging personal care and medical care into life at home and school
> - Planning with school
> - Providing for play and friends
> - Maintaining employment and finances
> - Caring for the household and the child
> - Responding to needs of siblings
> - Planning for emergencies
> - Deciding how to respond to symptoms
> - Planning for impending death
> - Planning for after death
>
> *Source*: Institute of Medicine (2003).

involved in caring for the sick child, as well as in keeping the household functioning. However, these responsibilities must be balanced with their needs to continue in school and participate in normal activities for their age. It is not surprising if they struggle with feelings of resentment and anger as all the family energy is focused on their dying sibling. Every effort should be made not to forget their individual needs.

Parents Grieving a Child's Death

Abraham Lincoln said, "You have not known grief until you have stood at the grave of your child" (Kane & Primomo, 2001, p. 162). Grief and mourning of parents who have lost a child possess some unique qualities beyond those discussed in Chapter 7 on grief. In particular, guilt is a frequent, unfortunate emotion in bereaved parents (Worden & Monahan, 2001). Guilt may arise over worry whether they made the right decisions in the child's care. They may feel responsible for the death and think that they made a mistake that caused it. It is not uncommon for surviving parents to feel guilt that they are alive while the child they were supposed to protect is dead.

After the death of a child, marriages are under greater stress. Parents may misunderstand and feel hurt by each other's grieving styles. One parent may be openly expressive, which threatens the other, who withholds emotions (Worden & Monahan, 2001). The expressive parent may conclude that the avoiding parent didn't care about the child. When neither parent is talking about the death, their surviving children are left with no way to mourn openly. Parents who do best are those who have found some meaning in the child's death, have ongoing support, and were able to give the dying child information and support. The family members are able to re-engage in life with less distressing persistent symptoms of grief. The death of a child tends to be a life-long sadness for surviving parents. Significant life events like birthdays, weddings, holidays, and graduations continue to be a reminder that the child is not present.

> *Parents who do best are those who have found some meaning in the child's death, have ongoing support, and were able to give the dying child information and support.*

 Planting the Seeds

The most powerful nursing intervention to help parents grieving over a child is active listening. Ask them to tell you about their child. Pay attention. Use reflection and summary. Urge them to reach out to their support network. Grief should not be borne alone.

CONCEPTS IN ACTION

Marty Chavez is 5 years old. She was diagnosed shortly after birth with a rare neurological disorder, which has caused her to be developmentally delayed. The family was told that Marty was unlikely to live beyond young childhood. She does not talk, seldom sleeps through the night, wears diapers, and cannot feed herself. Marty's mother had to quit her job to provide full-time care for her. Marty is able to smile and laugh in interactions with her parents and two healthy older siblings. The family is of modest means. Marty's father is a supervisor at the local post office.

Shortly after her fifth birthday, Marty takes a turn for the worse. She stops swallowing so that a PEG tube has to be inserted. More distressing is that Marty's happy personality deteriorates. She cries day and night. Muscle spasms erupt in her arms and legs. She kicks and hits whenever she is touched. The doctor recommends that she not be resuscitated if her heart stops. Marty's mother begins having frequent headaches and becomes forgetful. Her 11-year-old brother starts getting into fights at school. Her 14-year-old sister's grades start falling. Her father starts sleeping at a friend's house because he cannot rest with Marty's frequent screams.

- What are the family's needs? Consider all members.
- What are Marty's nursing needs?
- What kinds of services are needed if true palliative care is to be provided for this family?
- How would the situation be different and the nursing interventions changed if Marty were an adolescent? If she were 75 years old?

References

A New Language of Hope. (2002). *State Initiatives in End-of-Life Care*, 15, 5–8.

American Academy of Pediatrics. (2000). Palliative care for children. *Pediatrics, 106*(2), 351–356.

Armstrong-Dailey, A., & Zarbock, S. (Eds) (2001). *Hospice care for children*. New York: Oxford University Press.

Brown, C. (2001). Therapeutic play and creative arts: Helping children cope with illness, death, and grief. In A. Armstrong-Dailey and S. Zarbock, (Eds.), *Hospice care for children* (pp. 251–289). New York: Oxford University Press.

Brown, L., & Brown, M. (1996). *When dinosaurs die: A guide to understanding death*. Boston: Little, Brown & Co.

Buscaglia, L. (1982). *The fall of Freddie the leaf*. Thorofare, NJ: Charles B. Slack.

Christ, G. H. (2000). *Healing children's grief: Surviving a parent's death from cancer*. New York: Oxford University Press.

Davies, B., & Connaughty, S. (2002). Pediatric end of life care: Lessons learned from parents. *Journal of Nursing Administration, 32*(1), 5–6.

Doka, K. (Ed.). (2000). *Living with grief: Children, adolescents, and loss*. Philadelphia: Taylor and Francis.

Faulkner, K. (2001). Children's understanding of death. In A. Armstrong-Dailey & S. Zarbock (Eds.), *Hospice care for children*. New York: Oxford University Press.

Feeg, V. D., Miller-Thiel, J., & Will, J. (2001). Caring for children with life limiting illness and their families: Focus on pediatric hospice nursing. In A. Armstrong-Dailey & S. Zarbock (Eds.), *Hospice care for children* (pp. 68–99). New York: Oxford University Press.

Gibbons, M. B. (2001). Psychosocial aspects of serious illness in childhood and adolescence: Curse or challenge? In A. Armstrong & S. Zarbock (Eds.), *Hospice care for children* (pp. 49–67). New York: Oxford University Press.

Huff, S., & Joshi, P. (2001). Pain and symptom management. In A. Armstrong-Dailey & S. Zarbock (Eds.), *Hospice care for children* (pp. 23–48). New York: Oxford University Press.

Institute of Medicine. (2003). *When children die: Improving palliative and end-of-life care for children and their families*. Washington, DC: National Academies Press.

Kane, J., & Primomo, M. (2001). Alleviating the suffering of seriously ill children. *American Journal of Hospice and Palliative Care, 18*(3), 161–169.

Kastenbaum, R. (2000). *The psychology of death*. New York: Springer.

Lehna, C. (2001). Fathers' and siblings roles in families with children in home hospice care. *Journal of Hospice and Palliative Nursing, 3*(1), 17–23.

Oltjenbruns, K. (2001). Developmental context of childhood: Grief and regrief phenomenon. In M. Stroebe, R. Hansson, W. Stroebe, & H. Schut (Eds.), *Handbook of bereavement research* (pp. 169–197). Washington, DC: American Psychological Association.

Webb, N. B. (2000). Play therapy to help bereaved children. In K. Doka (Ed.), *Living with grief: Children, adolescents, and loss*. Philadelphia: Taylor and Francis.

Wolfe, J., Grief, H., Klar, N., Levin, S., Ellenbogen, J., Salem-Schatz, S. et al. (2000). Symptoms and suffering at the end of life in children with cancer. *New England Journal of Medicine, 342*(5), 326–333.

Worden, J., & Monahan, J. (2001). Caring for bereaved parents. In A. Armstrong-Dailey & S. Zarbock (Eds.), *Hospice care for children* (pp. 137–171). New York: Oxford University Press.

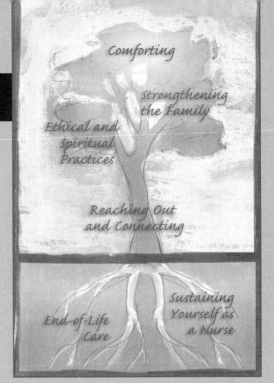

Comforting

Strengthening
the Family

Ethical and
Spiritual
Practices

Reaching Out
and Connecting

End-of-Life
Care

Sustaining
Yourself as
a Nurse

COMFORTING

CHAPTER 13

Understanding and Anticipating the Course of Terminal Disease

Philosophical Reflections

"From all the rest I single out you, having a message for you,
You are to die—let others tell you what they please, I cannot prevaricate,
I am exact and merciless, but I love you. There is no escape for you."

WALT WHITMAN, AMERICAN POET WHO NURSED DURING THE CIVIL WAR

("TO ONE SHORTLY TO DIE," IN READINGS FROM THE PRESIDENT'S COUNCIL ON BIOETHICS, 2003)

Learning Objectives

1. Discuss the tendency toward medical avoidance of end-of-life prognoses.
2. Identify physician and nurse roles in telling the truth about prognoses.
3. Explain generic signs of imminent death and those specific to the most common terminal disease processes.
4. Explain the predictable effects of a final common pathway involving end-stage organ failure.
5. Apply knowledge of disease course to the end-of-life nursing practice of anticipatory guidance.

This chapter begins Unit Six, which develops the reader's competence in physical comforting. In the End-of-Life Caregiving Model, the leaves represent comforting strategies to alleviate different kinds of physical distress. In order to comfort physically at the end of life, nurses need to be able to anticipate the course of illness. This chapter begins the unit by addressing the challenges of predicting the future course of disease and telling the truth about prognoses. The chapter also discusses anticipating the final course for the most common causes of mortality, the final common pathway of dying, and the nurse's end-of-life role in anticipatory guidance.

PROGNOSTICATION AND TRUTH-TELLING

In contrast to the words of Walt Whitman at the beginning of this chapter, professional norms in medicine lead physicians to avoid predictions and not to volunteer information unless questioned (Christakis, 1999).

Predicting the Future

Beginning in medical school, physicians learn not to talk about emotion-ridden matters. Doctors tend to believe that their predictions affect outcomes, so they are deliberately ambiguous or optimistic. They worry about destroying hope and creating self-fulfilling prophecies. Maintaining a positive attitude is strongly valued in contemporary America. With patients living with chronic illness and cancer, physicians tend to present the bright side and to use statistical generalizations rather than discussing individual fate. Grounded in an "ethic of beneficent silence," physicians tend to believe that optimism makes patients easier to manage and more trusting. "In American oncology practice, hope is primarily conveyed by physicians' commitment to provide patients with diagnostic and therapeutic information and to employ a dazzling array of high-tech therapies" (Christakis, 1999, p. 131). They choose euphemisms like "deposits" instead of "more cancer" and "interesting therapies" instead of "toxic therapies."

When physicians do prognosticate, they tend to minimize burdens of treatment and overestimate survival times (Christakis, 1999). Yet, the downside of "too much optimism near the end of life may mean patients never see the end coming, never prepare for it, and fight vainly against it" (Christakis, p. 178). Basta (2000) describes "a fate worse than death" when practitioners use invasive technology to "treat people to death," even after they have lost all cognitive functions. "Sustaining a life in a body that is irreversibly incapacitated and without a mind is no longer a miracle of medicine but a routine in American intensive care units" (Basta, 2000, p. 45). Too often, the focus is on maintaining physiological function when reason and experience indicate that it is impossible for medical intervention to achieve the desired physiological response. Failing to look honestly into the future, death catches physician, patient, and family unawares.

To better understand this failure in prognostication, it is important to also appreciate the contemporary medical preoccupation with aggressive life-saving measures. Physicians are socialized to battle disease and death; they have been taught to fight death down to the finish line. This "war" against death often requires emotional detachment from the patient who is suffering; the war may even require inflicting more suffering. Nurses are caught in the middle of this battle, frequently seeing that the battle has been lost, but still expected to maintain all the technologies of battle. And because the modern inclination is to fight death to the very end, truth sometimes gets lost in the battle.

Telling the Truth

Telling the truth is known as veracity and is a fundamental principle guiding health-care ethics. Truth often is concealed, however, when the practitioner fears that disclosure might cause harm or when the patient or family does not want to hear the truth. The Hippocratic Oath directs physicians to avoid saying anything that will upset the patient (Veatch, 2003). Although contemporary attitudes favor truth-telling, many physicians choose to disclose only partial truths to avoid the patient's distress. In addition, many cultural groups prohibit direct discussion of serious illness and a terminal prognosis with the patient. See Chapter 8, Cross-Cultural Competency at the End of Life.

Physicians have the responsibility for initially breaking the news that patients have a limited time left to live. They traditionally are considered to have the diagnostic and prognostic expertise to determine and disclose this information. This is a heavy burden for them, and frequently they do poorly in disclosing this information to patients. Lamont and Christakis (2003) propose the following protocol for providers delivering an end-of-life prognosis:

- *Preparation* involves research to clarify likely survival, alerting the patient ahead of time, arranging a private meeting, establishing what the patient feels and understands, and determining what the patient wants to know.
- *Content* involves telling the patient you have bad news, stating that simply, making optimistic statements that are true, and estimating survival based on published information about similar patients. For example, "I have bad news to share. The cancer has spread to your liver and bones, which means we can't cure it. But we can control the pain and any other symptoms. Patients in your situation live on the average 3 to 6 months."
- *Acknowledging* the patient's response by expressing empathy and assuring the patient that the physician will stay involved in care.
- *Closing* by summarizing the information, arranging for follow-up, and offering to discuss the news with anyone important to the patient.

Often nurses working collaboratively on an interdisciplinary team can facilitate the initial and ongoing process of disclosure. We encourage patients to ask their questions. We encourage physicians to stop and sit down and answer those questions.

Nursing patients who are facing death requires an ability to speak honestly with them. Three communication approaches are essential to speaking truth at the end of life. Each is identified with an example:

1. Asking difficult questions: "What did the doctor actually say about your condition? Did he give you a prognosis?"
2. Speaking the truth about losing functions: "You just can't expect yourself to keep up all the housekeeping and cooking. You need rest. Your anemia is getting worse."
3. Facing avoidance: "I know you want to try to build up your strength. But right now it is unsafe for you to go to the gym. Let's focus on what you can do despite the dizziness."

Because physicians emphasize the possibilities for each new intervention and try to project optimistic medicalized futures, patients and families often become extraordinarily preoccupied with maintaining medical regimens. As nurses, we "never use a sledgehammer to impose reality, but remain committed to telling the truth when invited" (Zerwekh, 1994, p. 33). Chapter 6 further explores the nurse's role in truth-telling.

 We never use a sledgehammer to impose reality, but remain committed to telling the truth when invited.

Prognostication is not an exact science, which makes truth-telling even more complex. The next section provides some insight into how to anticipate the final course of dying.

ANTICIPATING THE FINAL COURSE

To understand and be able to anticipate the hallmark events at the end of life, it is important to understand that some circumstances are predictable for all dying patients, and some are unique to specific disease processes.

General Guidelines

A terminal prognosis is more likely in patients whose disease is progressing clinically, who keep being hospitalized or seen in the emergency department, and who exhibit a striking functional decline. The Karnofsky Performance Status Scale is frequently used to rate functional decline; scores of 50% or below often indicate that the end of life is approaching (see Box 13-1). Reduction in nutritional status due to the terminal disease is also predictive of mortality.

Box 13-1 ■ **KARNOFSKY PERFORMANCE STATUS SCALE**

100%	Normal activity, no evidence of disease
90%	Normal activity, minor symptoms of disease
80%	Normal activity with effort, some disease symptoms
70%	Unable to perform normal activity or any active work, cares for self
60%	Needs occasional assistance with self care, but mostly independent
50%	Requires major assistance for self care, frequent medical care required
40%	Disabled and requiring significant assistance
30%	Severely disabled and needing active medical support
20%	Very sick, intensive medical support required
10%	Imminently terminal, rapid progress of fatal symptoms
0	Deceased

Source: Adapted from National Hospice Organization (1996).

In general, this comprises unintentional weight loss of more than 10% over the last 6 months and a serum albumin under 2.5 gm/dL. Patients are considered to have weeks to months to live when they are still alert, with declining disease course, growing weakness with functional impairment, and impaired nutritional status (American Academy of Hospice and Palliative Medicine, 2003). They often have days to weeks as their cognitive status becomes variable, confusion and/or restlessness is increasing, their disease course is advanced, and they are nearly bed bound. They may have hours to days when their consciousness is decreased or fluctuating, the clinical decline is rapid, oral intake and urine output are reduced, and they are unable to turn over in bed. They are within hours or minutes of death when there are periods of apnea, secretions are rattling in their throat, and the extremities are cold or mottled.

■
WWW. Internet Reference Box

See *www.victoriahospice.com* for explanation of the Palliative Performance Scale, developed by the Victoria Hospice. It incorporates a rating of ambulation, activity, evidence of disease, self care ability, nutritional intake, and consciousness to predict the end-of-life course effectively.

National Vital Statistics

Competent care at the end of life requires that nurses understand the final disease pathway for the most common causes of death. The top 10 causes of death for people of all ages in the United States are as follows:

1. Heart disease
2. Cancer
3. Cerebrovascular disease
4. Chronic lung disease
5. Unintentional injuries
6. Diabetes
7. Pneumonia and influenza
8. Alzheimer's disease
9. Kidney disease
10. Septicemia

For those aged 20 to 54, HIV disease moves to the top 10. From age 25 to age 64, chronic liver disease is a top killer (Anderson & Smith, 2005). In order of frequency, this section discusses the predictable terminal course of each of the following causes of death: heart, cancer, cerebrovascular disease, chronic lung disease including pneumonia, diabetes, Alzheimer's disease, kidney disease, liver disease, and HIV. Prognostic information in the following diseases is adapted from the National Hospice Organization (1996) guidelines and reported by the American Academy of Hospice and Palliative Medicine (2003).

Failure of the Heart

Some people with advanced coronary disease die quickly and without warning from arrhythmias. However, many live for prolonged periods of time with heart failure managed by medical and surgical interventions. It is therefore difficult to predict the end of life. The patient who is dying of advanced heart failure no longer responds to drug therapy, is not a candidate for further invasive procedures, and presents with significant symptoms due to the underlying pathophysiology.

The heart may fail due to many conditions, including myocardial infarction, coronary artery insufficiency, cardiomyopathies, myocarditis, diseases of the heart valves, congenital defects, pericarditis, systemic hypertension, and pulmonary hypertension (Porth, 2005). Manifestations of heart failure are due to reduced cardiac pumping ability, reduced blood flow to the kidneys, and activation of the sympathetic nervous system (elevated norepinephrine and epinephrine). In decompensated heart failure, stroke volume is reduced and the heart is working against great resistance in the constricted blood vessels. Vasoconstriction occurs due to the effects of sympathetic nervous activation and action of angiotensin II, which is activated by reduced renal circulation. Fluid is retained by the kidneys due to angiotensin II, which promotes aldosterone and ADH (antidiuretic hormone) production. Salt and water retention causes peripheral and pulmonary edema.

The ventricles become overstretched with excessive fluid volume (pre-load) because of increased venous return and diminished ventricular pumping ability. Treatment of advanced congestive heart failure involves reducing the high filling pressures with diuretics, angiotensin inhibitors like lisinopril, and beta-blockers like metoprolol to reduce vasoconstriction (Nohria, Lewis, and Stevenson, 2002). In the terminal phase, symptoms can no longer be controlled and/or patients may not tolerate the side effects of these drugs (Goodlin, 2003).

Prognosis worsens when the patient develops symptoms consistent with New York Heart Association Class IV in which patients cannot carry on any physical activity without discomfort (Porth, 2005). Symptoms may be present even at rest and include:

- Dyspnea at rest and on exertion
- Orthopnea and paroxysmal nocturnal dyspnea
- Angina
- Weakness, syncope, and exhaustion

Physical examination reveals inspiratory crackles, gallop rhythm, pitting edema in extremities, and distended neck veins. An ejection fraction of less than 20% predicts mortality. Decreased survival time can also be predicted by the presence of supraventricular and ventricular arrhythmias resistant to treatment, history of cardiac arrest, presence of HIV, history of syncope, and an embolic stroke of cardiac origin. The patient is considered terminal if he is not a candidate for invasive interventions or if these interventions have failed. Interventions include angioplasty, cardiac bypass (CABG), left ventricular assist devices, pacemaker, or defibrillator implant. With increasing frequency, patients dying of cardiac failure are being instrumentized and admitted to hospices with implanted defibrillators and ventricular assist devices.

Cancer

Normal cells are transformed into cancer cells through a process termed oncogenesis. The process involves inheritance of susceptible genes, immunological defects, and exposure to environmental agents such as viruses, radiation, and carcinogenic chemicals. Traditional cancer treatment involves surgical removal if the tumor is localized with defined margins, and radiation or chemotherapy, which target rapidly growing cells. Unfortunately, patients often arrive at the end of life with severe side effects of these treatments. Palliative care may include relief of radiation burns or other radiation-caused tissue damage. Likewise, patients may need relief of chemotherapy complications, such as stomatitis or bone marrow depression. Recent treatment includes biologic response modifiers, such as interferon and interleukin in selected cancers. Patients receiving these drugs near the end of their life may be suffering significant side effects. Commonly used in end-stage cancer treatment today are hematopoietic growth factors that increase the production of red blood cells (erythropoietin synthesized as Epogen or Procrit) and white blood cells (granulocyte colony stimulating factor synthesized as filgrastim or Neupogen). Continuing use of these extremely expensive drugs at the end of life can be a great cost burden on hospice.

Both radiation and chemotherapy are used palliatively for cancer patients at the end of life. Radiation controls pain and other symptoms at a specific site of tumor involvement. Chemotherapy can be selected for control of symptoms without the goal of prolonging survival. For instance, chemotherapy can reduce chest wall pain in breast cancer, chest pain in lung cancer, bone pain in prostate cancer, and pain from adenopathy in lymphoma (Prommer, 2004). However, chemotherapy-related toxicities can have a negative impact on quality of life and those burdens must be subdued.

Many terminal symptoms in dying cancer patients can be predicted based on the location of metastatic lesions. Pain is common due to the pressure from tumors on surrounding tissue, causing ischemia and nerve compression. Lymphatic spread causes pain and inflammation; enlarged lymph nodes can press on surrounding tissues as well as obstruct the gastrointestinal or urinary tracts. If the bone is involved, chemical mediators such as prostaglandins and bradykinins are released to cause pain. Bone breakdown places the patient at risk for pathological fracture and hypercalcemia. If the bone marrow is involved, there will be fatigue from low red blood cell production, bleeding from reduced platelet production, and infections from reduced white blood cells. Liver metastases cause hepatic failure and biliary obstruction causes jaundice. Brain metastases increase intracranial pressure and place the patient at risk for seizures. Thought processes deteriorate as masses of the brain enlarge. Metastases to the lungs impair airway clearance and cause multiple breathing problems. The patient with extensive metastatic disease is close to death when therapies are not slowing disease progression and their Karnofsky Peformance Scale is less than 50%.

The following sections briefly discuss the predictable course of the most common malignancies in the order of their likelihood of causing death: lung, colorectal, breast, prostate, pancreas, and non-Hodgkin's lymphoma.

LUNG

Lung cancer is the most common cause of cancer death in men and women. Eighty percent are non–small cell (adenocarcinoma, squamous cell, large cell) and 20% are small cell (oat cell), which is more aggressive (Krebs & Russell, 2001). Regional tumor spread includes the other lung, pleural cavity, pericardium, tracheal or esophageal obstruction, laryngeal or phrenic nerve involvement, or superior vena cava compression, which blocks blood return from the upper half of the body. Pancoast's tumor extends to the chest wall and causes shoulder pain radiating down the ulnar nerve distribution. The malignant cells can secrete hormones, including those that mimic the action of antidiuretic hormone (syndrome of inappropriate antidiuretic hormone or SIADH) to cause fluid retention and dilute serum sodium. Metastases occur early in the disease process and are common in the lymph nodes, brain, liver, bone, and adrenals of the patient with advanced disease (Kreb & Russell, 2001). Aggressive radiation and chemotherapies are often used late in the disease in an effort to secure periods of remission. Therefore, end-of-life care often involves management of radiation and chemotherapy complications and questions over the continuing use of hematopoietic growth factors.

COLORECTAL

Cancer of the bowel is the second leading cause of cancer death. The cancer spreads into layers of the bowel and invades surrounding structures. One quarter of patients already have metastases to the liver when they are diagnosed. Chemotherapeutic agents may be infused directly into the liver. Metastatic sites in order of frequency include the lymph nodes, liver, lung, brain, bone, and adrenal glands (Heidrich, 2002).

Extension of colorectal tumors is likely to cause obstruction of the bowel, ureter, or urethra. Surgery is used to resect or bypass obstructing lesions. Chemotherapy has minimal effect on metastatic colorectal malignancies.

BREAST

Breast cancer is the third cause of cancer death. Metastatic sites in order of frequency include the axillary lymph nodes, bone, lung, liver, pleura, and adrenals (Heidrich, 2002). Common complications of advanced breast cancer include malignant pleural effusions, compression of the spinal cord from tumor, and hypercalcemia caused by several factors including bony metastases. High dose chemotherapy is used to secure remissions, but may cause severe bone marrow depression. Endocrine therapies are indicated for patients whose breast cancer cells are positive for estrogen or progesterone receptors.

PROSTATE

Cancer of the prostate is fourth in causes of cancer death. It is the most frequently diagnosed malignancy in men. It is often diagnosed when it has spread into the pelvis, causing urinary obstruction. It frequently metastasizes to the bone, lungs, and liver. Advanced disease is treated by hormonal manipulation to stop the growth of androgen-dependent cells or by removal of the testes, which are the source of most androgens (Heidrich, 2002). Chemotherapy is tried for disease that does not respond to hormonal therapy.

PANCREAS

Pancreatic cancer is the fifth leading cause of cancer death; the prognosis is usually grave at diagnosis. It metastasizes regionally throughout the abdomen, causes jaundice due to biliary obstruction, and also travels to the lungs, bones, and brain.

Palliative surgeries are used to bypass obstructions of the bile ducts or bowel. Those with metastatic disease survive from 3 to 6 months. Pancreatic cancer cells are quite resistant to chemotherapy, which can only briefly prolong life. Radiation may control local disease.

NON-HODGKIN'S LYMPHOMA

Non-Hodgkin's lymphoma is the sixth leading cause of death from malignancies (Heidrich, 2002). Most commonly it presents with painless enlargement of nodes (adenopathy) in the cervical chain or supraclavicular region. Advanced disease involves lymphatic spread to organs in the chest and abdomen. Masses of the lymph nodes can cause pressure and obstruction wherever they are located. The disease metastasizes to the brain, bone, gastrointestinal tract, and bone marrow. Aggressive chemotherapy and interferon may still be considered palliative close to the end of life.

Cerebrovascular Disease

Most (70% to 80%) of strokes are caused by interrupted blood flow in a cerebral blood vessel, which causes ischemia. The less common and frequently fatal cause is hemorrhage of a cerebral vessel, the accumulating blood causes pressure on brain tissues. Immediately after a hemorrhagic or ischemic stroke, coma persisting past the first three days is a strong indicator of mortality. Likewise, the following predict death if they exist on the third day: age over 70, elevated serum creatinine, absent response to voice or pain, and an abnormal brainstem response. Once the disease has become chronic, poor survival is predicted based on older age; dementia; inability to toilet, dress, or bathe without assistance; poor nutrition; and the development of infections.

Chronic Lung Disease

Like heart disease, prognostication for those with chronic lung disease is extremely difficult. As a matter of fact, a recent study revealed that 83% of physicians did not discuss end-of-life plans with their patients (Newsbrief, 2004). This occurred despite the fact that 50% to 60% of COPD patients die within 5 years of diagnosis. The terminal stage is marked by increasing visits to the emergency department and hospitalizations for infections and failing respiratory function. Respiratory failure occurs when the lungs cannot oxygenate the blood (hypoxemia) and cannot eliminate elevated levels of carbon dioxide (hypercapnia). Carbon dioxide levels climb to a Pco_2 of 50 mm Hg or greater and, despite supplemental oxygen, the Pco_2 drops to or equals 55 mm Hg or lower with an oxygen saturation equal to or less than 88%. Hypoxemia causes deteriorating mental status and cyanosis; pulse and blood pressure are initially increased and then diminish as death nears. Hypercapnia has a sedative effect (carbon dioxide narcosis) and increases respirations and air hunger. In addition, deterioration of respiratory function leads to the following symptoms:

- Dyspnea at rest or with minimal exertion
- Cough
- Profound fatigue and weakness
- Inability to speak in full sentences

Physical examination reveals wet breath sounds, reduced level of consciousness, increasing confusion, resting tachycardia, and weight loss. The signs and symptoms of heart failure (cor pulmonale) develop.

Diabetes Mellitus

Mortality related to diabetes is due to end-stage renal disease, cardiovascular disease, and cerebrovascular disease. Diabetes is the leading cause of end-stage renal disease (Porth, 2005). Diabetics are at increased risk of these mortal conditions due to the impact of metabolic defects on selected body tissues, particularly the blood vessels.

Dementia

Patients with advanced progressive dementia due to Alzheimer's or multiple infarcts can live a long time until they finally develop complications that take their lives. They are considered close to death when they are functionally incapacitated and complicating conditions develop. Functional incapacity includes:

- Unable to ambulate, dress, or bathe without help
- Incontinent of urine and feces
- Unable to communicate meaningfully

Complications that predict likelihood of death drawing near include aspiration pneumonia, pyelonephritis, septicemia, multiple stage 3–4 pressure ulcers, recurrent fever despite antibiotics, and inability to maintain adequate nutritional intake with weight loss greater than 10% in 6 months and serum albumin less than 2.5 gm/dL. Special issues at the end of life are the patient's inability to make decisions for a period of years before death, loss of the capacity to chew and swallow food, and infection (Pahnke & Volicer, 2002).

Kidney Failure

End-stage renal disease is caused by a variety of chronic diseases including hypertension, diabetes, glomerulonephritis, and polycystic kidney disease (Porth, 2005). At the end of life, other advanced disease processes may also cause the kidneys to fail. Any condition that causes reduced circulation to kidneys can cause them to fail; heart failure and liver failure may cause kidney failure. The natural reduction of oral fluid intake in people close to death will eventually cause kidney failure. Likewise, invasion or obstruction of the urinary system by tumors will cause kidney failure.

A patient whose death is due to renal failure will be a person who is not a candidate for kidney transplant or dialysis, or whose complications or choice require discontinuing dialysis. The lives of dialysis patients are one third as long as patients without end-stage renal disease (End-Stage Renal Disease Workgroup, 2002). Nevertheless, there is a culture of denial within dialysis units that disregards the need for advance care planning and fails to address the palliative needs of patients and families. Many dialysis units actually prohibit the honoring of Do Not Resuscitate (DNR) directives (End-Stage Renal Disease Workgroup, 2002).

WWW.   Internet Resource Box

For more details regarding end-of-life challenges for those enduring dialysis, examine the Web site for promoting excellence in end-stage renal failure: *www.promoting excellence.org/esrd.*

Laboratory values associated with end-stage renal failure include a serum creatinine greater than 8.0 mg/dL and a creatinine clearance of less than 10 cc/min. Accumulation of nitrogenous wastes cause the symptoms of uremia, which include nausea and vomiting; neuropathy (muscle weakness, paresthesias, and paralysis); neuromuscular irritability (muscle twitching, tremulousness, and seizures); and uremic encephalopathy (reduced level of consciousness, delirium, and coma). Metabolic wastes accumulate in the skin to cause pruritus and uremic frost. The kidneys fail in their production of erythropoietin, causing anemia. Uremia contributes to platelet dysfunction, causing bleeding disorders. The patient becomes acidotic as hydrogen ions are not excreted. Potassium is not excreted, with resulting hyperkalemia. Because the kidneys are unable to eliminate fluids, edema and congestive heart failure result. The patient becomes hypertensive. Therefore, selected signs of terminal renal failure include:

- Oliguria with 24-hour urine output less than 400 cc
- Serum potassium over 7.0
- Fluid overload
- Confusion and diminishing level of consciousness
- Nausea and vomiting
- Pruritus
- Restlessness
- Uremic pericarditis
- Pain secondary to neuropathies

Liver Disease

The liver may fail due to advanced cirrhosis, usually caused by alcoholism or hepatitis. Functional liver tissue has been replaced by fibrotic tissue that is a result of chronic injury, inflammation, and repair (Iredale, 2003). Advanced cirrhosis caused by hepatitis can be treated by eliminating the virus using interferon, ribavirin, and lamivudine. Future treatments will seek to reverse the fibrotic process. Those who eventually need a liver transplant have a 75% 5-year survival rate. The terminal patient is a person who is not a candidate for liver transplant or whose transplant has failed. Liver failure causes many problems including encephalopathy, ascites, and bleeding.

Because the liver has lost its detoxifying capacity, neurotoxins accumulate to cause hepatic encephalopathy, which is manifested as progressive cognitive impairment leading to coma (Porth, 2005). Ammonia is one of those toxins; it is produced by bacterial degradation of proteins in the intestine. To improve mental status at the end of life, antibiotics may be given to reduce bowel bacteria, or lactulose may be administered to produce loose stools and a low bowel pH that inhibits ammonia production.

Venous circulation to the liver is blocked by bands of fibrous tissue so that blood backs up to cause portal hypertension (Porth, 2005). Major complications include ascites and the development of collateral channels to go around the obstructed liver and connect the portal vein with systemic circulation. In ascites, fluid builds up in the peritoneal cavity due to increased capillary pressure from portal hypertension, retention of salt and water by the kidney, and reduced colloidal osmotic pressure since the liver is failing to synthesize albumin, which normally maintains colloidal osmotic pressure. Massive fluid build-up is a challenge at the end of life. When diuretics fail, should the patient be subjected to repeated paracenteses? Those with a prognosis of several months are offered peritoneovenous shunts (Denver or LaVeen), which drain peritoneal fluid into the central venous circulation.

The most important clinical consequence of collateral venous channels is the development of esophageal varices. These develop in about 65% of patients with advanced cirrhosis (Porth, 2005). The liver fails to synthesize many clotting factors including prothrombin and fibrinogen, which renders the patient at risk for bleeding, particularly from those esophageal varices. Variceal bleeding causes death in half of the patients with varices.

Indicators of terminal condition include a serum albumin under 2.5 gm/dL and increased clotting time measured by a prothrombin time prolonged more than 5 seconds over control or an international normalized ratio (INR) greater than 1.5. The patient will have one or more of the following effects of hepatic failure that is unresponsive to treatment:

- Ascites
- Recurrent bleeding of esophageal varices
- Failure of the kidneys (hepatorenal syndrome)
- Bacterial peritonitis
- Hepatic encephalopathy

The prognosis is worsened in the face of progressive malnutrition, muscle wasting, active alcoholism, hepatic carcinoma, and hepatitis B.

Human Immunodeficiency Virus (HIV)

The human immunodeficiency retrovirus causes acquired immunodeficiency syndrome (AIDS), in which immunity is profoundly reduced through destruction of CD4 T lymphocytes and macrophages. The CD4 recognize infected cells and foreign antibodies, activate antibody-producing lympho-cytes, and orchestrate cell-mediated immunity in which infected cells and foreign antigens are destroyed (Porth, 2005).

When viral loads climb and CD4 counts drop, the immune system cannot resist the development of opportunistic infections and malignancies. HIV has become a chronic disease as antiretroviral drugs and drugs controlling oppor-tunistic infections have successfully prolonged life. A viral load of more than 100,000 copies and a CD4 count below 25 cells/mcL may predict a terminal condition if a patient is declining in function, choosing to forgo medication, antiretrovirals are no longer effective, or life-threatening complications have developed. Infections that do not respond to therapy are predictive of a poor prognosis. They include cryptosporidiosis, toxoplasmosis, mycobacterium avium complex bacteremia, progressive multifocal leukoencephalopathy caused by the JC virus, and toxoplasmosis. Life-threatening malignancies to which AIDS patients are most vulnerable include lymphoma of the central nervous system, systemic lymphoma, and visceral Kaposi's sarcoma. The ter-minal phase can be predicted by wasting that does not respond to treatment, renal failure without dialysis, diarrhea for 1 year, persistently low serum albu-min, age older than 50, symptomatic heart failure, and decision to forgo treat-ment. Box 13-2 identifies common late-stage symptoms of AIDS. These symp-toms are caused by progression of the disease itself, the effects of opportunistic infections, and side effects of medications. Fatigue, worry, and depression are present in almost all patients (Selwyn & Rivard, 2003).

In the period since highly active antiretroviral therapy (HAART) has been implemented, causes of death now are more likely to include hepatitis

---

Box 13-2 ■ SYMPTOM BURDEN OF PATIENTS WITH ADVANCED AIDS

Listed in order of frequency based on a study of more than 3000 U.S. patients:

- Fever, sweats, or chills
- Diarrhea
- Nausea or anorexia
- Pain, numbness, or tingling in hands/feet
- Headache
- Weight loss
- Vaginal discharge, pain, or irritation
- Sinus infection or pain
- Visual problems
- Cough or dyspnea

Source: From Selwyn & Rivard (2003).

B and C, various malignancies, and end-stage organ failure (Selwyn & Rivard, 2003). In addition, some patients fail to benefit from HAART due to lack of health-care access, nonadherence to treatment regimens, psychiatric illness or chemical dependency, intolerable drug toxicities, viral resistance despite therapy, or other coexisting diseases.

Preparation for death needs to coexist with the possibility that an effective antiretroviral regimen can be implemented. Challenging issues arise with dual goals of providing symptom relief and seeking to lengthen life for those living with advanced AIDS. Following are some of the related issues (Selwyn, 2003):

- Should highly active antiretrovirals (HAART) be discontinued, even in the presence of low CD4 and high viral loads? They may still be prolonging survival. However, their toxicities may be diminishing quality of life.
- Should prophylaxis against opportunistic infection be discontinued? An example is ganciclovir to maintain the sight in a dying person who has CMV retinitis.
- Should opportunistic infections be treated with specific anti-infectives that are costly and toxic, or should the symptoms be treated palliatively?
- If antiretrovirals are continued, they are known to interact with common antidepressants, benzodiazepines, and opioids. These should be used with great care and alternatives should be considered.
- Anorexia and weight loss should not be accepted without trials of medications that might reverse these manifestations, including megestrol acetate, steroids, testosterone, dronabinol, and recombinant human growth hormone.

Regardless of the specific disease process, the last hours or days of life often follow a remarkably similar pathophysiological pathway.

FINAL TERMINAL PATHWAY: MULTIPLE ORGAN FAILURE

As death draws close, a pattern of common physiological events becomes predictable. The patient progresses from countless preterminal disease processes, as previously described, to travel a final common pathway. Box 13-3 outlines the Pathophysiology of Dying Organs. This final pathway will eventually include cardiopulmonary failure and often includes renal or hepatic failure. The heart may fail due to many causes, including myocardial damage or the workload imposed by terminal pathologies such as pulmonary disease, pericardial or myocardial metastases, anemia, sepsis, or herniation of the brain onto the medulla. The lungs may fail due to many causes, including pulmonary disease, pneumonia, embolism, heart failure causing pulmonary edema, pleural effusion, or brain herniation. Cardiopulmonary failure causes hypoxemia and reduced perfusion of vital organs, resulting in progressive loss of capacity to remain conscious, think, communicate, and move. Comfort is impaired because of acute air hunger due to impaired gas exchange and ineffective airway clearance; the conscious patient will be acutely apprehensive. Death is imminent as cardiac output and low levels of oxygen in the blood will not support life. Blood pressure drops, peripheral cyanosis and mottling deepen, periods of apnea lengthen, and accumulating pharyngeal and pulmonary secretions produce a death rattle.

Kidney and liver failure are frequently associated events at the end of life; sometimes they are the initial cause as described earlier. At the very end of life, the kidneys fail when, due to any cause, there is reduced blood flow to the kidneys (prerenal failure) or obstruction to urine flow out of the kidneys (postrenal failure). Retention of sodium and water causes peripheral and pulmonary edema. The kidney no longer excretes nitrogenous wastes, so that creatinine and blood urea nitrogen accumulate. Capacities for thought and purposeful movement are impaired by accumulating toxic metabolites. Likewise, when the liver fails it no longer detoxifies toxic metabolites so that they accumulate to impair thought. Increased levels of aldosterone and antidiuretic hormone and reduced synthesis of albumin cause edema and ascites. When kidneys and liver fail, comfort is threatened by fluid build-up in the abdomen, lungs, and periphery.

The pathophysiological consequences of end-stage organ failure produce a predictable set of signs and symptoms that indicate that the following nursing diagnoses will be relevant for most patients at the end of their lives: ineffective tissue perfusion, disturbed thought processes, activity intolerance, impaired gas exchange, ineffective airway clearance, and ineffective breathing pattern. Reexamine Box 13-3 to understand the links between organ failure, signs and symptoms, and end-of-life nursing diagnoses. Ineffective tissue perfusion is the focus of resuscitative and restorative care. In contrast, palliative nursing focuses on the other end-of-life nursing diagnoses.

> *The pathophysiological consequences of end-stage organ failure produce a predictable set of signs and symptoms, which indicate that the following nursing diagnoses will be relevant for most patients at the end of their lives: ineffective tissue perfusion, disturbed thought processes, activity intolerance, impaired gas exchange, ineffective airway clearance, and ineffective breathing pattern.*

ANTICIPATING NURSING NEEDS

An essential skill for nurses working with patients at the end of life is being able to anticipate the disease course. Nurses able to predict the terminal course will be able to prepare the necessary interventions and to teach

Box 13-3 ■ PATHOPHYSIOLOGY OF DYING ORGANS

Basic Processes	Signs and Symptoms	Nursing Diagnoses
Lungs		
Hypoventilation, increased airway resistance to expiration, obstruction, secretions accumulating. Resulting hypoxemia and hypercapnia. Heart working harder to circulate diminishing levels of oxygen	Reduced endurance Reduced mentation Dropping level of consciousness Reduced breath sounds Bubbles, crackles, wheezes, rhonchi Accumulating secretion Tachypnea, apnea Dyspnea, orthopnea Pursed lips, accessory muscles Tachycardia Angina	Activity intolerance Disturbed thought processes Impaired gas exchange Ineffective airway clearance and breathing pattern Discomfort related to shortness of breath Death anxiety and fear
Heart		
Myocardial damage; causing heart failure. Without prior myocardial damage, heart eventually failing due to workload imposed at end of life	Reduced endurance Reduced mentation Tachycardia Arrhythmias Angina Oliguria	Activity intolerance Disturbed thought processes Pain related to angina Ineffective tissue perfusion Ineffective airway clearance and breathing pattern

(continued)

307

Box 13-3 ■ PATHOPHYSIOLOGY OF DYING ORGANS (CONTINUED)

BASIC PROCESSES	SIGNS AND SYMPTOMS	NURSING DIAGNOSES
Heart		
Diminished cardiac output, causing reduced perfusion of brain, kidneys, periphery. Blood backing up into pulmonary circulation to cause pulmonary edema. Blood backing up into vena cava, jugular, hepatic vein, general circulation	Hypotension Dusky nail beds Diminished peripheral pulses Cyanosis and mottling of extremities Dyspnea, tachypnea, orthopnea Distended neck veins Ascites Pitting peripheral edema	Discomfort related to edema, ascites, shortness of breath, angina Death anxiety and fear Crackles, rhonchi
Kidneys		
Accumulating nitrogenous wastes Hyperkalemia from failure to excrete potassium Acidosis from failure to excrete hydrogen ions Retention of sodium and water, producing peripheral and pulmonary edema	Reduced endurance Impaired mentation Pruritus, uremic frost Neuromuscular irritability Nausea and vomiting Deep and rapid respirations Bradycardia and cardiac arrest Pitting edema in dependent tissues Pulmonary edema	Activity intolerance Disturbed thought processes Discomfort related to edema, pruritus, neuropathies Death anxiety and fear

Liver

Liver		
Accumulating ammonia and other toxic metabolites, causing hepatic encephalopathy	Impaired mentation	Activity intolerance
Resistance to venous flow into liver, forcing fluid into lymphatic channels and then into peritoneal cavity	Peripheral and pulmonary edema	Disturbed though processes
Reduced detoxification of aldosterone and ADH, causing sodium retention	Edema, ascites	Discomfort related to edema and ascites
Reduced albumin synthesis, diminishing colloidal osmotic pressure	Peritonitis	Risk for infection
Diminishing filtration of intestinal blood by hepatic Kupffer cells so that more bacteria survive	Sepsis	Risk for bleeding
Portal hypertension, causing distention of venous channels in esophagus, stomach, intestine. Rupture, resulting in slow or massive bleeds	Hematemesis	
	Melena	
	Bleeding esophageal varices	
	Shock	

Source: Adapted from Zerwekh (2002).

309

patients and families what to expect. If we expect the patient to bleed from a malignant head and neck lesion likely to erode into the carotid, we make arrangements to manage this event in case it occurs. If we anticipate encephalopathy in a patient with failing liver, we anticipate necessary interventions. If the patient is at home, family members need extensive teaching and guidance.

Planting the Seeds

An essential skill for nurses serving patients at the end of life is being able to anticipate the disease course. Anticipatory guidance involves proactive nursing, not reactive nursing that waits for a crisis and then attempts to put out the fire when symptoms are out of control. Given a patient with a specific diagnosis, we anticipate a certain set of symptoms and nursing needs before we enter a room or make a home visit. We also need to anticipate future needs and prepare for them. In acute care, nurses are concerned to avoid life-threatening complications by identifying signs and symptoms early and having equipment ready. We seek to avoid crises leading to "failure to rescue." Likewise, in palliative care, nurses are concerned to avoid complications that are likely to cause new suffering. We look for early signs of these problems, and have supplies ready to handle them. We seek to avoid crises leading to "failure to comfort."

For example, consider a home visit to Catherine A., a 76-year-old widow living in the home of her 70-year-old sister, Maria. She has three married daughters living nearby whose goals are to "help Mama die in her own bed." Catherine suffered a right-sided CVA 2 years earlier, which left her with global aphasia, hemiplegia, and incontinence requiring a Foley catheter. She had been up in the wheelchair at the center of family activities until a second CVA just left her bedridden and dysphagic. Physical examination now reveals her to be somnolent, but able to respond to some commands. Her tongue is shiny and caked with white exudate, lungs are clear with diminished breath sounds throughout, breathing is irregular, hands are cool, blood pressure is 86/34, perineum is reddened and odoriferous, and feet are cold with nonpalpable pedal pulses. Her Foley is draining small amounts of dark amber urine with mucopurulent material. She is able to swallow small amounts of puddings and applesauce, but no clear liquids.

Nursing anticipatory guidance involves explaining the physical symptoms to the family and advising them what to expect, including the risk of infection. Because the family does not want active treatment, including antibiotics, but does want Catherine to be comfortable, the nurse has secured an order for both lorazepam (Ativan) and morphine sulfate liquid, which are stored in the kitchen cupboard to be used for restlessness or shortness of breath. After this new stroke, Catherine is completely bedridden. The family needs to be taught care of the completely immobilized patient. Teaching also focuses on palliative measures to relieve Catherine's existing stomatitis and poor perineal hygiene.

The nurse also thinks proactively to anticipate problems that might well arise with obstruction of the catheter. The family has to be taught to irrigate the Foley catheter if blocked, and an extra catheter and insertion kit are left in the home. The nurse also begins discussions with the family about the meaning of food and the difficulty of watching Catherine stop eating because that does mean that "the end is near." They ask about the benefits and burdens of tube feeding; with nursing guidance, they decide the burdens are too great. The discussion turns to sublingual and rectal drug administration, when Catherine can no longer swallow at all. The necessary medications are ordered and kept in the kitchen cupboard. Since Catherine's death may be imminent, the nurse reviews the signs that she may have only hours left. These include mottling of the extremities and death rattle due to pharyngeal secretions accumulating. Now that the family members recognize the implications of these signs, they decide that they will gather relatives at the bedside and say their farewells.

Concepts in Action

Arthur Kent is a 55-year-old patient with advanced AIDS. He has been living for 14 years with HIV, acquired through a sexual relationship with a man who died of AIDS 2 years ago. He is an only child and both of his parents are dead. He was born and raised north of Billings, Montana, and still has a cattle ranch in Montana that is run by a cousin. He has a Master's in Social Work and was working as a counselor with abused children and their families until his latest disease exacerbation. He had been taking a regimen combining several types of antiretroviral agents (HAART or Highly Active Antiretroviral Therapy). Drug complications have caused neuropathies in his feet, so consequently, he has problems walking quickly. Recently, his antiretroviral therapy has become ineffective against the virus so that his CD4 count is zero and viral load is high. He has started on a new drug regimen, but laboratory values have not improved. He takes trimethoprim-sulfamethoxazole (Bactrim) to prevent PCP pneumonia. He has had diarrhea for over a year, which has responded only partially to imodium loperamide (Lomodium) and dicyclomine hydrochloride (Bentyl). His weight loss has been dramatic, dropping from 172 to 123 pounds in 1 year. His appearance greatly distresses him. His appetite is severely diminished. Now he has developed a sore throat and laryngitis that have further restricted his

(continued)

CONCEPTS IN ACTION

intake of food and fluids. He can only speak in a whisper. A friend brought him to the emergency department when he complained of increasing pain in the neck and dizziness when standing. Last night he was admitted to the medical floor. He told the night nurse that he is not afraid of death, but is afraid of the suffering before death. Physical examination reveals an emaciated middle-aged man. His tongue is dry with fissures; there are yellow-white plaques in the back of his throat. Lungs are clear, but he is coughing up blood. Apical pulse is 96 and regular. BP 96/62 sitting and 72/30 standing. Skin is intact; on top of the hand his skin easily pinches between the nurse's fingers. Mr. Kent is afebrile. Peripheral pulses are present and there is no edema in the extremities. After a week in the hospital that included many tests, including CT, MRI, and biopsy of a laryngeal lesion, he has been rehydrated and is discharged. His new diagnosis is non-Hodgkin's lymphoma for which the doctors are recommending laryngectomy, radiation, and chemotherapy.

1. Compare Mr. Kent's condition with prognostic indicators for HIV discussed earlier.
2. Explain the medical culture that has led to recommendation of invasive therapies for the laryngeal mass.
3. Identify nursing diagnoses and goals for Mr. Kent. How do nursing goals change if Mr. Kent decides he wants continued aggressive medical and surgical intervention? How can both the goals of palliation and those focusing on intensive medical intervention be combined?
4. As Mr. Kent's home-health nurse, how might you sit with him to help him decide on options for future care? What words would you use? What questions would you ask?

References

American Academy of Hospice and Palliative Medicine (2003). *Pocket guide to hospice/palliative medicine.* Glenview, IL: AAHPM.

Anderson, R., & Smith, B. (2005). Deaths: Leading causes for 2002. *National Vital Statistic Reports, 53*(17).

Basta, L. (2000). *A graceful exit: Life and death on your own terms.* Xlibris Corp.

Christakis, N. A. (1999). *Death foretold: Prophecy and prognosis in medical care.* Chicago: University of Chicago.

End-Stage Renal Disease Workgroup. (2002). *Final summary report: Recommendations to the field.* Princeton, NJ: Robert Wood Johnson Foundation.

Goodlin, S. (2003). Report on consensus conference: Palliative and supportive care in advanced heart failure. *AAHPM Bulletin, 3*(2), 1, 21–22.

Heidrich, D. (2001). Malignancies. In K. Kuebler, P. Berry, & D. Heidrich (Eds.), *End of life care: Clinical practice guidelines* (pp. 165–179). Philadelphia: WB Saunders.

Krebs, L., & Russell, T. (2001). Lung cancer. In R. Gates & R. Fink (Eds.), *Oncology nursing secrets* (2nd ed., pp. 263–270). Philadelphia: Hanley & Belfus.

Iredale, J. (2003). Cirrhosis: New research provides a basis for rational and targeted treatments. *British Medical Journal, 327*(7407), 143–147.

Lamont, E., & Christakis, N. (2003). Complexities in prognostication in advanced cancer: "To help them live their lives the way they want to." *Journal of the American Medical Association, 290*(1), 98–104.

National Hospice Organization. (1996). *Medical guidelines for determining prognosis in selected non-cancer diseases* (2nd ed.). Arlington VA: National Hospice Organization.

Newsbrief. COPD Patients rarely discuss end-of-life plans with physicians (2004). *American Journal of Hospice and Palliative Care, 21*(1), 13.

Nohria, A., Lewis, E., & Stevenson, L. (2002). Medical management of advanced heart failure. *Journal of the American Medical Association, 287*(5), 628–640.

Pahnke, J., & Volicer, L. (2002). Caring for persons with dementia: A palliative approach. *Journal of Hospice and Palliative Nursing, 4*(3), 143–149.

Porth, C. (2005). Pathophysiology: *Concepts of altered health states* (7th ed.). Philadelphia: Lippincott, Williams & Wilkins.

Prommer, E. (2004). Guidelines for the use of palliative chemotherapy. *AAHPM Bulletin, 5*(1), 1–4.

Selwyn, P. (2003). HIV/AIDS in the new therapeutic era: Revisiting palliative care. *AAHPM Bulletin, 3*(2), 4–8.

Selwyn, P., & Rivard, M. (2003). Palliative care for AIDS: Challenges and opportunities in the era of highly active anti-retroviral therapy. *Journal of Palliative Medicine, 6*(3), 475–487.

Veatch, R. (2003). *The basics of bioethics* (2nd ed.). Upper Saddle River, NJ: Prentice-Hall.

Whitman, W. (2003). To one shortly to die. *The president's council on bioethics. Being human: Readings from the president's council on bioethics.* Washington, DC: U.S. Government.

Zerwekh, J. (1994). The truth-tellers: How hospice nurses help patients confront death. *American Journal of Nursing, 94*(2), 31–34.

CHAPTER 14

Comforting and the Essentials of Pain Relief at the End of Life

Philosophical Reflections

"I swore never to be silent whenever and wherever human beings endure suffering and humiliation."

ELIE WIESEL (1986), SURVIVOR OF THE NAZI DEATH CAMPS.

Learning Objectives

1. Define pain and contrast it with the definition of suffering.
2. Explain the challenges of pain control and how the subjectivity of the pain experience makes it difficult to control.
3. Identify the consequences of unrelieved pain in the dying and the effects on survival if pain is controlled.
4. Define "total pain."
5. Summarize the effects of culture, gender, and age on the pain experience.
6. Explain the barriers to comforting and identify those you have witnessed.
7. Identify essential dimensions of pain assessment.
8. Give an example of how selected comforting nursing interventions can relieve pain.
9. Explain how complementary therapies can be used at the end of life.

Comforting is the process of easing physical or emotional distress. Comforting is a vital dimension of caring for dying people and is illustrated as the leaves on the End-of-Life Caregiving Tree. The Caregiving Tree is rooted in self-care and branches out into all of the complex human needs at the end of life. The leaves covering and protecting the branches represent the numerous ways to relieve physical suffering for people at the ends of their lives. This chapter is the foundation for the knowledge essential to relieving physical discomfort. It defines pain, considers it as one dimension of suffering, and establishes nursing responsibility for its alleviation. Pain is examined as a pathophysiological process affected by complex psychosocial dynamics that must be addressed through a holistic interdisciplinary approach. The chapter identifies barriers to comforting, as well as forces that promote comfort, and it concludes by addressing pain assessment and detailing comforting nursing interventions.

The word pain is derived from the Latin word *poena*, which means punishment. The American Society of Pain Management Nurses (St. Marie, 2002) has created a conceptual definition of pain. Pain is subjective, which means it cannot be measured objectively. It is an intense feeling of discomfort, which usually indicates that tissue has been damaged; it includes physiological and behavioral responses. Pain is known to observers only through patient reporting. In this text, we define pain as whatever the patient says hurts.

WWW.   Internet Reference Box

The American Society of Pain Management Nurses can be contacted through *www.aspmn.org*. This organization publishes the journal *Pain Management Nursing*.

    " *Pain is whatever the patient says hurts. It is an intense feeling of discomfort, which usually indicates that tissue has been damaged.*

The Hospice and Palliative Nurses Association (HPNA, 2004) has identified the consequences of unrelieved end-of-life pain:

- Causing hopelessness and powerlessness in patients
- Causing hopelessness and powerlessness in families
- Consuming energy and attention of the dying
- Impairing social interactions
- Hastening death by increasing physiological distress, immobility, thromboemboli, and pneumonia

With better pain control, dying patients live longer and better. Pain shortens life. Relief of pain extends life. The position of the Hospice and Palliative Nurses Association is that:

All people, including vulnerable populations such as infants, children, and the elderly, facing progressive, life-limiting illness have the right to optimal pain relief. All healthcare providers have the obligation to believe the patient's report of pain (HPNA, 2004, pp. 62–63).

66 | *With better pain control, dying patients live longer and better. Pain shortens life. Relief of pain extends life.*

WWW.   **Internet Reference Box**

The Hospice and Palliative Nurses Association can be viewed at *www.hpna.org.*

PAIN AND SUFFERING

Pain is but one physical dimension of that complex psychic distress or human misery called "suffering." Suffering involves a threat to the person's integrity or survival as a whole person (Cassell, 1991). Morse proclaims, "nurses are the caretakers of suffering" (2001, p. 47). She identifies two opposing ways that people cope with suffering: enduring, which involves emotional suppression; and emoting, which entails emotional releasing. Enduring involves suppressing emotional response when the integrity of oneself is threatened. It is a natural response that permits the person to keep on functioning. Thus, a person who has just learned that her cancer has metastasized to her liver and brain may maintain a mask-like expression, going about "business as usual" with disinterest, focusing on the present to keep going. Occasionally, she may erupt emotionally over trivial concerns, but then she returns to enduring behavior to stay in control. Generally, when a person is enduring, he or she will not find it helpful to be touched or consoled by the nurse. He or she is blocking emotions and does not want them brought up. The caring response is silent presence, not empathetic statements.

By contrast, Morse describes emoting as confronting the meaning of the suffering. Associated behaviors include crying, screaming, moaning, and persistent talking about feelings. Posture may be stooped over and the face is described as drooping. The caring response from the nurse is empathy through active listening and caring touch, when culturally appropriate.

In response to suffering, many people move back and forth between enduring and emoting. They move from enduring to emoting when they acknowledge their suffering. They move from emoting back to enduring in order to be productive and get through the situation. These behaviors are determined by personality, understanding of the situation, and the norms of culture and religion.

⤙ Planting the Seeds

Pay careful attention to how your patients are coping with suffering. If their nonverbal cues indicate tight self control, do not assume that they will be helped by encouraging expression of feelings. The therapeutic response is to stand by and be available, but not intrusive. Help them maintain composure. If their nonverbal and verbal signs are openly expressive of suffering, listen and use empathetic responses like, "This must be terribly difficult for you."

66 | *Being accountable for pain relief involves believing and responding to our patients.*

Current Status of Pain Relief

Undertreatment of pain at the end of life is a serious health problem caused in part by its subjectivity, and in part by the fact that medical professionals fear overmedicating for pain.

One inherent problem with pain is its subjectivity. For those who are suffering, the pain is a dominant certainty, but for the observer, the presence of pain in another is elusive. "Thus, pain comes unsharably into our midst at once as that which cannot be denied and that which cannot be confirmed" (Scarry, 1985, p. 4). Too often, health professionals have "perceived the voice of the patient as an 'unreliable narrator' of bodily events, a voice which must be bypassed as quickly as possible so that they can get around and behind it to the physical events themselves" (Scarry, p. 6). Pain cannot be measured, is invisible, and is poorly expressed in language; as a result, it is frequently ignored. We can easily be in the presence of another person in pain and not see or hear it.

Since the middle of the 20th century, relief of pain has become peripheral to the attention and responsibilities of medical and nursing staff (Fagerhaugh, 1977). Contemporary medical practice focuses on the duty to preserve life and physiological functioning. The dominant mythology is that relieving pain will shorten life or suppress functioning. Being accountable for pain relief involves believing and responding to our patients. Unfortunately, many nurses and medical staff believe they know the patients' bodies and needs better than patients know themselves. Responding to pain can become an issue of power and control.

Likewise, many physicians fear prescribing treatments for pain, despite scientific evidence that opioids can be used safely. Fear of addicting patients and overmedicating them is deeply embedded in medical culture.

Despite a solid body of evidence regarding the possibilities of effective pain relief, there has been little improvement over the last 30 years (Pasero & McCaffrey, 2004). Medical literature provides clear evidence that the United States is suffering from an epidemic of undertreated pain (Rich, 2001).

Box 14-1 ■	**FIVE IMPORTANT INGREDIENTS FOR PAIN RELIEF**

1. Pain must be recognized.
2. The nurse needs the courage to be present.
3. The nurse often must be ready to do battle.
4. The nurse must be more empathetic than judgmental.
5. The nurse must be willing to educate himself or herself.

Source: From St. Marie, (2002), pp. 3–4.

Health-care team members do not hold each other accountable to relieve the suffering of their patients. For instance, a chart review of 195 patients in a large Midwestern medical center revealed that 77% of patients had been in pain, much of it poorly controlled (Paice, Muir, and Shott, 2004).

Pain control in nursing homes also continues to be poor; physicians underprescribe analgesics and nurses give less than what is prescribed. But the fact remains that pain does exist. For instance, more than 80% of people living with cancer develop pain before they die and the pain of cancer is greatly feared (Bruera & Kim, 2003). Dying people continue to suffer pain that could be relieved. The reasons for this failure to comfort are discussed in more detail later in this chapter. St. Marie (2002) has identified five important ingredients for pain relief. See Box 14–1.

THE DYNAMICS UNDERLYING PAIN

The pain of organic illness is never an isolated phenomenon. Pain is a holistic biopsychosocial phenomenon. When a person is living with pain at the end of life, all dimensions of the human experience are interwoven. Pain impairs the physical, psychological, social, and spiritual well-being of the individual. For instance, a person in persistent pain may become depressed and unable to interact with other people. He might cry out to God to explain his agony. Unrelenting physical pain may manifest itself in irritable behavior, hostility, and changes in eating and sleeping. It is common for people to withdraw and isolate themselves. Coping with their suffering becomes the exhausting, consuming center of their existence. Likewise, diminished psychological, spiritual, and social well-being will often aggravate the experience of physical pain. When a person is depressed and has withdrawn from others, pain is experienced more acutely. Cicely Saunders, founder of the modern hospice movement, first described this as the concept of *total pain* (Saunders, 1976). The person ends up suffering at many levels.

Because pain is a holistic biopsychosocial phenomenon, the interdisciplinary palliative team should include a range of disciplines: nursing, medicine, social work, spiritual counseling, physical therapy, and occupational therapy. The following sections describe major dimensions of the pain experience.

> " Pain impairs the physical, psychological, social, and spiritual well-being
> of the individual. . . . Likewise, diminished psychological, spiritual, and
> social well-being will often aggravate the experience of physical pain.

Pathophysiology of Pain

Pain generally implies that certain tissues have been injured. When tissues are injured, the body releases biochemical mediators, such as prostaglandins, histamine, serotonin, bradykinin, and the interleukins (St. Marie, 2002). These substances activate sensory nerve endings called nociceptors, which transmit the painful message through the peripheral nervous system. Nociceptive transmission occurs through the rapidly conducting A delta fibers and the slower conducting C fibers. Both ascend to the dorsal horn of the spinal cord where the sensory input is affected by neurotransmitters and other chemicals. Pathways ascend from the dorsal horn to transmit pain impulses to the brain stem, medulla, and thalamus. From the thalamus, fibers transmit pain (nociceptive) messages to the cerebral cortex, where pain is perceived, and the limbic system, which generates emotional reaction. Endogenous opioids (enkephalin, endorphin, dynorphin) inhibit pain transmission by binding to opioid receptors that are found in ascending and descending pain pathways.

Mediated by the cerebral cortex and limbic system, perception and emotional reaction to pain differ significantly between individuals. The pain of organic illness is never a phenomenon isolated to the physical. For instance, depression and physical pain are intertwined (Vastag, 2003). Recent medical research has demonstrated that serotonin and norepinephrine regulate emotional pain as well as physical pain sensation. It is well known that gender, age, and culture influence the pain experience.

Gender Differences in Pain Perception

Research has demonstrated that there are significant differences in the way men and women perceive and respond to pain. Vallerand and Polomano (2000) note that most studies reveal that women have a lower tolerance for pain and rate its intensity higher. For instance, after abdominal surgery, women report pain of greater severity than men.

Although they are more likely to experience and report pain, women are far less likely than men to receive adequate pain management (Hoffman & Tarzian, 2001). Their reports of pain are viewed less seriously, and they are perceived as better able to put up with the pain. When women complain of pain, they are often discounted and the pain is assumed to be due to emotional rather than physical causes.

Age Differences: Children and the Elderly

Pain is experienced differently at both ends of the age continuum.

challenges of pain relief among the Hmong people, who are migrants from Southeast Asia. Chapter 8 describes culturally sensitive end-of-life nursing.

Recent studies indicate that patients from minority racial and cultural groups are less likely to have their pain controlled (Lasch, 2000). These studies have documented that when mainstream and minority patients report the same amount of pain, physicians and nurses tend to be more responsive to the nonminority group. "African Americans in excruciating pain due to life-threatening illness or major surgery are denied effective pain medicine due to factors which ultimately center on race" (National Medical Association Panel, 2002).

Whether the patient is from mainstream or minority culture, it is often helpful to discern the meaning of pain for an individual whose pain is poorly controlled. For many, pain is an enemy to be eradicated. For some, it is a trial to be endured. For others, it is a punishment. One hospice patient posed particular challenges for the author. A founder of a dramatic troupe, he was dramatic in expressing his pain. He would cry in pain proclaiming, "It hurts! It hurts!" as he rocked back and forth in bed. Nevertheless, he refused to take any analgesics and would not cooperate with an acupuncturist. He also refused to speak to a spiritual counselor. Finally, another nurse tried to help him; she was able to remain calm in the face of his nonadherence with comforting interventions. Within days of his death, he told her that he perceived his pain as "Divine justice."

BARRIERS AND FACILITATORS OF COMFORT

Box 14-4, Barriers and Facilitators of Comfort, summarizes major factors that inhibit nurses' practice of comforting. First of all, *discomfort is peripheral to our attention.* Nurses are socialized to follow medical orders, monitor physiological function, and coordinate the countless expectations of the bureaucratic environments in which we work. Paying attention to pain and suffering often makes us feel vulnerable, and yet it is a responsibility that goes to the heart of our profession. "Recognizing the overwhelming urge to overlook the pain in the body in front of them, the introspective nurse must tap into the ability to stretch beyond his or her own reality. . . . Just as nurses have to overcome their own internal urge to overlook the patient's pain, they must convince a colleague (the prescribing physician) to overcome the same urges" (St. Marie, 2002, p. 3). Those of us who are experienced need to regain beginners' eyes and ears to hear the calls of those who are hurting.

> ❝ *Recognizing the overwhelming urge to overlook the pain in the body in front of them, the introspective nurse must tap into the ability to stretch beyond his or her own reality (St. Marie, 2002, p. 3).*

Secondly, we work in health-care systems that still do not hold physicians and nurses accountable for pain relief. This is still true despite the fact

| Box 14-4 ■ | **BARRIERS AND FACILITATORS OF COMFORT** |

BARRIER	FACILITATOR
1. Discomfort is peripheral to our attention.	We choose to pay attention.
2. We do not hold each other accountable for pain relief.	We are accountable and develop systems for accountability.
3. We doubt patients' claim that they are in pain.	We believe patients.
4. We admire people who silently endure.	We develop compassion for those who openly express pain.
5. We blame people for their suffering.	We are deliberately nonjudgmental.
6. We believe severe terminal pain is inevitable.	We never give up efforts to comfort.
7. We lack knowledge of pain and palliation.	We continually seek knowledge and look for clinical experts as our role models.
8. We feel powerless that our voices are not heard.	We choose to be patient advocates. We develop assertiveness skills to speak for those who cannot speak for themselves.
9. We are afraid to comfort.	We become aware of our fears, choose to stop nonproductive thoughts, find role models.
10. We fear opioids.	We use opioids wisely.

that the Joint Committee on Accreditation of Healthcare Organizations (JCAHO) has established pain intensity as the fifth vital sign and initiated standards that include patients' rights to pain relief, assessment and documentation of pain intensity and character, follow-up with pain management, staff education in pain relief, policies for appropriate use of effective analgesics, patient education, and addressing individual needs for pain control after discharge (Phillips, 2000; Rankin & Mitchell, 2000). Within health-care organizations, we must create a culture and develop systems that include reporting pain, handling pain, monitoring pain, and documenting effectiveness of pain interventions.

Third, we are socialized to doubt patients' claims of pain. We fear being deceived about the extent of suffering. Human beings readily doubt the suffering of others; expression of pain is often suspect. We doubt the reality of each other's pain and we judge those who express pain (Scarry, 1985). Even a few encounters with drug-seeking individuals can lead to our unfortunate categorizing of all who complain of pain as potential liars bent on deceiving us. Most are not. Keep in mind that pain is whatever the person experiencing it states that it is (McCaffery, 1979.).

Planting the Seeds

You can often tell the difference between drug seeking individuals and those who need drugs to relieve their pain. The first step is detailed assessment of their pain experience, which you must thoroughly document. Drug seekers not in pain tend to be vague and nonspecific about a pain complaint. Do not assume that terminally ill people who urgently ask for drugs at shorter intervals than ordered or who know a great deal about opioids are drug seekers. Their motivation is likely to be a desire for relief from pain rather than a desire to get "high."

Fourth, we admire those who silently suffer. Expectations of stoicism are deeply embedded in American culture and Western medical traditions. When we are young, we are told to "be strong" and not cry out when we receive injections or have blood drawn. Boys who cry when they are injured are taught to be quiet and "take it like a man." Those who express pain are considered weak and of diminished character. Stoics seek to maintain their indifference in the face of suffering. Nurses must develop compassion for those who openly express pain. Rather than respecting stoicism and silent suffering, nurses should encourage patients to express their pain accurately and not to suffer unnecessarily.

Fifth, in some cultures we blame people for their suffering. Remember that the Latin root word for pain is poena, meaning punishment. Many traditional religious faiths believe that people suffer due to their sins, as indicated by statements like "She'll get what she deserves," and "What goes around comes around." Even among some who hold secular beliefs, there is the assumption that people in pain must have done something wrong to deserve their hurting. Perhaps they ate too much of the wrong food. Perhaps they exercised too little. Perhaps they smoked tobacco or drank alcohol. Perhaps their bad attitude led to disease. We seek to find some fault to explain why some people suffer. It makes us feel safer if there is an explanation as to why someone else suffers. In contrast, nurses must choose to become deliberately nonjudgmental. This can only happen when we become aware of our judgmental assumptions and deliberately seek to suspend them whenever we find them surfacing in our thoughts.

Sixth and seventh, we assume that terminal pain cannot be controlled, revealing a continuing knowledge deficit. Nurses must be open to learning and should continually seek palliative education and clinical experts as our role models and teachers. We must never give up efforts to learn more ways to comfort our patients.

Eighth, nurses feel powerless to speak on behalf of patients in pain. Nurses must continually develop skills in advocacy, and should empower colleagues, followers, and students to speak for those who are hurting. People in pain often need nurses to be their advocates on the interdisciplinary team.

Ninth, we are afraid. Fear and avoidance are basic feelings held by nurses and physicians, and these feelings often become barriers to relieving pain (Zerwekh, 2002). Human beings manage fear by avoiding circumstances in which they feel helpless and vulnerable; avoidance maintains a perception of being in control. We confront our own vulnerabilities and fears when we acknowledge pain and suffering.

❝ | *We confront our own vulnerabilities and fears when we acknowledge pain and suffering.*

Tenth, many nurses and physicians suffer from opiophobia, fearing opioids themselves, afraid that they will cause addiction or suppress respirations. Chapter 15 is devoted to providing the reader with a solid understanding of opioids and evidence that they need not be feared. Knowledge alone, however, does not change practice when fear overwhelms practice judgment. Such severe fears of comforting are best managed by cognitive restructuring approaches, which involve deliberately restructuring destructive thoughts (Zerwekh, 2002). To challenge our fear of comforting with opioids, we must become aware of disturbing thoughts such as "I'm going to make this patient addicted if I give him any more." Question their validity by seeking evidence-based knowledge. Work on stopping the thought as soon as it clouds your mind. Find palliative role models, and seek to be accompanied by those expert colleagues when facing the feared situation. Palliative nurses learn from colleagues with clinical expertise, not from books and lectures alone.

❝ | *Palliative nurses learn from colleagues with clinical expertise, not from books and lectures alone.*

Consider the experience of Tony, who has been a surgical nurse for 6 years. In his hospital and on his unit, he has learned to use opioids sparingly. The other nurses have taught him to give as little as possible and stretch the interval between doses. He tells his patients that pain is expected after surgery and that pain medications might turn them into addicts. The surgeons use patient-controlled intravenous analgesia for the first 24 hours, then switch to acetaminophen with oxycodone, which is minimally effective and often causes heartburn and nausea. He has begun to wonder whether better acute pain relief might help his patients breathe more deeply, ambulate more quickly, and develop fewer complications. However, he is still afraid of giving opioids. Recently, five beds on his unit have been converted for palliative care. Following a 2-day palliative care course, Tony remained skeptical about the pain relief principles he had learned, but he sincerely wanted to help his dying patients. Therefore, he chose the following strategy:

1. Whenever a patient tells him the pain is severe, he is aware of his own skepticism and his own judgments like, "It can't be that bad. She's just complaining. She's too dependent on these drugs."
2. He challenges his own assumption, listens carefully to the patients, and responds with the best relief measures he has available.
3. When dealing with high opioid doses that frighten him, he seeks out the palliative-care nurse specialist to review the situation and go with him to the bedside, if possible.

Patient Barriers

In addition to barriers put up by health professionals, there are many barriers to patients themselves accepting pain relief (Ersek, 1999). Hesitant to distract physicians from disease treatment and fearing that pain is a sign that the disease is worsening, patients may be reluctant to report pain. They may decide that reporting pain is whining or complaining and seek to be a "good patient." Fearing addiction or worrying about opioid side effects or tolerance, they may hesitate to take medication. Some people will proclaim, "I'm just not the kind of person that takes drugs." For others, cost is a barrier to effective analgesics. Some patients expect themselves to be stoic and others are fatalistic in accepting their suffering. If pain relief involves painful injections, some patients will choose to endure pain rather than needles.

ASSESSING PAIN

Comforting requires the nurse to detect patient cues of distress (Morse, 2000). Assessing discomfort involves recognizing signs and symptoms based on a willingness to see, hear, and empathize with the patient's emotion and discomfort. The bedrock of pain assessment is asking patients about their pain and questioning them carefully about it. Essential components of pain assessment (see Box 14-5, Pain Characteristics Needing Assessment) are the determination of location, intensity, quality, pattern, aggravating factors, alleviating factors, and effects on life. Each characteristic is discussed in the following section, which concludes by proposing an acronym that can be useful to remember all of the components of pain assessment. Box 14-6 illustrates the Wisconsin Brief Pain Inventory, which is a practical clinical tool for ongoing pain assessment.

Location

It is essential to determine exactly where the pain is located and to examine that area physically, observing the site and palpating for tenderness. Many

Box 14-5 ■	PAIN CHARACTERISTICS NEEDING ASSESSMENT
CHARACTERISTIC	SAMPLE QUESTIONS TO ASK
Location	Where is your pain? Show me where you hurt. Can you point out the places where it hurts?
Intensity	How bad is your pain? Can you rate it for me on a scale from 0 to 10 with 10 being the worst pain you have ever had and 1 being no pain?
Quality	What words can you use to describe your pain? Examples might be dull, aching, cramping, twisting, burning, stabbing, shocking.
Pattern	Is your pain predictable? When is it worse and when is it better?
Aggravating Factors	What makes your pain worse? Examples might be movement, a certain position, toileting, or after eating.
Alleviating Factors	What relieves your pain and makes you feel better? What is the effect of medication?
Effects on Life	How is the pain influencing your life? Is it interfering with sleep or activity? How does it affect you emotionally or in your relationships? Is it affecting your spiritual life?

patients report pain in several locations. Failure to question and examine carefully can result in mistakes like giving morphine for shoulder pain due to bursitis or for abdominal pain related to constipation! When patients complain of hurting all over, consider that it may be due to psychosocial suffering, although such pain is sometimes due to myalgia, arthritis, or multiple metastases. Investigate the source. It is helpful in the patient record to have a simple diagram of the human body, front and back, to locate the pain.

Intensity

Patients should be asked to quantify their pain using a subjective rating scale. With a numerical scale, a horizontal or vertical line is anchored on one end with a zero meaning "no pain" and at the other end with a maximum of 5 or 10 indicating "severe pain." The patient assigns the severity of pain a number from 0 to 5 or 0 to 10. In the visual analogue scale, the line is drawn with "no pain" at one end and "severe pain" at the other end. The patient is

Box 14-6 ■ WISCONSIN BRIEF PAIN INVENTORY (SHORT FORM)

Study ID# _____   Hospital # _____
Do not write above this line
Date: _____/_____/_____
Time: _____
Name: _____
Last   First   Middle Initial

1) Throughout our lives, most of us have had pain from time to time (such as minor headaches, sprains, and toothaches). Have you had pain other than these everyday kinds of pain today?

1. yes   2. no

2) On the diagram, shade in the areas where you feel pain. Put an X on the area that hurts the most.

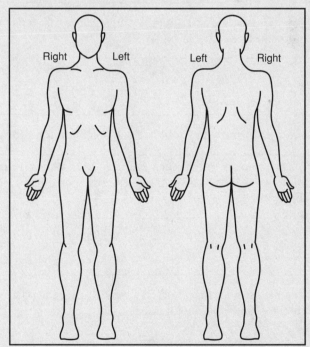

3) Please rate your pain by circling the one number that best describes your pain at its WORST in the past 24 hours.

0	1	2	3	4	5	6	7	8	9	10

No
pain

Pain as bad as
you can imagine

(continued)

Box 14-6 ■	**WISCONSIN BRIEF PAIN INVENTORY (SHORT FORM) (CONTINUED)**

4) Please rate your pain by circling the one number that best describes your pain at its LEAST in the past 24 hours.

0	1	2	3	4	5	6	7	8	9	10
No pain									Pain as bad as you can imagine	

5) Please rate your pain by circling the one number that best describes your pain on the AVERAGE.

0	1	2	3	4	5	6	7	8	9	10
No pain									Pain as bad as you can imagine	

6) Please rate your pain by circling the one number that tells how much pain you have RIGHT NOW.

0	1	2	3	4	5	6	7	8	9	10
No pain									Pain as bad as you can imagine	

7) What treatments or medications are you receiving for your pain?

8) In the past 24 hours, how much RELIEF have pain treatments or medications provided? Please circle the one percentage that most shows how much.

0%	10%	20%	30%	40%	50%	60%	70%	80%	90%	100%
No relief										Complete relief

9) Circle the one number that describes how, during the past 24 hours, PAIN HAS INTERFERED with your:

A. General Activity:

0	1	2	3	4	5	6	7	8	9	10
Does not interfere									Completely interferes	

Box 14-6 ■ (CONTINUED)

B. Mood

0	1	2	3	4	5	6	7	8	9	10

Does not
interfere

Completely
interferes

C. Walking ability

0	1	2	3	4	5	6	7	8	9	10

Does not
interfere

Completely
interferes

D. Normal work (includes both work outside the home and housework)

0	1	2	3	4	5	6	7	8	9	10

Does not
interfere

Completely
interferes

E. Relations with other people

0	1	2	3	4	5	6	7	8	9	10

Does not
interfere

Completely
interferes

F. Sleep

0	1	2	3	4	5	6	7	8	9	10

Does not
interfere

Completely
interferes

G. Enjoyment of life

0	1	2	3	4	5	6	7	8	9	10

Does not
interfere

Completely
interferes

Source: Pain Research Group, Department of Neurology, University of Wisconsin-
Madison. Used with permission.

Box 14-7 ■	**PAIN INTENSITY SCALES**

Visual Analogue Scale
Numeric Pain Rating Scale
Descriptive Words Pain Rating Scale

asked not to rate the pain with a number, but to mark the place on the line that represents the intensity of the pain. The FACES Scale, as mentioned earlier, uses cartoon faces with a smiling face at 0 and a grimacing face or a face with tears at the other end of the scale. See Box 12-4. The Verbal Rating Scale, another option, asks the patient to rate the severity of pain using descriptive adjectives that correspond to a numerical rating. See Box 14-7, Pain Intensity Scales.

Most patients are able to assign a number to rate the intensity of their pain, but some cannot understand the abstract concept that a smaller or larger number indicates less or greater pain. They may be able to use the verbal rating scale, however, to describe the range of pain: none, annoying, uncomfortable, dreadful, horrible, or agonizing (Abrahm, 2000). For children and the cognitively impaired, or those for whom language is a barrier, the FACES scale may be useful. When the patient cannot self report his or her pain using any of these subjective rating schemes, careful observation of functional clues indicates both success and failure to relieve pain. The nurse should take careful note of alterations in sleep, activity, mood, ability to relate, and ability to enjoy life. Nonverbal clues suggesting pain include irritability, withdrawal, grimacing, and moaning. These indicators should be compared with the patient's baseline behavior.

Quality

Vivid description of the quality of pain is helpful to determine the underlying cause. The McGill Pain Questionnaire (see Box 14-8) is a well-tested, widely used instrument to elicit patients' verbal descriptions of their pain. Pain can be categorized as somatic, visceral, and neuropathic. *Somatic pain* is described as aching and dull, increased by movement, and able to be localized to the injured area (Abrahm, 2000). Somatic pain arises from skin, bone, muscle, connective tissues, and blood vessels. This is the pain associated with arthritis and bone metastases. *Visceral pain* can be aching, but can also feel like squeezing and cramping. Visceral pain arises from the internal organs and lining of body cavities. Visceral pain can localize to superficial tissues and radiate to a larger area of skin or muscle. This is the pain of myocardial ischemia or liver metastases. *Neuropathic pain* is described as burning, shooting, tingling, or shock-like. It arises from damage to peripheral nerves. This pain is experienced in diabetic and AIDS neuropathies.

Box 14-8 ■ # McGILL PAIN QUESTIONNAIRE

Patient's Name _____ Date _____ Time _____ am/pm

PRI:S _____ A _____ E _____ M _____ PRI(T) _____ PPI ____
   (1-10)   (11-15)   (16)   (17-20)   (1-20)

1
FLICKERING ___
QUIVERING ___
PULSING ___
THROBBING ___
BEATING ___
POUNDING ___

2 JUMPING ___
FLASHING ___
SHOOTING ___

3 PRICKING ___
BORING ___
DRILLING ___
STABBING ___
LANCINATING ___

4 SHARP ___
CUTTING ___
LACERATING ___

5 PINCHING ___
PRESSING ___
GNAWING ___
CRAMPING ___
CRUSHING ___

6 TUGGING ___
PULLING ___
WRENCHING ___

7 HOT ___
BURNING ___
SCALDING ___
SEARING ___

8 TINGLING ___
ITCHY ___
SMARTING ___
STINGING ___

9 DULL ___
SORE ___
HURTING ___
ACHING ___
HEAVY ___

10 TENDER ___
TAUT ___
RASPING ___
SPLITTING ___

11 TIRING ___
EXHAUSTING ___

12 SICKENING ___
SUFFOCATING ___

13 FEARFUL ___
FRIGHTFUL ___
TERRIFYING ___

14 PUNISHING ___
GRUELLING ___
CRUEL ___
VICIOUS ___
KILLING ___

15 WRETCHED ___
BLINDING ___

16 ANNOYING ___
TROUBLESOME ___
MISERABLE ___
INTENSE ___
UNBEARABLE ___

17 SPREADING ___
RADIATING ___
PENETRATING ___
PIERCING ___

18 TIGHT ___
NUMB ___
DRAWING ___
SQUEEZING ___
TEARING ___

19 COOL ___
COLD ___
FREEZING ___

20 NAGGING ___
NAUSEATING ___
AGONIZING ___
DREADFUL ___
TORTURING ___

PPI
0 NO PAIN ___
1 MILD ___
2 DISCOMFORTING ___
3 DISTRESSING ___
4 HORRIBLE ___
5 EXCRUCIATING ___

BRIEF ___	RHYTHMIC ___	CONTINUOUS ___
MOMENTARY ___	PERIODIC ___	STEADY ___
TRANSIENT ___	INTERMITTENT ___	CONSTANT ___

E = EXTERNAL
I = INTERNAL

COMMENTS:

Pattern

Some pain may always be present and is termed baseline pain. Breakthrough pain may occur with activity, or as a result of underlying pathophysiology. The pattern should be documented because it assists in diagnosing the underlying cause. For instance, the pain of arthritis and bone metastases is aching and continual; it increases with movement. The pain of bowel obstruction comes and goes. The burning pain that can be a complication of breast surgery increases when the arm is extended and diminished when the arm is flexed (Abrahm, 2000).

Aggravating and Alleviating Factors

Thorough initial pain assessment requires determining those factors that make the pain worse, such as deep breathing or anxiety, and those factors that alleviate pain. For instance, if massage reduces the pain, the pathology is likely to be of musculoskeletal origin, rather than neuropathic (ELNEC, 2000). Likewise, determine and document drugs and other remedies that have worked and not worked. For instance, have heat, cold, or other traditional or alternative remedies brought relief? Ask about herbal products and over-the-counter drugs. A plan of care should include whatever works to bring relief, and should, obviously, avoid those factors that aggravate pain.

Effects on Life

As has been discussed, pain can impair all aspects of life quality: emotional, social, economic, and spiritual. Nurses are particularly concerned with enhancing patients' quality of living while dying. Therefore, we need to inquire about how the pain is interfering with everyday activities, such as work, movement, leisure activity, eating, sleeping, and relationships. Likewise, ask how the pain is affecting the person emotionally and spiritually. Inquire about depression, anxiety, fear, and enjoyment. What is the effect on the family? The following questions are useful to determine how pain may impact spiritual life (Abrahm, 2002):

- What are your religious beliefs about pain?
- Have your beliefs changed since you started to live with pain?
- Has there been any value to your living with pain?
- Has the pain affected your spiritual practice?
- Has the pain affected your spiritual beliefs or your relationship with God?

Investigating the effects of pain on the person's life assures the patient that we care about what they are enduring, and helps us to determine the actual extent of the pain experienced so that we can develop an effective plan

---

Box 14-9 ◼ W5 TO ASSESS PAIN

A straightforward acronym to remember for pain assessment is W5. This acronym includes five words: Where, Words, When, Worsens, Whole.

W1—*Where* is the pain located?
W2—*Words* to describe. Ask the patient to rate pain intensity and describe quality. Watch for nonverbal indicators.
W3—*When* does the pain occur? What is the pattern during the day?
W4—What *worsens* and relieves the pain? This identifies the aggravating and alleviating factors.
W5—*Whole* life. What effect is the pain having on the person's whole life?

---

of care. Box 14-9, W5 to Assess Pain, proposes an acronym that can be helpful to assess the total pain experience.

The initial pain history provides a baseline, but then the patient must be frequently reassessed. Patients must be urged to report changes in their pain. Rapid disease progression requires frequent reassessment in the last weeks of life. Pain ratings are now commonly charted at the same time as vital signs. But then we must take action to relieve the documented pain and comfort those who suffer. Box 14-10, Pain Management Outcome Measures, can be used to monitor pain management quality as part of hospital quality improvement efforts.

Box 14-10 ◼ PAIN MANAGEMENT OUTCOME MEASURES

1. Intensity of pain documented by a descriptive or numeric rating scale
2. Pain treated by a route other than intramuscular
3. Pain treated with regularly scheduled analgesics and other comforting interventions
4. Pain prevented and controlled to maximize function and life quality
5. Patients educated about pain management

Source: From Gordon et al. (2002).

COMFORTING NURSING PRACTICE

Nurses risk being in the presence of pain without seeing, hearing, or responding. We must re-train ourselves to be advocates for those suffering. "Understanding suffering, and the responses and needs of those who are suffering, rests squarely on the shoulders of nurses, and easing and alleviating suffering are the heart of nursing" (Morse, 2001, pp. 47–48). We are the largest group of health professionals and spend the most time at the sides of those in pain. We must choose to know patient experience and witness the presence of suffering. Witnessing requires seeing, hearing, acknowledging, documenting, and speaking out about pain. We must give voice to the burning, stabbing, and crushing experiences of patients so that their pain is not disregarded. We must not be silent. The American Society of Pain Management Nurses identifies five important ingredients for pain relief; see Box 14-1.

Comforting nursing interventions to relieve pain and other distress include developing a caring relationship, teaching, anticipating comfort needs, offering hands-on comforting, attending to stimulation and rest, initiating complementary therapies, and managing pharmacological therapies.

Developing a Caring Relationship

A caring nurse-patient relationship is vital to comforting patients in pain. Details of the practice of connecting and caring presence are contained in Chapter 6. As has been described, pain can be an isolating, power draining, and emotionally debilitating experience. Patients may have little energy to reach out to others. The relationship offered by the nurse needs to be a genuine encounter; the nurse's nonverbal and verbal behavior should communicate attention and receptivity. Persistence is essential because trust may develop very slowly, appearing only after the nurse has "proven" his or her reliability by persistently being present and implementing pain-relieving approaches that work. The expert nurse seeks to be available without being intrusive, offering to talk or just be there. A therapeutic relationship develops as we share our understanding of the patient's experience, and as patients validate and clarify what they are actually experiencing. This relationship with the nurse can help sustain the patient through the pain experience. Total pain can be eased significantly through experience of another's presence. Just as isolation and abandonment heighten pain, the presence of a caring person is calming and relieving. Here, one nurse explains her use of presence to ease the anxiety of a patient who had not relaxed despite significant opioid dosing:

> I sat at her side, quietly. She could no longer speak but had been moaning and rocking with distress all morning. I held her hand lightly and waited. After a while, she rested and fell asleep.

Teaching

Effective teaching is central to the goal of empowering the patient and family to learn to manage pain in the home environment. A teaching relationship begins with assessing the patient and family caregiver's concerns, knowledge, motivation, and ability to learn. The nurse must then determine realistic learning objectives based on his or her own knowledge of pain relief and on assessment of what the particular patient/family needs to learn. Because there are so many behaviors that must be learned in order to manage pain effectively, the teaching relationship needs to be extended over time. Objectives are not stated in terms of what the nurse teaches, but in terms of how the learner behaves following teaching. Sometimes, presenting the facts in a clear and systematic way may not result in learning because of emotional and cognitive barriers.

Strong emotions, including fear, are striking barriers to patients and families learning how to relieve pain (Zerwekh, 2002). Patients/families may not acknowledge the pain because of its association with progressive disease and loss of control. Patients may refuse to acknowledge pain or listen to nursing suggestions for its relief because they are protecting family from facing their condition; because their doctor told them they do not need so much medication; because they fear addiction; because they believe they must suffer for their sins; and for reasons that they cannot put into words. Likewise, impaired thought and attention render many dying patients unable to report their pain reliably or to manage their own comfort measures.

At the end of life, patients dying at home become reliant on family caregivers to administer pain relief. However, family resistance to comforting parallels patient issues around fear and avoidance (Zerwekh, 2002). In addition, family dynamics can be quite challenging. Family members may continue life-long abusive patterns. They may be impaired by mental illness or chemical dependency. They may refuse to have opioids in the house.

In challenging teaching situations, the nurse works with the interdisciplinary team to achieve the best possible outcomes. Individualized education that directly addresses patient misconceptions about pain treatment, along with development of strategies to control pain in order to address each person's own goals, is quite effective (Oliver, Kravitz, Kaplan, and Meyers, 2001). Often, patients need to develop and practice ways of negotiating with the physician even to receive satisfactory pain treatment in the first place. Nurses also help patients to develop these negotiation skills.

Anticipating Comfort Needs

Anticipating comfort needs is a hallmark of palliative nursing. With experience, the nurse becomes able to predict the likely disease course and anticipate possible signs and symptoms. If pain exacerbation is likely, the family is prepared for it. Likewise, the nurse plans ahead for dyspnea, bleeding, seizures, anxiety, and whatever other sources of distress are likely. A nurse explains:

We anticipate crises so that they are not crises. We walk through possibilities step-by-step. What would you do if he hemorrhages? What would you do if the pain gets bad and he can't swallow? We keep medications for crises in the home and teach the family how to manage.

Hands-on Comforting

Nurses comfort through hands-on nursing. We care for the body; we shave, turn, and care for the mouth and skin. "Skin is the locus of many comfort measures— a point of connection. . . . Sociologists point out that care of the skin and body is not high-status work, nor is it likely to be in a society that avoids images of dependency and the need for care" (Benner, Hooper-Kyriakidis, and Stannard, 1999, pp. 257–258). Yet hands-on comforting involves the skilled practice of basic nursing measures, such as positioning, dressing changes, and management of secretions to reduce discomfort. Here is a creative example of positioning to promote comfort:

> She and her husband had been sleeping in separate beds. He was afraid of hurting her and she was afraid that her swollen leg would hurt if they slept together. So we looked at the beds and bedroom and ways to arrange the beds. We put a single bed next to the double bed so there would be extra room. Then we got the two of them in and figured out a position with pillows so that she could have support for her leg and they could just cuddle.

Another nurse describes management of dressings and secretions to promote comfort:

> I cleaned and changed dressings and tried to organize his supplies. His caregiver was overwhelmed. He had a fulminating wound and there were secretions all over the place. I spent half of my time on my knees in order to dress his wounds. We got the secretions under control and I made the dressings more manageable. He became less anxious and his pain finally came under control.

Hands-on comforting also includes technological expertise when infusion pumps and access devices are used to infuse opioids A nurse describes this dimension of comforting.

> I did a lot of teaching until Doris became competent at managing the pump that infused the morphine into his epidural space. She knew how to turn it on and off. She could change the bags herself. We had to do quite a bit of trouble shooting with that pump. Joe's epidural catheter came around to his abdomen in front. We taught her to do the dressing changes around it and to watch for infection.

Attending to Stimulation and Rest

Attention to stimulation and rest is essential to comfort. Planning for and providing stimulation, distraction, rest, and retreat are vital comforting measures that require becoming attuned to the person's life. The nurse can help establish normal rhythms of day and night, rest and activity. In the technical environment, the nurse seeks to tame the disturbances of technology by controlling noise and light and intrusion. (Benner et al., p. 271). The contemporary challenge is that these nursing comfort measures can appear quite humble and ordinary to the point that organizational cultures ignore and eliminate them in favor of technological rituals.

In the home environment, patients and families need help to control visitors and telephone calls, and to ensure periods of uninterrupted rest and sleep. Likewise, meaningful activities should be planned as the patient wishes. For instance, an older patient may want to rest all day in order to get up for the Wednesday night bridge group with friends she has had for more than 30 years. A young dying woman may want to skip the nurse's next visit so that friends can take her to sit on the warm sand at the beach.

Complementary Therapies

At the end of life, expert nurses are open to using *complementary therapies*, such as music, herbs, or acupressure to complement mainstream palliative medicine. Complementary or integrative therapies include healing resources presently not considered part of conventional health care. Conventional health care is rooted in Western philosophy and is guided by scientific methods focused on treating disease (HPNA, 2003). Complementary methods are used in addition to, not as an alternative to, conventional palliative methods. These methods *complement* conventional medicine and are *integrated* in the conventional plan of care. Complementary therapies often are grounded in Eastern philosophy, emphasizing a holistic approach, the human experience of illness, and quality of life. In general, these therapies are less well studied than conventional approaches. Nevertheless, the National Center for Complementary and Alternative Medicine was established in 1998 as a division of the National Institutes of Health to support research. Palliative nursing roles regarding complementary therapies include:

- Gaining knowledge about specific types of complementary therapies, particularly their evidence base
- Informing patients and helping them decide about using these therapies
- Referring patients to qualified and respected complementary therapists
- Learning to utilize and incorporating selected types of complementary therapies in nursing practice to comfort

Box 14-11 identifies types of complementary and integrative therapies.

Box 14-11 ■	TYPES OF COMPLEMENTARY AND INTEGRATIVE THERAPIES

TYPE	EXAMPLES
Energy therapies that are intended to influence energy fields of body	Therapeutic touch Reiki Qi gong
Physical manipulation of body	Chiropractic Massage therapy Osteopathic manipulation
Biological therapies	Herbal therapies Dietary therapies
Mind-body interventions	Prayer Art, music, dance Hypnosis Meditation
Alternative medical systems in contrast to Western (allopathic) medicine	*Ayurvedic medicine*, traditional medicine of India that includes meditation, breathing, diet, exercise, massage, herbs, diet *Traditional Chinese medicine*, including herbs, massage, Qi gong, acupuncture *Homeopathy*, which uses small doses of minerals and plant extracts to strengthen the body's defense mechanisms *Naturopathy*, which incorporates diet, herbs, homeopathy, acupuncture, spinal manipulation, counseling, and physical therapies

■
WWW.   Internet Reference Box

The National Center for Complementary and Alternative Medicine Web site can be accessed at *www.nccam.nih.gov/health/whatiscam*.

A hospice nurse describes using imagery, one type of complementary technique, with a paralyzed young woman dying from multiple sclerosis:

She had difficulties with speech, with swallowing, with urination, with pain from muscle spasms. Since the pain was episodic, continuous opioids just knocked her out. The only thing she responded to for pain was imagery. I made imagery tapes with her. She would visualize her pain as a red spot and then I would have her visualize it getting light pink, then clear, and then blowing away in the breeze. Whenever she was having pain, she would ask for the tapes and the pain would go away.

Managing Pharmacological Therapies

Skilled end-of-life comforting requires that the nurse persistently work with the physician or nurse practitioner to try multiple pharmacological options as needed to comfort. The nurse communicates the need for analgesics and the experienced nurse actually makes recommendations for appropriate drugs. This requires balancing palliative success versus side effects of drugs. Fear of side effects must be overcome to permit competent adjustment of drugs. Organizing and reorganizing regimens and making major changes in regimens are essential end-of-life nursing competencies when the patient's condition is constantly changing. A nurse describes one visit, "Medication routes were changed, schedules adjusted, oxygen added, and personal care needs addressed." The knowledge foundational to managing palliative medications is discussed in Chapter 15, focusing on pharmacological pain management, and Chapter 16, focusing on relief of symptoms other than pain.

CONCLUSION

Pain and symptom management should be based on the following fundamentals:

1. Don't make assumptions. Believe the patient's report of pain and other symptoms.
2. Relieve the pain to the extent patients choose and in ways they can accept.
3. Repeatedly investigate physical, psychosocial, and spiritual dimensions of pain and evaluate the effectiveness of interventions.
4. Anticipate pain and other symptoms and relieve them before they reoccur.
5. Include nursing and complementary interventions.
6. Develop expertise in the use of palliative medication.
7. Choose the least complex intervention to keep end-of-life care affordable and manageable by patients and families at home.
8. Never give up hope of relieving discomfort. Keep trying different approaches.

CONCEPTS IN ACTION

Consider the plight of Maria, age 29, living with advanced AIDS. Maria's family emigrated from Guatemala when she was 14 years old. Maria's husband has already died of AIDS; she is living in a church-sponsored adult home after her parents and brother, fearful of contagion and feeling deep family shame, rejected her. She has lost one third of her body weight so that she currently weighs 85 pounds. Her vision is impaired due to CMV infection. Sitting for long periods and lying in one position cause significant neuromuscular pain. Invasive cervical cancer is causing pelvic, back, and leg pain. Poorly controlled diarrhea has caused painful rectal excoriation. Currently, she is being seen by a team of four infection-control specialists who practice at the county hospital.

1. What kind of pain would you expect Maria to describe? What questions would you ask her to assess her pain thoroughly?
2. What psychosocial dimensions of pain are relevant to Maria's case?
3. Are there any barriers to pain control that might be particularly likely with Maria?
4. Consider causes of Maria's discomfort. What hands-on comforting measures will be essential?
5. What complementary nursing measures might be especially helpful for Maria? Look up traditional Hispanic healing methods in a cross-cultural nursing text.

References

Abrahm, J. (2000). *A physician's guide to pain and symptom management in cancer patients.* Baltimore: Johns Hopkins.

Benner, P., Hooper-Kyriakidis, P., & Stannard, D. (1999). *Clinical wisdom and Interventions in critical care.* Philadelphia: WB Saunders.

Bernabei, R., Gambassi, G., Lapane, K., & Landi, F. (1998). Management of pain in elderly patients with cancer. *Journal of the American Medical Association, 279*(23), 1877–1883.

Bruera, E., & Kim, H. (2003). Cancer pain. *Journal of the American Medical Association, 290*(18), 2476.

Cassell, E. (1991). *The nature of suffering and the goals of medicine.* New York: Oxford University Press.

ELNEC (End-of-Life Nursing Consortium). (2000). *Pain management.*

Washington, DC: American Association of Colleges of Nursing.

Ersek, M. (1999). Enhancing effective pain management by addressing patient barriers to analgesic use. *Journal of Hospice and Palliative Nursing, 1*(3), 87–96.

Fagerhaugh, S., & Strauss, A. (1977). *Politics of Pain Management.* Menlo Park, CA: Addison-Wesley.

Hoffman, D., & Tarzian, A. (2001). The girl who cried pain: A bias against women in the treatment of pain. *Journal of Law, Medicine and Ethics, 29,* 13–27.

Hospice and Palliative Nursing Association (HPNA). (2003). Position paper: Complementary therapies. *Journal of Hospice and Palliative Nursing, 5*(2), 113–117.

Hospice and Palliative Nursing Association (HPNA). (2004). Position paper: Pain. *Journal of Hospice and Palliative Nursing, 6*(1), 62–63.

Huff, S., & Joshi, P. (2001). Pain and symptom management. In A. Armstrong-Daily & B. Zarbock (Eds.), *Hospice care for children* (pp. 23–48). New York: Oxford University Press.

Institute of Medicine. (2003). *When children die: Improving palliative and end of life care for children and their families.* Washington, DC: National Academy Press.

Lasch, K. E. (2000). Culture, pain, and culturally sensitive pain care. *Pain Management Nursing, 1*(Suppl. 1), 16–22.

McCaffery, M. (1979). *Nursing management of the patient with pain.* Philadelphia: Lippincott.

Miakowski, C. (2000). The impact of age on a patient's perception of pain and ways it can be managed. *Pain Management Nursing, 1*(Suppl. 1), 2–7.

Morse, J. (2001). Toward a praxis theory of suffering. *Advances in Nursing Science, 24*(1), 47–59.

National Medical Association (NMA) Panel (2002).

Oliver, J. W., Kravitz, R., Kaplan, S., & Meyers, F. (2001). Individualized patient education and coaching to improve pain control among cancer outpatients. *Journal of Clinical Oncology, 19*(8), 2206–2212.

Paice, J., Muir, J. C., & Shott, S. (2004). Palliative care at the end of life: Comparing quality in diverse settings. *American Journal of Hospice and Palliative Care, 21*(1), 19–27.

Panke, J. (2003). Difficulties in managing pain at the end of life. *Journal of Hospice and Palliative Nursing, 5*(2), 83–90.

Pasero, C., & McCaffery, M. (2004). Comfort-function goals. *American Journal of Nursing, 104*(9), 77–81.

Phillips, D. (2000). JCAHO pain management standards are unveiled. *Journal of the American Medical Association, 284*(4), 428–429.

Rankin, E., & Mitchell, M. (2000). Creating a pain management education module for hospice nurses: Integrating the new JCAHO standards and the AHCPR pain management guidelines. *Journal of Hospice and Palliative Nursing, 2*(3), 91–100.

Rich, B. (2001). Prioritizing pain management in patient care. *Postgraduate Medicine, 111*(3), 15–17.

Saunders, C. (1976). *Care of the dying.* London: Nursing Times.

Scarry, E. (1985). *The body in pain: The making and unmasking of the world.* New York: Oxford University Press.

St. Marie, B. (2002). *American society of pain management nurses: Core curriculum for pain management nursing.* Philadelphia: WB Saunders.

Vallerand, A., & Polomano, R. (2000). The relationship of gender to pain. *Pain Management Nursing, 1*(Suppl. 1), 8–15.

Vastag, B. (2003). Scientists find connections in the brain between physical and emotional pain. *Journal of American Medical Association, 290*(18), 2389.

Wiesel, E. (1986). Nobel Acceptance Speech. Oslo, Norway. Available through the Elie Wiesel Foundation for Humanity.

Zerwekh, J. (2002). Fearing to comfort: A grounded theory of constraints to opioid use in hospice care. *Journal of Hospice and Palliative Nursing, 4*(2), 83–90.

CHAPTER 15

Medicating for Pain at the End of Life

Joyce Zerwekh and Dionetta Hudzinski

Philosophical Reflections

"Suffering enforces isolation. It ruptures a person's sense of wholeness, fracturing his or her personhood."

Gregory & English, 2001, p. 21

Learning Objectives

1. Identify and explain essential principles for using palliative analgesia at the end of life.
2. Identify the effects and side effects of nonopioid analgesics.
3. Identify the therapeutic and side effects of opioids.
4. Examine three common fears that physicians and nurses may have about using opioids and identify evidence that counters those fears.
5. Identify the common opioids and those best used at the end of life.
6. Explain the different opioid routes and approaches to determining effective dosages.
7. Identify the effects of adjuvant medications commonly used to relieve pain.
8. Describe the use of analgesics for neuropathic pain, bony metastases, and elderly patients.
9. Explain six nursing responsibilities in the use of palliative medication at the end of life.

Chapter 14 defined pain, addressed the challenges in its relief, described comprehensive pain assessment, and identified independent nursing actions that provide comforting. Because the severity of end-of-life pain usually requires drug therapy, this chapter provides a sound foundation for understanding the drugs that are used to provide comfort. Pain relief is symbolized by the leaves on the End-of-Life Caregiving Tree. The numerous leaves represent the multiple ways that physical suffering can be relieved. In order to explain drug therapy for pain, this chapter first introduces essential principles for using analgesics to control terminal pain. It then examines nonopioid analgesics, opioid analgesics, adjuvant drugs, and the collaborative nursing role in medicating for pain. The chapter also explores published clinical practice guidelines as resources to change institutional pain management practice.

BASIC ESSENTIALS OF MEDICATING FOR PAIN AT THE END OF LIFE

Medicating for pain should be guided by certain essential concepts. Analgesics should be carefully adjusted to individual need, balancing therapeutic and side effects. Individuals vary dramatically in their response to opioids; genetic differences determine how they metabolize the drugs (Fine, Miaskowski, and Paice, 2004). There is no certainty of the degree of pain relief that can be expected given a specific amount of medication. Therefore, it is essential to monitor the degree of pain and the extent of relief continually in order to be successful in relieving terminal pain. At the end of life, it may be necessary to make frequent adjustments in drugs, dosage, and interval when underlying disease processes change and escalate. The following three basic essentials are summarized in brief.

 It is essential to monitor the degree of pain and extent of relief continually in order to be successful in relieving terminal pain.

In Brief: Scheduling of Analgesics

Analgesics should be scheduled around the clock (ATC) to maintain continuous blood levels and prevent recurrence of pain. When pain medication is given p.r.n. (as needed, only when the patient complains) after the pain becomes dominant, the pattern of pain relief becomes a roller coaster with episodes of suffering alternating with episodes of relief.

Long-acting preparations are preferable to short-acting (immediate release) preparations in order to sustain blood levels. Taking medication every 12 hours permits long periods of rest. This is the reason for a growing number of sustained or controlled-release (CR) opioids now on the market. In addition to receiving long-acting opioids, patients also need orders for breakthrough pain, which requires supplementary immediate-release (IR) opioids.

In Brief: Routes of Administration

Using the least invasive route for analgesic administration is a fundamental principle for contemporary palliative care. The first choice of route of administration for control of terminal pain should be oral because it is easiest to manage and also highly effective. We now understand that most patients can be kept comfortable without needing injections or infusions. It does take a larger amount of a drug to be effective by mouth than if it is given by injection, but opioids taken by mouth are well absorbed and able to maintain a constant blood level.

> 66 | *Using the least invasive route for analgesic administration is a*
> | *fundamental principle for contemporary palliative care.*

In Brief: The Three-Step Ladder

The World Health Organization has established a three-step ladder as an international guide to pain relief. See Figure 15-1, The Three-Step Ladder. The first step is to use a nonopioid analgesic and perhaps an adjuvant medication. Adjuvants include corticosteroids, antidepressants, anxiolytics, anticonvulsants, muscle relaxants, anesthetics, bisphosphonates, and other agents that target underlying causes of pain. When pain persists, the second step is to add an opioid for mild-to-moderate pain. Perhaps include a nonopioid or perhaps add an adjuvant medication. When pain continues or is accelerating, the third step is to add a strong opioid for moderate or severe pain, as well as nonopioid and adjuvant medications as needed. Box 15-1 summarizes Effective Use of Analgesics.

Figure 15-1 The Three-Step Ladder.

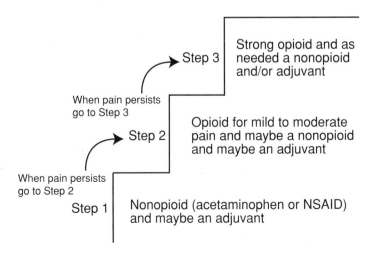

Step 3 — Strong opioid and as needed a nonopioid and/or adjuvant

When pain persists go to Step 3

Step 2 — Opioid for mild to moderate pain and maybe a nonopioid and maybe an adjuvant

When pain persists go to Step 2

Step 1 — Nonopioid (acetaminophen or NSAID) and maybe an adjuvant

| Box 15-1 ■ | EFFECTIVE USE OF ANALGESICS |

1. Individualize plan for each patient
2. Monitor effects and side effects
3. Keep adjusting and readjusting as needed
4. Schedule around-the-clock, not p.r.n.
5. Anticipate breakthrough pain and ensure medication available
6. Give by mouth as much as possible
7. Use nonopioids, opioids, and adjuvants according to the WHO ladder.

NONOPIOID ANALGESICS

Nonopioid analgesics are used for mild pain at the end of life and in combination with opioids for mild-to-moderate pain. The nonopioid analgesics include acetaminophen (Tylenol) and the nonsteroidal anti-inflammatory drugs (NSAIDS). NSAIDS include a wide variety of preparations such as aspirin, ibuprofen (Motrin, Advil), and the COX-2 NSAIDS (Celebrex). There are also nonopioid analgesics, such as capsaicin cream, that provide relief of mild pain when they are absorbed through the skin.

Acetaminophen relieves pain and reduces fever; it does not have the prominent anti-inflammatory effect of the NSAIDS. Unlike the NSAIDS, it does not impair platelet aggregation or cause gastrointestinal problems. The most serious side effect of acetaminophen is liver dysfunction when taken in doses higher than 4000 mg (AAHPM, 2003). Acetaminophen has a ceiling effect, which means that a patient gets no added relief beyond taking 4000 mg daily (Abrahm, 2000). Acetaminophen is commonly mixed with an opioid to treat mild-to-moderate pain. As pain accelerates and the intake of these acetaminophen/opioid compounds increases, there is a risk of liver toxicity. Some of the most commonly used compounds are 5 mg oxycodone with 325 mg acetaminophen (Percocet), 5 mg oxycodone with 500 mg acetaminophen (Tylox), and 5 mg hydrocodone with 500 mg acetaminophen (Vicodin). As pain worsens, it is not uncommon for a patient to keep increasing his dosage. For example, a patient taking two Tylox every four hours around the clock will end up with an acetaminophen dose of 2×500 mg $= 1000$ mg per dose $\times 6$ doses in a day $= 6000$ mg acetaminophen a daily, a toxic dose. Obviously, such compounds are inappropriate to manage accelerating pain.

NSAIDS reduce the secretion of the biochemical mediator prostaglandin. Prostaglandins activate the sensory nerve endings that transmit painful messages. NSAIDS inhibit an enzyme called cyclooxygenase (COX), which is essential to prostaglandin production. Most NSAIDS inhibit both COX-1 and COX-2. COX-1 is present in the stomach and kidney. COX-2 is present only in inflamed tissues. Prostaglandins released during the inflammatory process in bones and joints result in pain at the site of inflammation. Therefore, when NSAIDS are given, bone and joint pain diminish. NSAIDS are especially useful to reduce the pain of bony metastases.

Unfortunately, beneficial prostaglandins are also reduced with COX-1 suppression. Prostaglandins that protect the blood vessels, kidney, and stomach are diminished. NSAIDS can impair renal function because prostaglandins maintain normal renal arterial flow. NSAIDS cause gastrointestinal symptoms in approximately 10% of patients, including nausea and epigastric distress, as well as the danger of bleeding ulcers. Another dangerous effect is inhibition of platelet aggregation, particularly risky in those whose platelets have been impaired by chemotherapy or anticoagulants. Some elderly patients have troubling neurological effects when they take NSAIDS; they may become confused, have headaches, or complain of dizziness. NSAIDS can cause retention of salt and water in people with heart or liver disease and bronchospasm in people with asthma (Abrahm, 2000). Patients who are on NSAIDS over a period of months need to be evaluated for impaired renal function and checked for occult fecal blood. When terminally ill patients are on NSAIDS and also on corticosteroids for symptom relief, they are at significantly greater risk for gastrointestinal bleeding. Patients on anticoagulants should not receive NSAIDS. See Table 15-1, Characteristics of Selected NSAIDS. The gastritis and gastric ulcers associated with NSAIDS can be prevented by administering agents that reduce gastric acid secretion, like cimetidine (Tagamet) and omeprazole (Prilosec).

The more costly COX-2 inhibitors reduce inflammation without the adverse effects on platelets and with less gastric complications. But they have been associated with adverse cardiovascular complications, including stroke and myocardial infarct.

Just as high acetaminophen dosages may become a risk, aspirin overdose is a threat when patients take higher and higher doses of compounds with aspirin. For example, the combination of oxycodone 5 mg and aspirin 325 mg in Percodan becomes toxic when the patient in severe pain takes escalating amounts. Three Percodan tablets taken every 3 hours equals 975 mg aspirin × 8 or 7800 mg aspirin in a 24-hour period. Doses much beyond 6000 mg daily cause toxic salicylism, ranging from tinnitus and ataxia to delirium and coma (Abrahm, 2000).

Planting the Seeds

NSAIDS are remarkably effective to reduce inflammatory pain, particularly in bony metastases. Remember the two most common side effects that require watchful nursing: GI bleeding and renal insufficiency. Watch stools for guiac/occult blood and lab values for elevations in BUN and creatinine. Question NSAID orders for patients receiving steroids and those with allergies to aspirin, bleeding disorders, kidney failure, gastritis, and gastric ulcers.

Table 15-1

CHARACTERISTICS OF SELECTED NSAIDS

Name	Dosing Schedule	Starting Dose	Maximum Dose	Feature
Salicylates				
Aspirin	q 4–6 h	650 mg	6000 mg/day	Suppository available
Choline	q 8–12 h	500 mg	4500 mg/day	Less GI toxicity
Magnesium				No platelet effect
Trisalicylate (Trilisate)				
Propionic Acids				
Ibuprofen,	q 4–8 h	400–600 mg	3200 mg/day	
(Motrin, Advil, Nuprin)				
Naproxen (Naprosyn)	q 12 h	500 mg	1500 mg/day	Suppository available
Acetic Acids				
Indomethacin (Indocin)	q 8–24 h	75 mg	200 mg	GI bleeding & CNS toxicity
				Suppository available
Pyrrolo-pyrrole				
Ketorolac (Toradol)	q 4–6	IV/IM 30–60 mg p.o. 10 mg	IV/IM 120 mg p.o. 40 mg	Risk of renal & GI complications if long-term use
COX-2 Inhibitors				
Celecoxib (Celebrex)	q 12	100 mg	400 mg	Risk of cardiovascular complications

Source: From Coyle (1995); and AAHPM (2003).

Topical nonopioid analgesics, such as capsaicin cream and aspirin cream, can also have a role in pain relief at the end of life (St. Marie, 2002). Capsaicin is derived from hot peppers; it can relieve postoperative neuropathic pain and post-herpetic neuralgia. Capsaicin cream can be applied to the skin three to four times daily. It causes burning and erythema, which may sometimes require discontinuing therapy. Creams with aspirin and ibuprofen are available over the counter, but their use is unproven.

OPIOID ANALGESICS

Opioids are the most important pharmacological tool for controlling moderate-to-severe pain at the end of life. An opioid is defined as any drug that has actions similar to morphine. The word "narcotic" is no longer used in the medical literature because of its lack of precision. Opioid drugs act at the body's opioid receptors in the central nervous system (Porth, 2004) to produce analgesia, reduce anxiety, and increase a sense of well-being. Thus, they diminish both the perception of pain and the resultant suffering. Opioid drugs mimic the effects of the endogenous opioids, which include the endorphins, enkephalins, and dynorphins. Table 15-2 identifies

Table 15-2

COMMONLY USED OPIOIDS

DRUG	TRADE NAMES AND COMPOUNDS	INDICATIONS/ WHO STEPS
Morphine sulfate	MS Contin, Roxanol, Kadian, Avinza	Step 3
Hydromorphone	Dilaudid	Step 3
Oxycodone	OxyContin	Step 3 alone
	Combinations: Percocet, Percodan, Tylox	Step 2 in combinations
Methadone		Step 3
Oxymorphone	Numorphan suppositories	Step 3
Codeine	Immediate release and combinations	Step 2
Hydrocodone	Combinations: Vicodin, Lortab, Hycodan	Step 2
Meperidine	Demerol	Acute pain only No role at end of life Risk of toxic metabolite accumulation

commonly used opioids, including morphine, hydrocodone, oxycodone, and methadone.

Opiophobia

Physicians and nurses often hesitate to prescribe and administer opioids at the end of life for three prominent reasons: fear of patient addiction, fear of legal repercussions, and fear of depressing respirations.

Fear of Addiction and Pseudo-addiction

The myth that opioids commonly cause addiction just will not go away; this inaccurate assumption is buried deep within the belief systems of physicians and nurses. It is important to understand what addiction really is. Addiction is characterized by compulsive use of a drug to regulate one's mood, not to relieve pain. Box 15-2 defines addiction and related terms. The addicted person becomes preoccupied with obtaining and using the drug for the psychological effect. Continued use reduces quality of life.

Box 15-2 ■ **ADDICTION AND RELATED TERMS**	
Adapted from definitions developed by the American Academy of Pain Medicine, the American Pain Society, and the American Society of Addiction Medicine	
Addiction	A chronic, neurobiologic disease.
	Genetic, psychosocial, and environmental factors influence development and symptoms.
	Characterized by one or more of the following behaviors: impaired control over drug use, compulsive use, continuing use despite harm, and craving for the drug.
Physical dependence	Withdrawal syndrome specific to a drug class that is produced by abruptly stopping the drug, rapidly reducing the dose, decreasing blood level, and/or administering an antagonist. Some call this "physical addiction" and contrast it with "psychological addiction."
Tolerance	Adaptive state in which exposure to a drug causes changes that result in diminished drug effects over time.

Source: From Savage et al. (2003).

This psychological addiction should not be confused with physical dependence (or physiological addiction), in which the body's cells have adapted to the presence of the opioid. Stopping an opioid taken over several days to several weeks will result in a physiological withdrawal syndrome. Everyone who needs opioids for severe pain over a prolonged period will become physiologically dependent and need to be withdrawn gradually to avoid withdrawal symptoms. In fact, people who have needed opioids for pain rarely develop compulsive cravings for the drug to alter their mood (psychological addiction). The actual risk of addiction, characterized by a craving to use opioids to get "high," is minimal. In two classic *New England Journal of Medicine* studies, the likelihood of addiction in medical patients receiving opioids for pain was 0.1% and 0.03%, respectively (Angell, 1982; Porter & Jick, 1980). The typical addict simply does not start out as a pain patient. Known drug addicts suffering pain need carefully supervised and adjusted opioids to experience relief.

66 | *Known drug addicts suffering pain need carefully supervised and adjusted opioids to experience relief.*

To gain a perspective on why drug addiction is so feared, it is valuable to look at history. Before 1914, physicians commonly prescribed opioids to relieve the suffering of drug addicts. In other words, physicians maintained their patients' habits legally. In 1914, Congress approved the Harrison Narcotic Act, initially designed to develop a system for the orderly marketing and prescribing of opioids (Brecher, 1972). Its intention was to tax those who produce and sell narcotics, and it required that physicians keep records. In practice, it was interpreted by law enforcement officers to mean that a doctor could not prescribe opioids to an addict to maintain his addiction because addiction was a "moral failure," not a disease. Physicians were soon arrested for helping addicts obtain drugs, and criminals trafficking in drugs became wealthy. Addicts were punished and imprisoned, as they are now. Those addicted resorted to degrading and criminal acts to pay for their supply of drugs.

Criminalization of addiction has, in effect, imposed extraordinary suffering on the patients who are living in pain in the United States. The association of opioids with crime and moral failure persists as the foremost barrier to relieving terminal pain.

66 | *The association of opioids with crime and moral failure persists as the foremost barrier to relieving terminal pain.*

Undertreated patients in pain frequently manifest the symptoms of pseudoaddiction in which they seek additional medications, higher dosages, and more frequent drug administration. Frequently, they may be disparaged as "drug seekers" whose pain "can't be that bad." Pseudoaddiction is the false labeling of a patient as "an addict" because he is seeking opioids to relieve pain. Such patients in pain are reduced to begging and demanding and other behaviors that may be labeled as inappropriate and may estrange health-care professionals. They are the people whose pain is so poorly controlled that its presence preoccupies them. When hospitalized, they can't stop watching the clock to anticipate when their next dose of opioid is ordered. The nursing responsibility is to recognize the meaning of these pseudoaddictive behaviors, and to call for better pain management. The solution is comprehensive planning for pain relief, more medication, better medication, and scheduling to prevent breakthrough pain. Patients should not experience a roller coaster of suffering and relief, but rather be receiving medication to achieve a constant level of analgesic that maintains a comfortable plateau.

❧ Planting the Seeds

When your colleagues are afraid of addicting patients, first be sure that they understand the difference between physical dependence and psychological addiction. Anyone taking opioids over a week or more will have flu-like symptoms if the drug is stopped abruptly. Explain the evidence that people in pain need opioids for pain relief and that studies have repeatedly shown that pain patients rarely become psychologically addicted, which involves taking opioids to get "high," not to get pain under control. Persons with addiction take their opioids to escape life, whereas persons with pain take their opioids to live life more fully.

In the past, dying patients were often given small doses of opioids, with long intervals between to prevent building up tolerance and having to increase the doses continually. Current evidence indicates, however, that tolerance—defined as loss of opioid effectiveness implicating a need to increase the dosage to achieve the same level of pain relief—is less common than previously understood (AAPM & APS, 1997). The phenomenon of tolerance does not prohibit long-term use of opioids. When pain increases in cancer patients receiving a constant opioid dose, it is usually due to disease progression, not increasing tolerance to opioids. Moreover, most opioids have no upper dosage limit, so that tolerance does not become an issue. The argument that there is a ceiling for morphine was once used as a rationale for withholding the drug until the pain became "really bad."

❧ Planting the Seeds

Labeling patients as "addicted" or "drug seekers" or "manipulative" can get in the way of caring for persons in pain. It clouds critical thinking and professional judgment. Accept what patients state about their pain. If there is a concern about whether the patient is telling the truth, confront it head on, in an honest caring exchange with the patient. Discuss the incongruities that you see. Many times this will uncover deeper issues that need to be dealt with before the pain can be relieved. This type of compassionate, caring interaction can facilitate building a trusting relationship, rather than an adversarial one.

Fear of Legal Repercussions

Physicians and nurse practitioners may fear being sanctioned for prescribing large quantities of opioids. In contemporary America, opioids are being diverted from medical use to illegal use through deceptive claims by persons seeking prescriptions for nonmedical purposes, improper dispensing by pharmacies, prescription forgery, doctor shopping, and theft. Fear of opioid diversion has resulted in states and law enforcement agencies adopting policies that restrict the access of suffering people to pain relief in order to reduce drug abuse. Policies include states restricting pharmacies that can dispense, limiting those who can prescribe opioids, requiring multiple copy prescription forms, and defining opioids as treatments of last resort (Examples of Balanced and Unbalanced Policy, 2002).

In fact, physicians who prescribe high volumes of opioids for extended periods are usually clinicians highly knowledgeable in the management of chronic and terminal pain; a very small number are either ignorant or criminal. Physicians are being targeted by overzealous law enforcement, and a growing number of physicians are restraining their opioid prescribing because of fear of investigation (Doctors Behind Bars, 2004). A joint public policy statement from the American Academy of Pain Medicine, the American Pain Society, and the American Society of Addiction Medicine (2004) notes that poor medical practice is evidenced both when (1) providers fail to recognize and provide appropriate treatment for the disease of addiction; and (2) when they persistently fail to use opioids to treat pain. The organizations note that a distinction must be made between those who are deliberately complicit in drug diversion or other illegal activities, and those who inappropriately prescribe opioids due to lack of knowledge regarding pain and addiction.

66 | *Poor medical practice is evidenced both when providers fail to recognize and provide appropriate treatment for the disease of addiction; and when they persistently fail to use opioids to treat pain.*

To remain safe from suspicion of wrong-doing, nurses and physicians must collaborate to complete thorough, well-documented patient assessments and evaluations of response to therapy. The physician or practitioner's clinical judgment indicating the rationale for opioid selection, dosage, and interval for each individual case must be recorded. The chart should explain what they are doing, why opioids are indicated, whether there are alternatives, and patient follow up. Nurses work in a supportive role to ensure that opioids are prescribed and used in ways that protect everyone's license. The American Academy of Pain Management identifies 10 tips to avoid legal repercussions when prescribing opioids. See Box 15-3.

> " *To remain safe from suspicion of wrongdoing, nurses and physicians must collaborate to complete thorough, well-documented patient assessments and evaluations of response to therapy.*

Physicians and nurses can also be held responsible for undertreating pain. For example, a nurse in North Carolina refused to administer prescribed opioids to a terminally ill patient because she believed it would lead to addiction. The family brought a lawsuit against her and her nursing home employer and was awarded $7.5 million in compensation for the patient's months of suffering (Rich, 2001). Likewise, a jury in California awarded a family $1.5 million against a physician and hospital for failure to relieve severe pain that the jury concluded was tantamount to elder abuse (Rich, 2001). Pain must be carefully assessed and treated; there are legal repercussions for careless ordering or administration of excessive or inadequate opioid analgesics.

Fear of Respiratory Effects

Contradicting long-standing medical assumptions, the evidence now reveals that respiratory depression caused by opioids tends to occur primarily in the

---

Box 15-3 ■ TEN TIPS TO SURVIVE OPIOID PRESCRIBING

1. Obtain a thorough history and physical. Screen patients for substance abuse.
2. Chart everything.
3. Require patient consent to just one provider prescribing for pain.
4. Require patient consent to use just one pharmacy.
5. Get a second opinion from a specialist.
6. Prescribe long-acting opioids. Stabilize opioid levels to minimize need for short-acting breakthrough medication.
7. See patients regularly. Do not allow refills and avoid telephone orders.
8. Determine minimum dose to sustain quality of life.
9. Order a urine drug screen to rule out drug diversion and check for illicit substances.
10. Receive regular opioid analgesic education.

patient receiving opioids for the first time (Pasero & McCaffery, 2002). Opioids given to the opioid naïve patient depress the respiratory centers in the brainstem. Nevertheless, even in the opioid naïve patients, the presence of pain counteracts the respiratory depressant effect of opioids (American Academy of Pain Medicine and American Pain Society, 1999). In other words, pain is an antidote to opioid-induced respiratory depression. Withholding opioids from a patient in pain because of fear of suppressing respiration is therefore inexcusable. Physicians and nurses frequently avoid adequate opioid medication at the end of life because they fear shortening the patient's life by slowing respirations until respiratory arrest occurs. A recent study revealed, however, that hospice patients receiving escalating doses of opioids at the end of life had no different survival time than those whose opioid dose stayed stable (Thorns & Sykes, 2000). In a terminal patient receiving regular opioids to control pain, life comes to an end with respiratory arrest because of the disease process, not because a nurse administered an opioid to relieve suffering in the last hours.

66 | *In a terminal patient receiving regular opioids to control pain, life comes to an end with respiratory arrest because of the disease process, not because a nurse administered an opioid to relieve suffering in the last hours.*

 Planting the Seeds

Careful assessment and titration are to the prevention of unnecessary sedation and respiratory depression. Increase the dose slowly in incremental percentages (by 25% if pain rating is 4 or lower on a 0-to-10 scale; 50% if pain rating is 5 or higher) based on the most current assessment findings and the half-life and duration of action of the opioid being given. Keep in mind that (a) you can always add more drug, but once you give it you cannot take it back; and (b) sedation will almost always precede respiratory depression. Sedation alerts us that the opioid may suppress breathing.

In the opioid naïve patient and whenever you are rapidly increasing opioid dosages to "get on top of the pain," opioid dosage must be carefully titrated to the level of pain. Although the presence of pain is an antidote to respiratory effects, monitor level of sedation in the patient who has never received opioids and is initially receiving parenteral opioids, because sedation is a sensitive indicator of the chance of respiratory depression (Pasero & McCaffery, 2002). Respiratory status and sedation should be monitored every 1 to 2 hours during the first 24 hours after initiating opioid infusions. Respiratory depression is clinically relevant when there is a reduction in both respiratory rate and depth. When somnolence and respiratory depression develop in the dying patient receiving opioid infusions who is not close to death, opioid dose should be titrated down to a level that continues to control pain.

Remember that respiratory depression is rarely a worry in patients receiving regular opioids for more than a week. They will become tolerant to both the respiratory depressant and sedative effects. When dying patients who are on continuous opioid therapy become somnolent with diminishing response to physical stimulation, the cause will be the underlying disease process.

Side Effects of Regular Opioid Administration

The following sections address opioid side effects that require careful monitoring and management. It is important to realize that individuals can vary dramatically in their sensitivity to the adverse effects of opioid analgesia.

66 | *Individuals can vary dramatically in their sensitivity to the adverse effects of opioid analgesia.*

Constipation

All opioids reduce gastrointestinal secretions and peristalsis. Therefore, constipation is a universal risk in patients receiving opioids around the clock, and it does not get better over time. Constipation is too often ignored, sometimes leading to impaction, abdominal pain, anorexia, and even vomiting. All patients receiving continuous opioid analgesics should be receiving a regularly scheduled stool softener, such as docusate sodium (Colace) and a stimulant laxative such as bisacodyl (Senekot). See Figure 15-2, Bowel Management Algorithm.

66 | *Constipation is a universal risk in patients receiving opioids around the clock, and it does not get better over time.*

Nausea and Vomiting

Nausea and sometimes vomiting are common initially with opioid administration but will rapidly resolve in most patients. Morphine directly stimulates the chemoreceptor trigger zone in the medulla and slows gastric emptying. If nausea continues, anti-emetic drugs like metoclopramide (Reglan) that also promote gastric emptying should be added to the drug regimen. Persistent nausea and vomiting can sometimes be reduced by switching to another opioid (Cherny at al., 2001).

Sedation and Impaired Cognition

When patients first receive opioids, most experience some degree of sedation. Those with severe sleep deprivation because of unrelieved pain may

Bowel Management Algorithm

Step 1: (choose one)
- Docusate Sodium 250 mg daily to bid
- Fruit Paste 1-2 Tablespoons daily
- Docusate Sodium plus senna 1-4 tablet(s) tid

Step 2: (if no BM in any 48-hour period, add one of the following)
- Biscodyl 10-15 mg PO daily
- Milk of Magnesia 30-60 ml PO daily
- Laculose 15-60 ml daily (or in equally divided doses bid-tid)

Step 3: (if no BM by 72 hours)
- **Perform rectal exam to rule out impaction**
Try one of the following:
- Biscodyl rectal suppository 10 mg PR
- Magnesium citrate 8 oz PO
- Mineral oil 30-60 ml PO
- Fleet enema PR
- Warm saline enema PR

If a fecal impaction is present:
- Manually disimpact if stool is soft enough
- Consider pretreatment of patient with analgesic or anxiolytic
- Soften stool with mineral oil retention enema
- Follow up with enema of choice until clear
- Increase intensity of daily bowel program
- If rectal pain or discomfort, use hemorrhoid ointment or suppositories,warm sitz baths, also consider use of Tucks rectal wipes.

NOTE: DO NOT implement in neutropenia, thrombocytopenia without physician consultation.

Figure 15-2 Bowel Management Algorithm. (Copyright Dionetta Hudzinski.)

sleep on and off for days once the pain is relieved. Most patients find that sedation disappears within a week. Patients who nap when alone but are easy to arouse and readily communicate are not suffering from sedation due to opioids. If opioids were the cause, they would not be able to awaken. For those who continue to be troubled by sedative effects, another opioid drug may have less sedative effect. A small number of patients may need a cerebral stimulant such as caffeine drinks or methylphenidate hydrochloride.

Other causes of sedation may include progressive disease and the sedative effects of other drugs. Frequently, patients receiving opioids over time complain of mental dullness, but research reveals minimal or no significant measurable impairment in cognitive functioning (Ersek, Cherrier, Overman, and Irving, 2004). Fears of rendering a person unable to think clearly should not hinder appropriate use of opioids.

Planting the Seeds

When a patient complains of sedation that is disturbing to them, it deserves careful evaluation and treatment. Many patients, when given the choice between pain and mild sedation that cannot be reversed without reversing some pain relief, will chose sedation. But it is their choice and we must respect whatever choice they make. Their choice may change over time and we need to be ready and willing to change course with them. Occasionally, family members will be disturbed by the patient's level of sedation, and will discourage or withhold analgesics. Listening and careful education are the keys to managing this problem successfully.

Neurotoxicity

Opioid-induced neurotoxicity, which impairs the central nervous system, can occur in patients who are receiving high opioid doses or prolonged administration, as well as in those with reduced kidney function (Bruera & Kim, 2003). Manifestations include delirium, agitation, muscle twitching (myoclonus), and heightened sensitivity to pain. It is managed by investigating and reversing other possible causes, switching to another opioid, reducing dosage and adding adjuvant medication, hydration, and sedation with a drug like lorazepam (Ativan) or midazolam (Versed). Patients receiving meperidine (Demerol) are at highest risk of neurotoxicity, due to the neurotoxic effects of the metabolite normeperidine. Meperidine (Demerol) is not indicated for persistent chronic pain because of this neurotoxic metabolite.

Other Effects

Opioids have no major effect on blood pressure or on cardiac rate or rhythm (Hardman, Limbird, and Gilman, 2001). Other side effects sometimes reported include initial urinary retention, itching, sweating, and dry mouth. Itching is caused by histamine release. In those cases, an alternative drug should be used. Antihistamines are useful but can cause unacceptable sedation.

Preferred and Less Preferred Opioids

Codeine is the preferred opioid to treat mild-to-moderate pain. Morphine, oxycodone, hydromorphone, levorphanol, methadone, and fentanyl are currently the preferred opioids to treat severe pain. Meperidine should not be used for terminal pain.

Codeine

Codeine is a weak opioid that is very effective in relieving mild-to-moderate pain, especially when given in combination with a nonopioid like Tylenol (Tylenol #3 = acetaminophen 300 mg and codeine 30 mg). It is less than one sixth as potent as morphine so that codeine 190 mg p.o. is considered equivalent to Morphine 30 mg p.o. Codeine relieves pain of medium intensity and is highly effective in suppressing coughing.

Morphine Sulfate (MS)

Morphine is the gold standard among opioid drugs; it is the prototype to which all other opioids are compared. It is the best-known opioid. More is understood about morphine than the other opioids. Morphine works well when given by mouth, but it does lose potency through digestion and passage through the liver. Therefore, it takes 30 mg of morphine by mouth to be equivalent to a 10 mg injection. Remember that 3:1 ratio. So if your patient has been receiving 60 MS IV in a 24-hour period, that is equivalent to 180 mg by mouth in a 24-hour period. Nurses in all settings participate in decisions to convert patients from parenteral to oral medication and need to understand parenteral to oral conversions. Inexpensive immediate-release tablets are available so that patients can take 30 mg every four hours to total 180 mg daily. For long-term management of terminal pain, the patient will maintain a constant blood level on a long-acting, controlled-release morphine preparation, such as Oramorph SR or MS Contin. MS Contin is available in a variety of dosages from 15 mg to 200 mg tablets, which are given every 12 hours. The patient needing 180 mg daily could take a 30 mg and a 60 mg tablet twice daily. The emphasis is on switching from high technology and high cost, to making the medication manageable and low cost for patient and family caregivers.

Morphine sulfate is also available in preparations that can last up to 24 hours (Avinza and Kadian), in oral solutions (Roxanol liquid), and in suppositories (RMS). Twenty-four-hour duration has advantages for patients who may not reliably take or receive medication more often. Oral liquids and suppositories work when swallowing tablets has become at problem. Subcutaneous and intravenous morphine infusion should be reserved only for those patients with extreme pain that has become unmanageable through other routes of administration.

Oxycodone

Oxycodone is a strong oral opioid not available in parenteral form. To put it in perspective, 20 mg oxycodone p.o. is considered equivalent to 30 mg morphine p.o. It is available in a short-acting form that lasts 3 to 4 hours, a long-acting form (Oxycontin) that last 12 hours, and in combinations such as Percocet (combined with acetaminophen) and Percodan (combined with aspirin). Effects and side effects are comparable to morphine. Oxycodone is chosen as an alternative to morphine.

Hydromorphone (Dilaudid)

Hydromorphone is the most potent opioid in parenteral and oral form that is available in the United States. Oral hydromorphone is four times stronger than oral morphine. The use of 7.5 mg hydromorphone p.o. is considered equivalent to 30 mg morphine p.o. Parenteral hydromorphone is five to eight times more potent than morphine (Thwaites, McCann, and Broderick, 2004). Potent amounts of hydromorphone can be concentrated in small amounts of fluid, making it especially useful for patients with severe pain to be relieved with hydromorphone infused in small volumes given intravenously or subcutaneously. Over half of patients receiving doses greater than 20 mg/hour for more than 15 days may exhibit neurotoxic effects (agitation, myoclonus, seizures). Hydromorphone is most frequently chosen because of its high potency that can be delivered in small fluid infusions for extreme pain.

Levorphanol (Levo-Dromoran)

Levorphanol is a potent opioid available in 2 mg tablets and in 2 mg/mL for injection. Effects and side effects are similar to morphine. Levorphanol has been less commercially developed than the other strong opioids. Levorphanol 4 mg p.o. is equivalent to levorphanol 2 mg IM and morphine 30 mg p.o.

Methadone

Before long-acting morphine was available, methadone was used in the early days of the American hospice movement because of its effectiveness and long duration (Blues & Zerwekh, 1984). It has been rediscovered recently because it is inexpensive and is well absorbed orally (Bruera & Kim, 2003). Methadone binds to opioid receptors and possesses some unique pharmacological qualities that reduce neuropathic pain. It causes less myoclonus, constipation, and dry mouth than other opioids. The main disadvantages are a prolonged half-life leading to potential accumulation with possible sedation, significant interactions with other drugs, and highly variable equianalgesia, which means that the dose that is equivalent to morphine is highly variable.

For instance, when the patient is receiving low doses of morphine, a one-to-three ratio or two-to-three ratio is reliable so that 10 mg or 20 mg of oral methadone is considered equivalent to 30 mg of morphine. When the patient is receiving high doses of morphine, however, methadone is more potent so that 1 mg methadone may be equivalent to 10 or even 20 mg morphine. Methadone can be administered orally, sublingually, rectally, and parenterally.

Fentanyl

Fentanyl is a potent, fast-acting opioid analgesic useful in end-of-life pain management through the application of long-lasting transdermal patches (Duragesic patch) or rapid-acting buccal absorption with lozenges on a stick (Actiq). The transdermal patches provide a stable absorption rate of 25, 50, 75, or 100 mcg/hour over a 3-day period. Transdermal fentanyl is chosen to manage stable pain when it has been relieved inadequately with other drugs or routes of administration, or when gastrointestinal symptoms prevent oral intake. It is also useful when compliance or adherence to a dosing schedule is a problem; it can also be used when drug diversion within the household is an issue or concern. In that case, one patch is dispensed at a time. The lozenges relieve acute breakthrough pain. Fentanyl dosage is calculated in micrograms, not milligrams. Side effects of fentanyl are the same as other opioids.

Meperidine (Demerol)

Meperidine is effective for the relief of acute pain, but it is unacceptable for chronic and terminal pain. There are four main reasons why meperidine should have no role at the end of life: First of all, meperidine has a toxic metabolite, normeperidine, that can cause agitation, myoclonic jerking, and seizures. Second, meperidine lasts only about 2 hours. Therefore, around-the-clock relief requires extraordinarily frequent dosing. Third, meperidine is very poorly absorbed by mouth. It takes six 50 mg tablets to equal the same analgesia as a single 75 mg injection. Fourth, patients taking monoamine oxidase (MAO) inhibitors for depression are vulnerable to fevers, seizures, and death if given with meperidine. Meperidine should be used only to manage acute surgical or procedural pain.

Opioid Administration

During the early days of the American hospice movement, home visiting nurses were pioneers in developing alternative routes for analgesia when the patient stopped taking medication by mouth. See Box 15-4. When the oral route no longer works, opioids can be administered through the oral mucosa, rectally, transdermally, or by infusion.

If the patient can no longer swallow or is persistently nauseated, it is now well established that medication can be absorbed through the oral or

---

Box 15-4 ■ ANALGESIA INNOVATION IN THE EARLY HOSPICE MOVEMENT

Early home visiting hospice nurses were in the forefront of the movement to seek alternatives to painful injections, which were traumatic for patients and the family caregivers trying to administer them. Before central venous lines with Hickman or Portacath access, the intravenous route would malfunction and require frequent painful venipuncture or cutdown procedures. When the patient could no longer swallow, we concocted suppositories out of crushed tablets and margarine. We took morphine tablets designed to be diluted for injection and tried them under the tongue. They worked. When infusions were absolutely essential to control pain, we found that the subcutaneous route, which had been abandoned previously in favor of intravenous, was effective and much easier for families to manage.

---

rectal mucosa. Sublingual or buccal opioids may be given regularly every 3 to 4 hours with doses equivalent to the parenteral rather than the oral route because absorption is directly into the bloodstream. Oral transmucosal fentanyl lozenges on a stick (Actiq) have been developed specifically for breakthrough pain and are available in a range of strengths from 200 mcg to 1600 mcg. Concentrated solutions of morphine (Roxanol 20 mg/cc) or oxycodone (Intensol) are preferred because small volumes can deliver large amounts of analgesic. Rectal suppositories or sustained-release tablets inserted rectally are also an option, with dosage usually equivalent to that for oral medication, but absorption through the rectal mucosa is variable. Venous drainage from the lower rectum flows into the systemic circulation, bypassing the opioid degradation by the liver (Abrahm, 2000). Other mucosal routes include absorption through the vagina and through an ostomy stoma.

Transdermal fentanyl patches (Duragesic) are very expensive and should be chosen only when the oral route is unacceptable. The transdermal (TD) patches work well for stable pain and are applied to the skin of the upper torso every 72 hours. Many patients prefer patches because they do not have to remember to take pills. Fentanyl patches contain a lipid-soluble analgesic in a drug reservoir attached to a rate-limiting membrane. The fentanyl slowly diffuses through the membrane into the fat of the subcutaneous tissue, where it is gradually absorbed through the capillaries into the systemic circulation. Transdermal patches are not easily titrated when pain is out of control or rapidly escalating. If this occurs, it is best to remove the patch and titrate upwards using an immediate-release preparation until pain is once again stable. Then, readminister the patch at the higher dose. Patches can take up to 16 hours or more to produce significant analgesia, and their effects last approximately 16 hours or more after their removal. Effectiveness is limited when cachexia has reduced the fat depot through which fentanyl can be absorbed. Likewise, fevers can increase drug absorption, resulting in over-dose. Monitor the patient with a fever carefully and consider switching to an immediate-release preparation until the patient is stable.

Subcutaneous or intravenous infusions are a last resort when the other routes have been demonstrated to be ineffective, or when immediate deliv-ery of high opioid doses is necessitated by a new source of extreme pain (such as vertebral collapse due to metastases). Subcutaneous infusions are easier and safer than intravenous doses when the client is receiving care at home. High doses can be delivered by infusion pump, through a 27 gauge "butterfly" needle inserted subcutaneously on the anterior chest or abdomen. These are changed with few complications every 5 to 7 days by patients or families. Hydromorphone (Dilaudid) and morphine are usually well absorbed and nonirritating (Abrahm, 2000). When high opioid doses are needed, highly concentrated hydromorphone is available (Dilaudid HP 10 mg/cc) so that small volumes of fluid can deliver large amounts of pain relief. Occasionally, when site integrity is an issue with more concentrated doses, dexamethsone can be added to the solution; as an adjunct, it also has a role in reducing the pain. Intravenous opioid infusions should be reserved for acute pain management in the hospital. The patient should be switched to simpler routes when going to a skilled nursing facility, inpatient hospice, or home.

Opioid Dosing and Dosages

No evidence supports the universal selection of one opioid drug over another (Fine, Miaskowski, and Paice, 2004). When patients are started on strong opioids by mouth, the usual practice is to begin with immediate-release analgesic for the first 2 or 3 days and to titrate the dose for comfort. Immediate-release morphine is given every 4 hours and has a peak effect in about 1 hour. To get on top of poorly controlled pain, it may be necessary to escalate dosage rapidly. Occasionally, dosing hourly is necessary to achieve rapid pain relief and better control. This requires careful assessment of the pain and sedation levels. When a particular 4-hour dose fails, the next dose might be increased by one half (AAHPM, 2003). There-fore, if a patient is receiving 10 mg MS and that fails to relieve the pain, the next dose should be titrated upward (by 50%) to 15 mg.

When the pain is controlled and the dosage stabilized, the 24-hour dose is determined and the patient is switched to a long-acting opioid. If analgesics like MS Contin or OxyContin, which last 12 hours, are chosen, determine the dose by dividing the 24-hour dosage in half. Thus, a patient receiving oxycodone 30 mg every four hours would have a 24-hour total of 30 × 6 doses in 24 hours = 180 mg/24 hours. A switch to OxyContin requires divid-ing 180 mg ÷ 2 = OxyContin 90 mg p.o. q 12 h. As pain increases, the dosage of long-acting opioid can be increased by 25% to 50%, but the dosage fre-quency should not be altered. When pain does not respond to careful opioid titration, reassessment of the pain and potential etiologies can indicate the addition of adjuvant drugs to target the underlying causes of the pain. Pain that is difficult to manage with opioids often stems from psychosocial and spiritual distress.

Planting the Seeds

Titrating opioid drugs, changing dosage forms, and switching between drugs first requires calculating the daily 24-hour total the patient is receiving. So, if you are giving MSIR 15 mg every 4 hours, multiply that by 6 to calculate the 24-hour total, which is 90 mg of morphine in 24 hours. Now, to switch to MS Contin, given every 12 hours and therefore twice daily, divide the 24-hour intake by 2. That would be 90 ÷ 2 = 45 mg MS Contin. The 24-hour intake is always your reference point.

Initial palliative-care guidelines advised persistent use of a single opioid, as long as it worked. This approach involves gradually escalating opioid doses as pain escalates. Now some experts are finding that stopping the initial opioid, even though it continues to be effective, and replacing it with an equivalent dose of an alternative opioid has made it possible to keep doses lower, reduce side effects, and still effectively control pain (Bruera & Kim, 2003; Cherny at al., 2001).

Switching Opioids

Switching opioids and opioid routes requires an understanding of equivalent dosages. See Table 15-3, Equianalgesic Opioid Starting Doses. Although the initial conversions between different drugs for opioid naïve patients are better known, the equivalent dosages are quite variable for patients who have been taking opioids for some time. It is useful to remember that the

---

Table 15-3

EQUIANALGESIC OPIOID STARTING DOSE EQUIVALENTS

DRUG	EQUIVALENCE TO MS 30 MG PO	ORAL-TO-INJECTABLE RATIO	EQUIVALENCE TO MS 10 MG IV
Morphine	30 mg	3:1	10 mg
Oxycodone	20–30 mg	No parenteral form available	
Hydromorphone (Dilaudid)	7.5 mg	5:1	1.5 mg
Methadone	20 mg	2:1	10 mg

equivalent oral dose for morphine 30 mg is oxycodone 20 mg and hydromorphone 7.5 mg. Morphine 30 mg by mouth is equivalent to 10 mg IV or SC. That is a three-to-one ratio that compares the strength of oral to parenteral morphine. In contrast, hydromorphone (Dilaudid) 7.5 mg is equivalent to 1.5 mg injectable. That is a five-to-one ratio comparing the strength of oral to parenteral hydromorphone.

Transdermal fentanyl (Duragesic) dosage is determined by first calculating the 24-hour total of opioids previously received. Duragesic patches are calibrated in micrograms (mcg). Patches delivering 25, 50, 75, and 100 mcg/hr are available. Equivalence of Duragesic and oral morphine is determined by ranges so that:

- 90 mg MS (24-hour dose ranging from 45 to 134 mg) = 25 mcg/hr patch
- 180 mg MS (24-hour dose ranging from 135 to 224 mg) = 50 mcg/hr patch

For each 90 mg (ranging from 45 to 134 mg) of MS daily, another 25 mcg/hr patch is added. Therefore, a patient receiving MS 30 mg every 4 hours is receiving 30 mg × 6 = 180 mg daily, which would convert to an equivalent 50 mcg patch. See Table 15-4, Equianalgesic Fentanyl and Morphine.

As kidneys and/or the liver fail, opioids may accumulate with adverse consequences, such as neurotoxicity and increased sedation. Lowering dosages may help. Some clinicians propose artificial hydration to forestall renal failure and thus reduce the possibility of myoclonus and delirium.

Managing Breakthrough Pain

Breakthrough pain is a temporary increase in pain that rises above the baseline level where the patient is well controlled with around the clock opioid dosing. It may be caused by activity or occur just before the next dose of

Table 15-4

EQUIANALGESIC FENTANYL AND MORPHINE

PATCH DOSE IN MCG/HOUR	MS ORAL IN MG/DAY	MS IM/IV IN MG/DAY
25	45–134	8–22
50	135–224	23–37
75	225–314	38–52
100	315–404	53–67
125	405–494	68–82
150	495–584	83–97

Box 15-5 ■   CALCULATING BREAKTHROUGH OPIOID DOSES

When incident pain or end-of-dose failure occurs in a patient receiving an around-the-clock opioid dose that usually keeps him comfortable, breakthrough opioid doses are necessary. The dosage of breakthrough immediate-release morphine should be in the range of 10% to 15% of the 24 hour total:

- First determine the patient's 24-hour opioid dose. A patient receiving MS Contin 75 mg every 12 hours receives 150 mg in 24 hours.
- Now take 10% of the 150 mg to equal a low breakthrough dose of 15 mg.
- Now take 15% of the 150 mg to equal a high breakthrough dose of 22.5 or 23 mg.
- The breakthrough dose would range from 15 to 23 mg immediate-release oral morphine sulfate.

Source: From McCaffery & Pasero (2003).

controlled-release opioid is due (McCaffery & Pasero, 2003). Nurses should expect and plan for breakthrough pain, and patients should be instructed to keep a pain diary to understand when breakthrough incidents are occurring. This pain is treated with PRN supplemental oral "rescue" doses of fast acting opioids, such as immediate-release morphine (MSIR), oxycodone (OxyIR), or hydromorphone (Dilaudid); the breakthrough drug should be the same opioid as that used for around-the-clock dosing. The amount of breakthrough dose is based on 10% to 15% of the patient's 24-hour opioid requirement. When breakthrough medication needs accelerate, increase the dosage of around-the-clock long acting opioid. Box 15-5 illustrates Calculating Breakthrough Opioid Doses. With an onset of five minutes, oral transmucosal fentanyl (Actiq) is an excellent response to sudden severe breakthrough pain. It would seldom be used as a routine breakthrough order, but is appropriate for sudden extreme pain, such as a pathological fracture.

 The breakthrough drug should be the same opioid as that used for around-the-clock dosing.

ADJUVANT MEDICATIONS

An adjuvant medication is added to the analgesic regimen for its primary effect that is not directly analgesic, but instead targets an underlying pain mechanism, such as inflammation or anxiety. In severe pain, adjuvants are used in conjunction with both opioid and nonopioid analgesics. Adjuvants commonly used at the end of life include the corticosteroids, antidepressants, anxiolytics, anticonvulsants, muscle relaxants, anesthetics, and bisphosphonates.

Corticosteroids

Corticosteroids, such as dexamethasone (Decadron) and prednisolone (prednisone), are frequently used for their anti-inflammatory effect. They inhibit synthesis of prostaglandins and diminish edema. In particular, steroids reduce malignant bone pain and control many symptoms of expanding tumors, particularly those due to spinal cord compression and increasing intracranial pressure. Side effects, such as vulnerability to infections or hyperglycemia, are due to the steroid effects on immune mechanisms and metabolism. See Box 15-6, Complications of Prolonged Corticosteroid Use. Long-term use poses high risks of these complications; short-term use at the very end of life often provides significant relief of distress, with minimal worry about adverse consequences.

Antidepressants

The older tricyclic antidepressants, such as amitriptyline (Elavil) and desipramine (Norpramin), or nortriptyline (Aventyl), inhibit the reuptake of norepinephrine and serotonin at the level of the presynaptic neuron. Thus, more norepinephrine and serotonin are left circulating; the result is a pronounced reduction in neuropathic pain, which is burning and shooting discomfort due to nerve involvement. The tricyclics take weeks to reverse depression, but they take only days to reduce pain. They also are useful to induce sleep. Sometimes their anticholinergic side effects can cause trouble, however: dry mouth, dry eyes, blurred vision, urinary retention, constipation,

---

Box 15-6 ■   COMPLICATIONS OF PROLONGED CORTICOSTEROID USE

GI ulcerations: Prevented by concurrent administration of omeprazole (Prilosec) or misoprostol (Cytotec).

Suppressed immunity to infection: Candidiasis (thrush) in mouth or esophagus. Prevented by administering ketoconazole.

Mood changes: Euphoria, depression, agitation, psychosis.

Hyperglycemia: May require insulin.

Redistribution of fat: Moon face, alteration in body image.

Muscle weakness: May require physical therapy if not close to death.

Source: From Abrahm (2000).

postural hypotension, and arrhythmias. Nortriptyline has fewer side effects and is better tolerated, particularly in the elderly (Fine, Miaskowski , and Paice, 2004).

▓ ﾞﾑ Planting the Seeds

To decrease side effects and increase patient tolerance when starting a patient on a tricyclic antidepressant for pain, it is sometimes best to start out low (i.e., 10 mg at bedtime) and increase by 10 mg every 3 days until pain is relieved or intolerable side effects occur. The effective dose can vary from patient to patient.

It is not yet clear whether the newer selective serotonin reuptake inhibitors (SSRIs), including drugs like fluoxetine (Prozac), paroxetine (Paxil), and sertraline (Zoloft), are effective to control neuropathic pain. Related drugs with slightly different mechanisms of action include venlafaxine (Effexor), bupropion (Wellbutrin), and mirtazapine (Remeron). Their effectiveness with pain is also uncertain.

Anxiolytics

Benzodiazepines remain the linchpin for relief of anxiety, which often aggravates pain at the end of life. Remember that many of these drugs have "pam" or "lam" as the suffix: diazepam (Valium), alprazolam (Xanax), lorazepam (Ativan), and midazolam (Versed). Sedation is the primary adverse effect of the benzodiazepines. In high doses, blood pressure and respirations may be diminished. Respiratory suppression is a risk when benzodiazepines are combined with opioids. In addition to benzodiazepines, several other anxiolytics are commonly used at the end of life, particularly buspirone (BuSpar) for acute anxiety and zolpidem (Ambien) to induce sleep.

Anticonvulsants

Neuropathic pain can also be relieved with adjuvant anticonvulsants. Currently, gabapentin (Neurontin) is considered a strong choice (Fine, Miaskowski, and Paice, 2004). It is well tolerated by patients; dizziness and somnolence are the most common side effects. Older agents that have been used extensively include phenytoin (Dilantin), carbamazepine (Tegretol), and valproic acid (Depakote). They are associated with more serious side effects, including hepatic toxicity and agranulocytosis. For instance, carbamazepine is highly effective but associated with bone marrow depression that limits its use in patients with cancer.

Muscle Relaxants

Benzodiazepines are commonly prescribed for muscle spasms. A wide variety of skeletal muscle relaxants are also available to combat muscle spasms, including baclofen (Lioresal), carisoprodol (Soma), cyclobenzaprine (Flexeril), methocarbamol (Robaxin), and orphenadrine (Norgesic). Because of their significant sedative and central nervous system effects, these drugs should be reserved for short-term use with acute muscle spasm or injury (Abrahm, 2000).

Bisphosphonates

This class of drugs includes alendronate (Fosamax), etidronate (Didronel), and pamidronate (Aredia). They decrease the pain of bony metastases and can prevent pathological fractures by diminishing bone reabsorption.

Anesthetics

Anesthetics are useful for neuropathic pain that has not responded to opioids, anticonvulsants, and antidepressants. They are given parenterally by specially trained anesthesiologists. Local anesthetics can be injected to block spinal, peripheral, and sympathetic nerves. Anesthetics and steroids can be injected into the spinal space or nerve roots. To eradicate refractory pain, nerves can actually be destroyed (neuroablation) with heat or cold, or a chemical agent like glycerol. This may impair normal sensation and motor function.

In contrast to these invasive approaches, topical anesthetics can be useful for specific indications: lidocaine ointment and patch, and lidocaine and prilocaine cream (EMLA). Lidocaine gel and ointment can also be used to relieve similar nerve-related pain. EMLA anesthetizes the skin before intrusive medical procedures, such as bone marrow aspiration or lumbar puncture. The cream is applied and covered with a semipermeable dressing 1 hour before the planned procedure.

▪ ૐ Planting the Seeds

When pain is resistant to management, possible undiscovered sources of pain should be identified by thorough psychosocial, spiritual, and head-to-toe physical assessment. For instance, in a patient with metastatic cancer, investigate beyond the obvious as she writhes and cries out with extreme abdominal and back pain. Are there unresolved emotional or spiritual issues? Could she be constipated? Is her bladder extended from urinary retention? Could she have a pathological fracture? What else could be going on?

COMMON PAIN CONTROL CHALLENGES

Some of the most common pain challenges include pain from nerve damage, pain of bony metastases, and pain in the drug-addicted patient.

Neuropathic Pain

First-line management for neuropathic pain is actually different from the WHO 3-step ladder (Fine, Miaskowski, and Paice, 2004). The incidence of neuropathic pain is increasing as a result of nerve-damaging chemotherapeutic drugs, such as cisplatin and vincristine. Neuropathies experienced at the end of life also include those due to invasion or pressure from malignant tumors, postoperative neuropathies, diabetic neuropathy, and HIV-associated neuropathy. Medications used to manage neuropathic pain include gabapentin (Neurontin), lidocaine patch, tricyclic antidepressants, and opioids. The opioid of first choice is tramadol (Ultram). It acts like an opioid and also inhibits the reuptake of norepinephrine and serotonin, just like the tricyclic antidepressants. Side effects are similar to the opioids, but seizures are an additional risk.

Pain of Bony Metastases

Pain of bony metastases can be particularly challenging to manage. Opioids alone do not control this pain that frequently immobilizes the patient. The most common cancers, such as breast and prostate, have a tendency to metastasize to the bone, causing dull aching or throbbing, and breakthrough pain with activity (Sabino & Mantyh, 2005). Prostaglandins and endothelins are released by the cancer cells, sensory neurons are destroyed, and pain is caused by bone breakdown (osteoclastic activity). NSAIDS, corticosteroids, bisphosphonates, or calcitonin reduce pain by targeting these underlying pathological processes. NSAIDS and corticosteroids reduce the inflammation associated with bone injury. NSAIDS inhibit prostaglandins synthesized when bones are injured. Calcitonin and the bisphosphonates, such as pamidronate (Aredia), inhibit breakdown of bone. Radiation is often used to control bony metastases. One can achieve lasting relief from bone pain by using external beam radiation and intravenous administration of radioactive strontium chloride 89, which is deposited in bony metastatic sites to destroy cancer cells (Abrahm, 2000).

Pain in Substance Abusers

Whenever you suspect that a patient is currently abusing drugs, seek interdisciplinary consultation with substance abuse experts to assess and develop a treatment plan. Keep in mind that drug abuse is a chronic disease and relapse is common, but all dying people deserve to have their suffering relieved. Assessment of patients for possible aberrant use of drugs requires a nonjudgmental stance that begins with sweeping questions to discern attitude toward drugs, what they mean in daily lives, and how they are used to cope (Passik & Kirsh, 2005). Yes/no questions should be avoided in the effort to determine how central drugs are to the patient's life. Dying patients in pain, who also have a history of drug use, will tell you the truth if they believe that your goal is to comfort them and not to condemn.

Nursing the dying drug abuser requires compassion and a sophisticated understanding of the culture and behaviors associated with drug abuse. The following guidelines may be helpful to guide nursing management of pain in a dying drug abuser (Kuebler, Berry, and Heidrich, 2002):

1. Focus on reducing suffering.
2. Involve the interdisciplinary team.
3. Propose that one physician, one pharmacist, and one primary nurse coordinate care and communicate with each other regularly. This prevents splitting and manipulating.
4. Realize that higher initial opioid doses will be needed to overcome the pain.
5. Understand that long-acting opioids are less likely to contribute to dysfunctional behavior.
6. Recognize and expect dysfunctional drug-related behavior, such as lying and manipulation.
7. Set clear limits on drug availability and diversion possibilities.
8. Contract with the patient to establish shared goals to control pain and clear expectations of how the patient will cooperate to achieve this.
9. Reassess frequently.

> 66 *Remember that drug abuse is a chronic disease, that relapse is common, and that all dying people deserve to have their suffering relieved. Nursing the dying drug abuser requires compassion and a sophisticated understanding of the culture and behaviors associated with drug abuse.*

Patients who have recovered from drug and/or alcohol addiction, perhaps having been "clean and sober" for years, may have great difficulty agreeing to use controlled substances to reduce their end-of-life suffering. They require persistent, respectful efforts to understand and accept these drugs so that they may live fully until they die. Emphasize that they will be using an opioid like a person with diabetes uses insulin to live; there is no shame in that type of "dependence." In contrast to their past experience when alcohol or illegal drugs reduced control over life and degraded its quality, opioids carefully adjusted will increase their control over life and improve quality. Keep making these contrasts. Invite your patient to consider a trial of opioids, followed by an evaluation of the effects.

NURSING RESPONSIBILITY IN THE ADMINISTRATION OF ANALGESICS

Based on thorough pain assessment, independent nursing measures to control pain include developing a caring relationship, teaching, anticipating comfort needs, offering hands-on comforting, attending to stimulation and rest, and initiating complementary therapies (see Chapter 14). This section focuses on nursing management of pharmacological therapies, which requires close collaboration with those who prescribe. Whereas physicians, physician assistants, and nurse practitioners order the drugs, nurses become the managers and coordinators of the therapies for inpatients and for those living at home who need ongoing consultation and advocacy. It is the nurse's job to coordinate the pain relief effort and ensure clear communication between all parties. When collaboration with a physician, physician assistant, or nurse practitioner is stressful and challenging, examine Box 15-7 to identify effective steps to collaboration (Griffie, 2003):

The nurse assumes five collaborative responsibilities in the administration of analgesics to control terminal pain:

1. Helping patients accept opioids
2. Regularly reassessing pain and monitoring analgesic effects and side effects
3. Balancing pharmacological effects

Box 15-7 ■ FIVE STEPS TO FOSTER COLLABORATION WITH PHYSICIANS, PHYSICIAN ASSISTANTS, AND NURSE PRACTITIONERS

1. Organize information to present a thorough pain assessment.
2. Focus on the patient's goal for pain relief.
3. Evaluate the pain treatment plan and make suggestions for change based on your knowledge of analgesics and consultation with other team members with palliative expertise. Suggestions might include breakthrough doses for escalating pain, increasing routine dosages, shortening dosing intervals, changing routes, adding analgesics, and considering nonpharmacological approaches.
4. Use current research and your agency's accepted guidelines as evidence to back up your suggestions.
5. Review your plan.
6. If you are expecting resistance, practice with a colleague your presentation of information to the physician or other provider.

Source: From Griffie (2003).

4. Trying multiple options
5. Anticipating needs

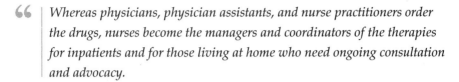

Whereas physicians, physician assistants, and nurse practitioners order the drugs, nurses become the managers and coordinators of the therapies for inpatients and for those living at home who need ongoing consultation and advocacy.

Helping Patients Accept Opioids

Just like physicians and nurses, many patients and families fear opioids. They fear addiction and side effects. They fear losing mental clarity. They fear not having anything left to control the pain when it gets "really bad." Morphine can be seen as an enemy, not a friend (Zerwekh, Riddell, and Richard, 2002). Some patients fear acknowledging their pain. The list of fears is endless. Assume that most patients fear taking opioids, and overcome the fear using the following strategies:

1. Question them to elicit their worries. Try to uncover hidden fears. Fashion your teaching accordingly. Refer patients for emotional and spiritual counseling if deep-seated denial, guilt, or anger is leading to refusal of medication.
2. Explain the extraordinarily low incidence of addiction.
3. Make the analogy of a diabetic needing insulin or a patient with heart failure needing a diuretic.
4. Explain that dosages can always be increased. They don't have to take as little as possible now in order to have medication work later.
5. Explain how side effects are managed and that drugs can be rotated if necessary.
6. Help them to clarify the teachings of their faith community. In general, Christian, Muslim, and Jewish teachings support the use of opioids to relieve suffering. (Abrahm, 2000).

Regular Pain Reassessment and Monitoring of Analgesic Effects and Side Effects

Effective pain relief requires regular and thorough reassessment of pain and response to analgesics. Chapter 14 examines comprehensive pain assessment. Document regular reassessment of pain, analgesic effects, and side effects in the patient record. Too often this involves only the use of a subjective 0 to 10 rating scale. As long as pain is not completely controlled, nursing assessment of pain must include the essential components: location, intensity, quality, pattern, aggravating factors, alleviating factors, and effects on daily living. Monitoring of analgesia goes beyond determination of pain relief to evaluate presence of side effects, such as nausea in the person with a new morphine prescription or myoclonus in a patient with rapidly escalating doses. The experienced nurse understands the manifestations of pain, its pathophysiology, and the pharmacology of analgesics so that she is able to interpret the terminal pain experience. Consider this example of an expert hospice nurse questioning pain and analgesia in a patient:

> She was agitated and stiff as a board. They had her restrained and thought it was over-medication. The private duty nurses were withholding the ordered MS Contin. Yet every time we increased the morphine, all the symptoms disappeared. I believed that rest-lessness was occurring because of the pain. Yet asking her if she was in pain was not working because this was a woman who did not believe that she should complain. I taught the night nurses to observe the reaction when they medicated her as ordered. She became calm and oriented.

Balancing Pharmacological Effects

In home, nursing home, and hospital, nurses need flexible medical orders that permit nursing judgment to alter drug regimens to maximize comfort and minimize side effects. The American Pain Society and the American Society for Pain Management Nursing support the use of "as needed" range orders that identify adjustments in doses based on individual responses. These must include a dosage range and a fixed time interval, such as "MS 2 to 8 mg IV q 2h PRN pain."

WWW.   Internet Reference Box

For more information about range orders, consult the American Pain Society site: *www.ampainsoc.org/advocacy/range.htm.*

For some patients, the nurse can feel like she is walking a tightrope to minimize cognitive and perceptual effects while still giving enough analgesia to assure pain relief. Many expert nurses describe this as "a balancing act." When patients are still functioning in most of the activities of their daily life, some will choose a degree of discomfort rather than experience mental dullness. Although some patients complain of feeling "out of it" or too groggy when they take opioids, remember that research reveals minimal thought impairment in most patients (Ersek et al., 2004). Flexible medical orders are very helpful to keep adjusting the analgesic dose to balance maximum relief with minimal cognitive side effects. A nurse describes a frail elderly patient who experienced unusual and dramatic cognitive effects:

> I got her an order for 30 mg MS Contin every 12 hours, which is just a baby dose compared to most patients. Her family would cut those pills in half or quarters because she said it made her crazy in

the head. She became disoriented and forgot they had indoor plumbing. She was up at night trying to get to the outhouse. Her son rescued her a couple of times by bringing her in from outside. I explained the danger of cutting up those pills.

To achieve greater pain relief and minimize side effects, nurses try multiple options.

ᘒ Planting the Seeds

Caution patients and families that sustained-release opioids should not be cut, broken, crushed, or chewed. These drugs are specially compounded to be long acting. If they break them apart, they will convert the drug into a high dose of immediate-release drug.

Trying Multiple Options

Hospice and palliative-care nurses often initiate new ways to manage pain. This involves organizing and reorganizing regimens, as well as recommending major changes. Sometimes nurses organize ways that patients and families can adhere to medication regimens as prescribed. Sometimes they propose changes in the existing medication regimen: changes in timing, dosage, or route. Sometimes they collaborate with the physician to add a medication. Frequently, they suggest independent nursing interventions, such as music, touch, or imagery. Perhaps they refer to a social worker or spiritual counselor to allay the emotional and spiritual dimensions of pain. An expert hospice nurse explained multiple options:

> You always come back with some option. Take pills in a different way or time. Come back and ask if there is a different way I can think through to sequence their medication. We are making a little custom suit every time we go on a visit. Tailor the plan to where they are with physical and psychological comfort.

Another nurse describes organizing the regimen during the first home visit:

> You go in and the house is in chaos. The patient is doubled over in pain. He can't get out of bed. You teach them care of the bedridden. Get other team members to come in. Organize around the clock dosing. Within 2 hours everything is calmed down and the morphine is ordered. He's gotten the first dose and is falling asleep.

66 | *We are making a little custom suit every time we go on a visit. Tailor the plan to where they are with physical and psychological comfort.*

Anticipating Analgesic Needs

Anticipating and preventing pain before it ever occurs is a hallmark of quality nursing care at the end of life. That is the premise underlying around-the-clock dosing instead of waiting for the pain before medicating. Nurses need to understand the underlying pathophysiology to anticipate which patients are likely to experience escalating pain. That is always a threat with metastatic cancer. Certainly pain can be anticipated in patients with a history of myocardial ischemia (angina). With each end-stage process, nurses and physicians work together to have analgesic orders that consider the possibility of pain and cover the need for pain relief. Maintaining analgesia levels can be a problem when a patient at home can no longer take oral medicines or experiences an exacerbation of pain. However, you can plan ahead to stay on top of the pain in anticipation of such a time. Make a plan with the family, which often includes having a "crisis kit" with sublingual or rectal opioids available.

IMPLEMENTING CLINICAL PRACTICE GUIDELINES

Clinical practice guidelines are the foundation for any program to improve pharmacological pain relief. Between 1992 and 1996, the Agency for Health Care Policy and Research (AHCPR) (now known as the Agency for Healthcare Research and Quality—AHRQ) sponsored development of a series of 19 clinical practice guidelines. In 1992, the AHCPR published *Acute Pain Management* and in 1994, *Cancer Pain Guidelines*, providing great help for practitioners dealing with patients in pain. Although the AHCPR guidelines for acute and cancer pain are considered outdated at this point, the ABCs of pain management outlined in these guidelines still hold true today and represent the backbone of all present guidelines:

> Assess and screen for the presence of pain regularly
> Believe the patient's report of pain
> Choose the appropriate intervention, analgesic and/or adjuvant
> Deliver the intervention in a coordinated and timely fashion
> Evaluate the efficacy of the interventions given
> Educate yourself, patient, and family regarding the management
> of pain
> Fine-tune the pain plan as often as needed.

Since 2000, multiple pain guidelines have been published and are more representative of current practice:

> *Cancer Pain: Treatment Guidelines for Patients*, 2001, National Comprehensive Cancer Network and the American Cancer Society.
> *Clinical Practice Guidelines for Quality Palliative Care* 2004, National Consensus Project for Quality Palliative Care.
> *The Management of Chronic Pain in Older Persons*, 2002, The American Geriatrics Society.
> *Guidelines for the Assessment and Management of Chronic Pain*, 2004, The Wisconsin Medical Society Task Force on Pain Management.

Model Guidelines for the Use of Controlled Substances for the Treatment of Pain, 1998, Federation of State Medical Boards of the United States.

Clinical guidelines allow room for individual adaptation to various practice settings. They simply provide a jumping-off point for organizational policies and procedures. Practical application of the various pain guidelines has given rise to development of algorithms for pain and symptom management. An algorithm is a branching decision-making tree that assists the practitioner in making treatment decisions for a variety of pain etiologies and other symptoms, such as constipation (Figure 15-2). Review Figure 15-3, Algorithms for Pain Management Plan.

Figure 15-3   Algorithms for Pain Management. (Copyright Dionetta Hudzinski.)

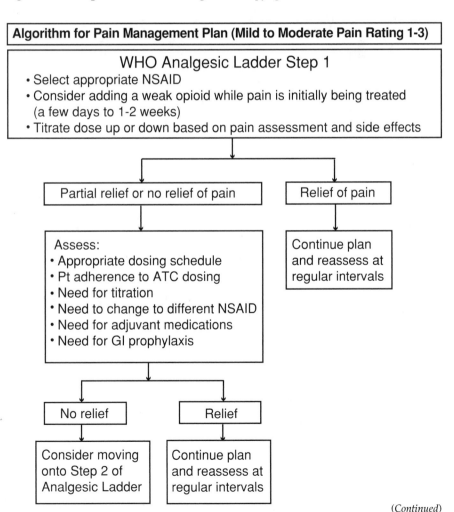

Algorithm for Pain Management Plan (Mild to Moderate Pain Rating 1-3)

WHO Analgesic Ladder Step 1
- Select appropriate NSAID
- Consider adding a weak opioid while pain is initially being treated (a few days to 1-2 weeks)
- Titrate dose up or down based on pain assessment and side effects

Partial relief or no relief of pain

Relief of pain

Assess:
- Appropriate dosing schedule
- Pt adherence to ATC dosing
- Need for titration
- Need to change to different NSAID
- Need for adjuvant medications
- Need for GI prophylaxis

Continue plan and reassess at regular intervals

No relief

Relief

Consider moving onto Step 2 of Analgesic Ladder

Continue plan and reassess at regular intervals

(Continued)

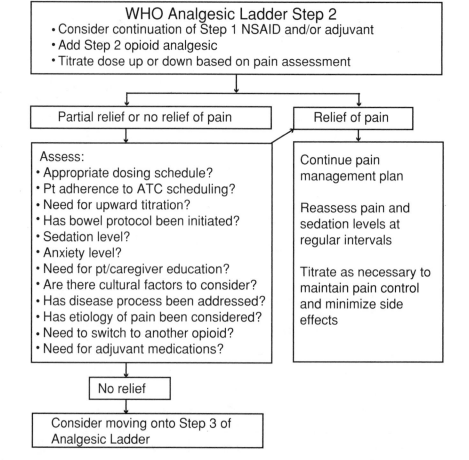

Algorithm for Pain Management Plan (Moderate to Severe Pain Rating 4-6)

- Has progression of disease been addressed?
- Are psychological and spiritual needs being addressed?
- Are there caregiver barriers or knowledge/skill issues to address?
- Functional status and quality of life assessment?
- Anxiety level? Sedation level?
- Is pain constant or intermittent?
- Have non-pharmacologic interventions been initiated?
- What are the patient's wishes and goals?

Physician-Nurse-Pharmacist Consultation
- Share assessment findings
- Discuss appropriate interventions
- Develop pain management plan and appropriate interval for reassessment

WHO Analgesic Ladder Step 2
- Consider continuation of Step 1 NSAID and/or adjuvant
- Add Step 2 opioid analgesic
- Titrate dose up or down based on pain assessment

Partial relief or no relief of pain

Relief of pain

Assess:
- Appropriate dosing schedule?
- Pt adherence to ATC scheduling?
- Need for upward titration?
- Has bowel protocol been initiated?
- Sedation level?
- Anxiety level?
- Need for pt/caregiver education?
- Are there cultural factors to consider?
- Has disease process been addressed?
- Has etiology of pain been considered?
- Need to switch to another opioid?
- Need for adjuvant medications?

Continue pain management plan

Reassess pain and sedation levels at regular intervals

Titrate as necessary to maintain pain control and minimize side effects

No relief

Consider moving onto Step 3 of Analgesic Ladder

Figure 15-3 (*Continued*)

Algorithm for Pain Management Plan (Severe Pain Rating 7-10)

Assessment:
- Has an in-depth pain assessment been done?
- Has progression of disease been addressed?
- Are psychological and spiritual needs being addressed?
- Are there caregiver barriers or knowledge/skill issues to address?
- Functional status and quality of life assessment?
- Anxiety level? Sedation level?
- Is pain constant or intermittent?
- Have non-pharmacologic interventions been initiated?
- What are the patient's wishes and goals?
- Is there a need for an alternate route of administration?
- Would pt benefit from initiation of steroids or other adjuvant meds?
- Has a medication review been done to avoid polypharmacy?

Physician-Nurse-Pharmacist Consultation
- Share assessment findings
- Discuss appropriate interventions
- Develop pain management plan and appropriate interval for reassessment

WHO Analgesic Ladder Step 3
- Consider continuation of Step 1 NSAID and/or adjuvant
- Discontinue Step 2 opioid analgesic
- Add Step 3 opioid analgesic
- Titrate dose up or down based on pain assessment

Partial or no relief	Relief of pain

Assess:
- Appropriate dosing schedule?
- Pt adherence to ATC scheduling?
- Need for upward titration?
- Has bowel protocol been initiated?
- Sedation level?
- Anxiety level?
- Need for pt/caregiver education?
- Are there cultural factors to consider?
- Has disease process been addressed?
- Has etiology of pain been considered?
- Need to switch to another opioid?
- Need for adjuvant medications?

Continue pain management plan

Reassess pain and sedation levels at regular intervals

Titrate as necessary to maintain pain control and minimize side effects

No relief

Continue reassessments with upward titration
Consider alternate routes of administration
Consider consultation with pain specialist
Consider new etiology or advancing disease
Consider adding or changing adjuvants

Figure 15-3

CONCEPTS IN ACTION

You are assigned to care for J.B., who is a 69-year-old male, diagnosed with advanced prostate cancer with bone metastases. His prognosis is weeks to months, and he is referred to the palliative team for management of his pain and symptoms. During shift report you are told that in spite of "huge" amounts of drugs, his pain remains out of control. The patient has been nauseated and vomits every time he changes position. His last bowel movement was 5 days ago; bowel sounds are present but hypoactive. His abdomen is distended and nontender. Lungs are clear and oxygen saturation is running at 96%–98% room air. Respirations are 16/minute. He has been agitated and irritable, refusing to get out of bed to sit in the chair. His last solid food was 2 days ago, but he does take sips of fluids.

After report, you find J.B. lying in a fetal position with the sheet pulled up tightly to his chin. His fists are clenched, eyes are tightly shut, and his brow is deeply furrowed. When you ask him about his pain, all he can say is, "It hurts all over and I'd rather die than keep going like this." He rates his pain on a scale of 0 to 10 as "way past 10."

You go to the medication administration record (MAR) to determine what analgesic he is getting and when he can have another dose. You find the following orders:

- Acetaminophen 500 mg PO every 6 hours (4 doses charted as given in the past 24 hours)
- Darvocet N 100 mg PO 1 tab every 6 hours (3 doses charted as given in the past 24 hours)
- Demerol 75 mg IM every 4–6 hours (6 doses charted as given in the past 24 hours)
  1. Referring to the Algorithm for Pain Management (Figure 15-13), how would you investigate his discomfort?
  2. What combination of medications would be most appropriate for this patient's pain, based on his diagnosis?
  3. Which alternative route of administration would be most appropriate at this time?
  4. Refer to the Bowel Management Algorithm, Figure 15-2. What actions would you take to treat his constipation?
  5. What actions should be taken for his nausea at this time?
  6. How might you communicate your assessment findings and recommendations for changes in the pain plan to the physician to get the best response?

References

AAPM, & APS (American Academy of Pain Medicine and the American Pain Society). (1997). Use of opioids for the treatment of chronic pain. A consensus statement.

AAHPM (American Academy of Hospice and Palliative Medicine) (2003). *Pocket guide to hospice/palliative medicine.* Glenview, IL: AAHPM.

Abrahm, J. (2000). *A physician's guide to pain and symptom management in cancer patients.* Baltimore: Johns Hopkins University.

Angell, M. (1982). The quality of mercy. *New England Journal of Medicine, 306,* 98–99.

Blues, A. & Zerwekh, J. (1984). *Hospice and palliative nursing.* Orlando, FL: Grune & Stratton.

Brecher, A., & Editors of *Consumer Reports.* (1972). The Consumers Union report on licit and illicit drugs. *Consumer Reports Magazine.*

Bruera, E., & Kim, H. (2003). Cancer pain. *Journal of the American Medical Association, 290*(18), 2476–2479.

Cherny, N., Ripamontik C., Pereira, J., Davis, C., Fallonk, M., McQuay, H., et al. (2001). Strategies to manage the adverse effects of oral morphine: An evidence-based report. *Journal of Clinical Oncology, 19*(9), 2542–2554.

Doctors Behind Bars: Treating pain is now risky business. (19 October, 2004). *New York Times,* pp

Ersek, M., Cherrier, M., Overman, S., & Irving, F. (2004). The cognitive effects of opioids. *Pain Management Nursing, 5*(2), 75–93.

Examples of Balanced and Unbalanced Policy. (May, 2002). *State Initiatives in End-of-Life Care, 14,* 4.

Fine, P. G., Miaskowski, C., Paice, J. A. (2004) Meeting the challenge in cancer pain management. *Journal of Supportive Oncology, 2*(6Suppl. 4), 5–22.

Gregory, D., & English, J. (1994). The myth of control: Suffering in palliative care. *Journal of Palliative Care, 10*(2), 18–22.

Griffie, J. (2003). Addressing inadequate pain relief. *American Journal of Nursing, 103*(8), 61–63.

Hardman, J., Limbird, L., & Gilman, A. (2001). *Goodman and Gilman's the pharmacological basis of therapeutics* (10th ed.). New York: McGraw-Hill.

Kuebler, K., Berry, P., & Heidrich, D. (2002). *End-of-life-care: Clinical practice guidelines.* Philadelphia: WB Saunders.

McCaffery, M., & Pasero, C. (2003). Breakthrough pain. *American Journal of Nursing, 103*(4), 83–84, 86.

Pasero, C., & McCaffery, M. (2002). Monitoring sedation. *American Journal of Nursing, 102*(2), 67, 69.

Passik, S., & Kirsh, K. (2005). Managing pain in patients with aberrant drug-taking behaviors. *Journal of Supportive Oncology, 3*(1), 83–86.

Porter, J., & Jick, H. (1980). Addiction rare in patients treated with narcotics. *New England Journal of Medicine, 302*(2), 123.

Porth, C. M. (2004). *Essentials of pathophysiology.* Philadelphia: Lippincott Williams and Wilkins.

Public Policy Statement on the Rights and Responsibilities of healthcare Professionals in the Use of Opioids for the Treatment of Pain (2004). A consensus document from the American Academy of Pain Medicine, the American Pain Society, and the American Society of Addiction Medicine.

Rich, B. (2001). Prioritizing pain management in patient care. *Postgraduate Medicine, 110*(3), 15–17.

Sabino, M., & Mantyh, P. (2005). Pathophysiology of bone pain. *Journal of Supportive Oncology, 3*(1), 15–24.

Savage, S., Joranson, D., Covington, Scholl, S., Heit, H., & Gilson, A. (2003). Definitions related to the medical use of opioids: Evolution towards universal agreement. *Journal of Pain and Symptom Management, 26*(1), 655–667.

St. Marie, B. (2002). *Core curriculum for pain management nursing*. Philadelphia: WB Saunders.

Thorns, A., & Sykes, N. (2000). Opioid use in last week of life and implications for end-of-life decision making. *The Lancet, 356*(9227), 398–399.

Thwaites, D., McCann, S., & Broderick, P. (2004). Hydromorphone neuroex-

citation. *Journal of Palliative Medicine, 7*(4), 545–550.

Zerwekh, J., Riddell, S., & Richard, J. (2002). Fearing to comfort: A grounded theory of constraints to opioid use in hospice care. *Journal of Hospice and Palliative Nursing, 4*(2), 83–90.

CHAPTER 16

Management of Physical Nonpain Symptoms

Philosophical Reflections

"It is up to us to use our positions in the healthcare system to ensure that effective palliation occurs. We have the ability to mandate our patients' physical comfort throughout their lives. I challenge you to examine your practice and environment; if barriers exist to promoting patient or family comfort, speak up and demand changes."

PATRICK COYNE, CLINICAL NURSE SPECIALIST, 2003

Learning Objectives

1. Explain unique qualities of symptom assessment when comfort is the focus.
2. Identify essential components of symptom assessment.
3. Identify the goal-setting process essential to relieving symptoms.
4. List pain and symptom management guidelines.
5. Name comforting independent nursing interventions and give an example how each might be used in symptom control.
6. Describe pharmacological and nonpharmacological management of common end-of-life physical symptoms.
7. Develop a system to recall common end-of-life physical symptoms.
8. Evaluate the role of palliative sedation when other palliative strategies fail.
9. Develop a plan to advocate for dying patients suffering from unrelieved physical symptoms.

Managing symptoms at the end of life is symbolized by leaves on the End-of-Life Caregiving Tree. These leaves illustrate the multiple efforts that caregivers bring forth to relieve various physical symptoms. Knowledge about contemporary symptom management is rapidly expanding, and there is much we can do to comfort the dying. This chapter describes the process of assessing nonpain symptoms and setting goals for symptom relief at the end of life. The chapter then sets forth symptom management guidelines for nursing interventions to relieve symptoms; these guidelines create a foundation for management of symptoms including fatigue, fever, infection, dehydration, skin breakdown, cognitive impairment, malnutrition, dyspnea, death rattle, constipation, diarrhea, and impaired urinary function. The chapter examines palliative sedation when symptom-control fails. The chapter concludes with the assertion that the nurse must become an advocate for patients with unrelieved symptoms.

SYMPTOM ASSESSMENT AND GOALS

Assessing symptoms thoroughly and identifying symptom-relief goals will help to achieve the highest possible quality of life in a person's final months, weeks, days, and hours. Patients themselves define what quality of life they desire and nurses listen. It is important not to impose our own ideas about what level of comfort is or is not acceptable.

 Assessing symptoms thoroughly and identifying symptom-relief goals will help to achieve the highest possible quality of life in a person's final months, weeks, days, and hours. Patients themselves define what quality of life they desire and nurses listen.

Comfort

Nurses and physicians tend to think we know what is happening in the patient's body. We tend to doubt a patient's complaints and rely on objective tests to tell us what is true. However, suffering cannot be confirmed or denied by a blood test or scanned by the most expensive technology. Comfort is always the overriding goal; so assess symptoms with the goal of comfort in mind. Nevertheless, comfort and discomfort are subjective concepts and are therefore tricky to assess. Focusing on comfort in your symptom assessment means attending to the lived experience of the patient and how he or she defines comfort. Comfort is highly individualized. Sometimes a patient's other needs, such as denial or control, will be stronger than the desire for physical comfort. A patient might choose to sacrifice physical comfort in order to participate fully in family interaction. Another might desire to have all physical distress controlled. Comfort should always be the overriding concern in end-of-life physical assessment. Before implementing tests, ask the question, "How will the results assist in providing comfort and meeting the patient's wishes?" Is this blood draw, that rectal exam, or the proposed lung scan really going to help comfort the person or meet his or her goals? If the patient is experiencing new sources of discomfort, investigate the cause unless the burdens of diagnosis outweigh any palliative benefit. Comfort is the priority, particularly when death is imminent.

Assessment of nonpain symptoms (and discomfort produced by them) is approached similarly to pain assessment. As with pain, the bedrock of assessing symptoms such as fatigue or nausea, is questioning patients carefully. Essential components of nonpain symptom assessment include determination of intensity, quality, pattern, aggravating factors, alleviating factors, and effects on life. The Edmonton Symptom Assessment System (ESAS) is a particularly useful tool that documents severity of pain, fatigue, nausea, depression, anxiety, drowsiness, appetite, well-being, and shortness of breath. After completing a thorough symptom assessment, the next step in achieving comfort for the patient is to enumerate specific comfort goals.

WWW. Internet Resource Box

A variety of symptom assessment tools are available through the Practical Ethics Center Web site at the University of Montana: *www.promotingexcellence.org.*

> ❝ *As with pain, the bedrock of symptom assessment is asking patients about symptoms and questioning them carefully. Essential components include determination of intensity, quality, pattern, aggravating factors, alleviating factors, and effects on life.*

Goals of Comfort Care

Setting goals begins with the first assessment and continues with each encounter. Goals change during the variable course of illness. Goals of comfort care are determined by discovering those symptoms that (1) the patient finds most troubling, (2) are most likely to respond to intervention, and (3) have interventions that the patient finds acceptable. Prioritize goals in order of importance to the patient and ease of treating to achieve comfort (Abrahm, 2000). Also consider the desires of the family, physician, and nurse, which may need to be reconciled to develop an effective plan of care. End-of-life symptom management goals must be individualized and are often formulated as a result of ongoing negotiation. Even if the patient generally has been an assertive decision-maker, his voice usually weakens as disease progresses. Various family members may speak up and take various positions. Likewise, physicians are accustomed to being powerful decision-makers and having their opinions dominate. Without their cooperation in prescribing palliative medication, no plan for comfort care can succeed. Nurses must seek to uncover the wishes of the patient and to identify goals that all can share.

Consider this generic example of how to arrive at goals of comfort care. A hospice nurse does an initial assessment of the patient and identifies how the hospice program can help. She suggests possible goals that can be realized through hospice care, considering what the team can realistically achieve. She identifies pain and nausea relief, counseling for the caregiver's depression, spiritual support by the hospice chaplain, and assistance with physical caregiving by the home-health aide. She uses language that is understandable and will be heard by the stressed patient and family. The nurse observes interpersonal dynamics carefully to begin understanding family patterns. The family's ability to communicate clearly and problem-solve will determine its ability to manage the challenges of end-of-life care. Chapter 11 addresses the influence of family dynamics on caregiving. The nurse seeks to synthesize goals of the patient, family members, physician, and hospice team into a workable focus. It is difficult to merge goals with conflicting ideas and divisive emotions. For example, one family member insists on a nursing home whereas another wants to keep her loved one at home. In the presence of such conflict, the nurse seeks to maintain a calm presence that continually refocuses all parties on maintaining comfort and dignity for the dying person. The immediate hospice goal is not to tackle long-standing family troubles, but to bring everyone together to honor and comfort the dying family member.

66 | *Nurses seek to maintain a calm presence that continually refocuses all parties on maintaining comfort and dignity for the dying person.*

Consider Martha, for example. She has suffered for several years while receiving aggressive treatment for her ovarian cancer. A comfort assessment reveals three major complaints causing her discomfort: weakness, worsening dyspnea, and nausea. The weakness cannot be reversed, although she can be helped to conserve her energy. The dyspnea can be managed with medications she is willing to accept. She rejects debulking surgery to reduce her bowel obstruction but does accept palliative medication for nausea. One younger daughter lives nearby and understands that her mother is close to death. An older daughter arrived yesterday from a city 2100 miles away; she has not returned home for 8 years, and there is obvious tension with her younger sister. Since arriving, she has been sitting at the bedside, encouraging her mother to eat and drink. She also has been trying to convince her mother to try some alternative therapies only available in Mexico. Martha's physician has encouraged her to try another round of chemotherapy that has a small chance of working.

Even as she walks through the door, the nurse is engulfed by the tension in the home as both sisters are yelling at each other. She resolves to be a calming presence, using touch and slowing down her own speech. She breathes deeply to stay centered. The nurse first completes a physical assessment, observes tense family interaction, and listens carefully to each daughter's position. Then she sits down with Martha and her two daughters to develop a priority list of comforting goals about which they all can agree: no trip to Mexico, no surgery, no chemotherapy, no forced eating, relief of symptoms, but rejection of all opioids as "dope." The nurse agrees that the hospice team will work with the family to achieve Martha's symptom management goals, despite the constraint she has imposed on drug selection. At her next home visit she will do some more teaching about the effect of opioids. The daughters continue to disagree, but not about appropriate symptom relief. As always, the nurse has to be careful not to impose her own agenda. The goals identified determine the interventions chosen; as the goals change, the interventions will also be modified.

GUIDELINES FOR NURSING INTERVENTIONS

Relief of terminal symptoms is guided by the pain and symptom management fundamentals initially identified at the conclusion of Chapter 14, which emphasized pain relief. Although this chapter addresses nonpain symptoms, the palliative fundamentals are the same for all symptoms, pain and nonpain, and include the following:

1. Don't make assumptions. Believe the patient's report of symptoms.
2. Relieve the symptom to the extent patients choose and in ways they can accept.
3. Repeatedly investigate physical, psychosocial, and spiritual dimensions of pain and evaluate the effectiveness of interventions.
4. Anticipate symptoms and relieve them before they recur.
5. Include nursing and complementary interventions.
6. Develop expertise in the use of palliative medication.
7. Choose the least complex intervention to keep end-of-life care affordable and manageable by patients and families at home.
8. Never give up hope of relieving discomfort. Keep trying different approaches.

Include comforting independent nursing interventions as you work at the bedside of those close to death. These comforting nursing responses to suffering include the following:

- Developing caring relationships
- Teaching
- Offering hands-on care
- Promoting stimulation and rest
- Incorporating complementary therapies
- Providing anticipatory guidance
- Managing pharmacological therapies

Examples of some of these are incorporated into discussion of specific symptoms below. Anticipatory guidance and choice of pharmacological therapies are examined specifically here.

ANTICIPATORY GUIDANCE

Anticipatory guidance is an essential dimension of planning to relieve end-of-life symptoms. It involves predicting the course of illness and complications of therapies in order to anticipate challenges that will face the patient and family. Anticipating likely problems, the nurse teaches them what to expect and guides them to prepare for possible symptoms. Anticipatory guidance can replace turmoil with undisturbed calm. For inpatients, equipment and drugs are on hand to anticipate exacerbation of symptoms or new complications. At home, families and other caregivers should be prepared to manage predictable problems. They should be able to say, "We were expecting that and we were prepared." Anticipatory guidance is more likely to succeed when a family's coping style is oriented toward problem-solving and planning ahead. It is less likely to be successful when family members have lived their lives from crisis to crisis.

66 | *Anticipatory guidance can replace turmoil with undisturbed calm.*

Normalizing is one dimension of anticipatory guidance. Normalizing involves making the end-of-life course as normal as possible. Instead of unexpected and terrifying, the final symptoms before death should be made normal, predictable, and controllable. A nurse might say, "She might have some breathing difficulties after a while. That's normal. We are going to be ready in case that occurs. You'll have the needed medicine in the home, and we're going to go over everything to be sure there is no crisis."

66 | *Instead of unexpected and terrifying, the final symptoms before death*
     | *should be made normal, predictable, and controllable.*

Managing Pharmacological Therapies

Physicians and nurse practitioners prescribe the drugs that make symptom control possible. Nurses become the managers of those therapies. For patients at the end of life, it is essential that nurses continually assess the effectiveness of therapies, work collaboratively with prescribers, and have the knowledge to make recommendations for changes. Control of symptoms should involve choosing the simplest technologies, preferring the oral or sublingual medication route instead of injections. Such methods are more readily managed by patients and families without continual professional intervention. They permit a patient to die without attachment to multiple devices and lines. As technologies accumulate around a person, the patient can be overlooked as a focus of attention. Oral medication and minimal technology is also more affordable. Nevertheless, contemporary hospices are having continual difficulty keeping interventions simple and low-tech once complex technologies have been implemented. Complex technology should be chosen only if it is the only method available to relieve symptoms.

Management of Common Symptoms

Symptoms that commonly cause distress at the end of life include fatigue and impaired mobility, infection and fever, impaired fluid balance, impaired skin integrity, impaired thought, risk for hemorrhage, imbalanced nutrition, ineffective breathing pattern and airway clearance, impaired bowel elimination, and impaired urinary elimination. Each is discussed in the sections that follow.

▦ ࣷ Planting the Seeds

Use a systematic approach as you learn to anticipate end-of-life physical symptoms and their assessment. First, remember to expect and investigate whether problems affecting the whole body (fatigue, fever, dehydration, and skin breakdown) have developed. Then proceed from head to toe. Beginning with the head, assess the presence of cognitive changes. Next, move to the mouth and impairments related to digestion. Then, move to the chest and examine the patient for respiratory alterations. Then, consider the gut and predictable impairments in bowel and bladder function. Use this systematic approach to remember symptoms and their management.

Fatigue and Impaired Mobility

Progressive fatigue, immobility, and self-care deficits are inevitable with a slow downhill terminal course. Assess intensity, quality, patterns, aggravating factors, relieving factors, and effects on life. For example, a patient reports that he is exhausted "all of the time except for a couple of hours after breakfast." He rates his fatigue as 9 on a 1 to 10 scale. It is worsened by attempting any housework, like washing the dishes, and relieved only by napping and drinking several cups of coffee. Coffee provides just brief relief. He is unable to carry out any everyday activities. His goal is to have enough energy for short visits with good friends and family.

Palliation goals may include identifying and correcting underlying reversible conditions, such as depression, electrolyte abnormalities, drug side effects, and anemia (Berger, Portenoy, and Weissman, 2002). Some patients may wish to receive psychostimulants, such as methylphenidate (Ritalin, Concerta), to boost their energy for a while. Subcutaneous injections of epoetin alpha (Epogen, Procrit) may increase hemoglobin and hematocrit in selected terminally ill patients, but the high cost needs to be balanced with the quality of life achievable.

Nurse interventions for fatigue at the end of life include strategies to promote sleep, improving nutrition when possible, reducing the burden of other symptoms, and managing decreased energy. When death is not yet near, the nurse can help the patient cope with fatigue and weakness by recommending assistive equipment, emphasizing priority activities, and referring to occupational and physical therapy. The nurse can encourage periods of rest and activities to restore emotional energy, such as spending time with family, surrounding oneself with nature, listening to music, or meditating. One nurse gives us an example:

> They were still going out to concerts and playing bridge with friends. She was exhausted and nauseated and short of breath. When I made my home visit, she couldn't stop crying, "I'm so tired. I can't do anything. I feel wretched." Beginning then and over the next few visits, we talked about letting go of the energetic life she once lived, resting more, and focusing on those activities that mattered most. I talked about her experience as normal for someone with such advanced disease. This made sense to her and she slowed down and started feeling a lot better. She decided that each day she would take a nap before and after visiting with one of her closest friends.

Ideally, patients and their families should prepare for the day when the person is first chair bound and then bed bound. But anticipation of increasing dependency is highly threatening. For many, acceptance of weakness and diminished self-care abilities is tantamount to giving up, so many people will object to planning for such an eventuality. For instance, some patients living alone will reject the idea that they will eventually need a caregiver. Others object to the idea of needing a hospital bed in their home. In the United States, we pride ourselves on self-help and feel shame in asking others for help. The nurse respects the patient's choices and points out the advantages and availability of help. Sometimes a crisis must occur, such as an episode of incontinence or a fall, before the person acknowledges need.

When fatigue and progressive immobility lead the person to be bedridden, the nursing role is to teach caregivers to care for an immobilized patient. The nurse must quickly teach nursing fundamentals, including turning, positioning, bathing, mouth care, skin care, bowel and bladder management. Equipment and supplies must be ordered to make that possible. Preparing the environment and teaching the family is a common focus of home-health and hospice nurses. An expert nurse explains this work:

> I'm giving them the tools that they need to make this work. I'm teaching them to do the physical care for someone who is no longer able to care for himself. I train them in bowel management and what to do with skin care and how to position him.

Infection and Fever

Dying people are highly susceptible to infection. Their immunity is compromised, making them prone to the usual pathogenic organisms, as well as invasion from opportunistic protozoa or fungi. As the dying person becomes immobilized with associated stasis, urinary and pulmonary infection threatens. Microbial invasion is also more likely with the damage to skin and mucous membranes that comes with catheterization, venipuncture, and other invasive procedures. At the end of life, the decision to investigate and treat infection is challenging when the goal is comfort. Common infection sites include the respiratory tract, urinary tract, mouth, skin, venous access sites, and perianal area. Do the patient and family choose diagnosis and active treatment, which will involve invasive procedures such as blood culture, sputum culture, x-ray, serologies, or spinal tap? Will antibiotics relieve discomfort associated with the infectious process, or will they prolong an uncomfortable dying process? It is best that discussion about using antibiotics be undertaken with patient and/or family well before infection occurs. The nurse can help patient, family, and the health-care team clarify benefits and burden of diagnosis and treatment. They may choose to treat the infection if the patient's wish is to keep fighting for life, or if unfinished business remains, such as a family member who has not yet said good-bye. Often a terminal infection is untreatable, despite vigorous investigation and treatment. When the dying has been long and lingering with an overwhelming symptom burden, the patient and/or family often welcome the final infection.

Remember that comfort is the goal when a dying patient develops a fever. Avoid cooling measures that are uncomfortable and cause shivering. Encourage fluids and wet cloths that are comforting. The subjective discomforts of fever can usually be relieved with antipyretics such as aspirin, acetaminophen, and ibuprofen. Aspirin suppositories are useful when people can no longer swallow.

 Will antibiotics relieve discomfort associated with the infectious process, or will they prolong an uncomfortable dying process?

Impaired Fluid Balance

Most dying people reduce their oral intake of fluids before they die, because of weakness, anorexia, depression, cognitive impairment, nausea and vomiting, dysphagia, and bowel obstruction. The hospice movement has challenged the assumption that hydration is good for all patients, and that dehydration causes suffering at the end of life (Zerwekh, 1997). Dehydrated hospice patients are usually quite comfortable. Too often, funding mechanisms drive decisions about whether to hydrate a dying patient. In the hospital, the need for intravenous fluids becomes a justification for billing insurers (Dalal & Bruera, 2004). In contrast, current hospice funding mechanisms make parenteral fluids difficult to finance. Many hospices have blanket policies against hydration, which they have not found to be palliative.

 The hospice movement has challenged the assumption that hydration is good for all patients, and that dehydration causes suffering at the end of life (Zerwekh, 1997, 2004).

Fluid and electrolyte balance in the dying patient is poorly understood. Dying people who are dehydrated have surprisingly normal blood chemistries. Classic laboratory findings associated with volume depletion are simply not found in the dying. The most consistent change in those close to death is azotemia with elevated urea, creatinine, and uric acid levels (Ellershaw, 1995).

Physical signs of fluid deficit include tachycardia, postural hypotension, reduced skin turgor, and dry mucous membranes, but these signs can also be present at the end of life in people who are well hydrated (Dalal & Bruera, 2004). Patients' greatest complaints are thirst and dry mouth, but many end-stage disease processes and medication side effects contribute to this discomfort. It is surprising that thirst and dry mouth are not correlated with specific fluid and electrolyte changes. Fluid deficits at the end of life are sometimes associated with cognitive impairment and altered behavior.

Water requirements of dying patients are reduced due to age, diminished body weight, lower insensible losses (perspiration), and lower output. We now understand that the water requirement for a dying patient is in the range of 800 to 1000 mL daily (Dalal & Bruera, 2004) in contrast with approximately 1500 to 2500 mL in a nondying adult. Of course this varies with weight.

> We now understand that the water requirement for a dying patient is in the range of 800 to 1000 mL daily (Dalal & Bruera, 2004).

Box 16-1 ■ BENEFITS AND BURDENS OF ARTIFICIAL HYDRATION

BENEFITS	BURDENS
May reduce disorientation, myoclonus, and restlessness.	Increased urine output so need for catheterization or incontinence care.
Will relieve reversible imbalances such as hypercalcemia.	Increased GI fluid so more vomiting.
Readily corrects fluid losses from diarrhea and diuretic effects.	Increased pulmonary secretions so more coughing and congestion.
May prevent neurotoxicity due to high opioid doses.	Increased edema and ascites.
Appears to provide a human need and can be a symbol of nurturance.	Maintaining the line may be painful and preoccupy family and caregivers.
Appears to meet a minimum standard of care, adhered to by agencies and physicians.	Often requires restraining patient. "Medicalizes" end of life. May prolong suffering.

Source: From Dalal & Bruera (2004); and Zerwekh (1997).

Box 16-2 ■	BENEFITS AND BURDENS OF DEHYDRATION

BENEFITS	BURDENS
Reduced urine output with less need for bedpan, urinal, commode, catheter, incontinence care.	Religious and cultural objections.
Less vomiting, especially with obstructed bowel.	Delirium due to opioid toxicity will not be relieved.
Reduced respiratory and pharyngeal secretions.	Confusion and nausea due to hypercalcemia will not be relieved.
Less edema and ascites.	
Increased ketones and endogenous opioids as natural anesthetic/analgesic.	
No need to restrain patient to permit technology.	
No preoccupation with maintaining the line.	

Source: From Dalal & Bruera (2004); and Zerwekh (1997).

In truth, the decision to hydrate a dying patient should be individualized and based on a balance of benefits and burdens. See Box 16-1, Benefits and Burden of Artificial Hydration, and Box 16-2, Benefits and Burdens of Dehydration. There is evidence that hydration can be beneficial for some dying patients. Intravenous or subcutaneous infusions can sometimes correct fluid and electrolyte imbalances, stabilizing the patient's condition. Hydration reduces disorientation and restlessness in some terminal patients; this has been clearly demonstrated in those experiencing neurotoxicity from high opioid doses. Some palliative-care programs are now routinely providing small-volume hydrating fluids by subcutaneous infusions (Lanuke, Fainsinger, and DeMoissac, 2004).

At the same time, hydration can be a burden for dying people. Consider its potential to exacerbate unfortunate fluid accumulation. If the kidneys have not shut down, more fluid circulating to the kidneys builds up in the bladder to increase urine output. This will require catheterization or frequent changes of diapers and linens in the weakened, comatose, or incontinent person at the end of life. The amount of fluid in the gastrointestinal tract will increase, exacerbating vomiting in a patient already troubled by this. In the presence of end-stage heart, liver, and/or kidney failure, fluid moves out of the blood into tissues and third spaces. Therefore, excessive fluid given to dying people with end-stage organ failure often goes where it cannot be useful and may aggravate symptoms. If the patient has a tumor, hydration can expand the edematous layer around it, aggravating symptoms due to pressure. Parenteral fluids can worsen edema, ascites, and fistula or wound drainage. In addition, many clinicians have observed increased respiratory secretions in the hydrated patient with pneumonia or pulmonary edema. All of these ill effects appear to be associated with large-volume fluid replacement.

> *In the presence of end-stage heart, liver, and/or kidney failure, fluid moves out of the blood into tissues and third spaces. Therefore, excessive fluid given to dying people with end-stage organ failure often goes where it cannot be useful and may aggravate symptoms.*

"Gentle hydration," approximately 1 liter of fluid daily, has been proposed as a strategy to keep a patient hydrated without causing fluid overload. In the hospice and palliative-care setting, fluids should be given by subcutaneous infusion; this process is called hypodermoclysis and avoids the risk of complications and the need for technical skill associated with intravenous therapy. It is inappropriate to use in patients with bleeding disorders or generalized edema. A butterfly needle is inserted subcutaneously in the thighs, outer arm, and abdomen of bedridden patients, or the abdomen and upper chest of ambulatory patients (Dalal & Bruera, 2004). Common electrolyte fluid solutions can be administered continuously by gravity at a rate of 40–60 mL/hour in the bedridden patient. An alternative is administering fluids overnight at a rate of perhaps 80 mL/hour or in two or three bolus infusions of 500 mL at a time. Localized edema is occasionally noted. Box 16-3 identifies advantages of the subcutaneous route for fluid administration.

Rectal administration of fluids (proctolysis) is also an inexpensive, low-tech method of infusion (Dalal & Bruera, 2004). A 22 French nasogastric catheter is inserted to about 40 cm and saline or tap water is infused several times a day. Fluids may leak out of the rectum and large volumes

---

Box 16-3 ■	**ADVANTAGES OF SUBCUTANEOUS FLUID INFUSION**

Inexpensive
Lasts 5 to 7 days
Minimal technical skill to initiate and maintain
Minimal pain with needle insertion
Lower incidence of adverse reactions than IV access
Minimal need for restraint to avoid needle reinsertion

Source: From Dalal & Bruera (2004).

can have an enema effect. This route should be reserved for circumstances in which the IV and subcutaneous routes are not feasible, such as in developing countries.

Contrary to the medical impulse to administer fluids, artificial hydration should not be initiated without clear indication that it will benefit the individual patient. What may be a benefit for some patients will be a burden for others. Even presuming hydration can improve level of alertness, an improved level of alertness may actually intensify suffering and interfere with the natural analgesia that seems to occur near death. Hospice professionals continue to note that for most patients close to death, hydration offers no benefit. Dehydrated patients die comfortably most of the time (Zerwekh, 1997 & 2003). Nurses are ideally situated to ask clarifying questions about the benefits and burdens of hydration for the individual.

> *Contrary to the medical impulse to administer fluids, artificial hydration should not be initiated without clear indication that it will benefit the individual patient.*

 Planting the Seeds

When considering artificial hydration, ask the following questions to clarify the best intervention:

1. What is the overall benefit of hydration for this patient? Is there any objective reason to think that hydration will or is making her feel better?
2. Is there reason to believe that any specific symptoms will be relieved or are being relieved by hydration?
3. Are some symptoms currently being aggravated by artificial hydration? Is hydration likely to cause symptoms in this individual?
4. Does end-stage organ failure place this patient at risk of fluid accumulations in tissues in third spaces? Is this already occurring?
5. Is there reason to think that fluids will improve the patient's alertness? Is this what the patient wants?
6. Might fluids diminish delirium in this patient?
7. What are or might be the psychosocial complications of the infusion technology? Is there or might there be distress about the needle insertion or attachment to lines? What are or will be the effects of the technology on the family? Is it or might it be causing caregiver stress? What about financial burden? Will it preoccupy caregivers when the focus should be on the person?

Keep in mind that a patient or his surrogate decision-maker have a right to give informed consent about any invasive procedure, including artificial hydration. If fluids are ordered, patients need to approve that order based on the best current information. Likewise, if fluids are not ordered, patients have a right to question why not. Nurses are often in a position to explain possible benefit or harm. When family members disagree among themselves, nurses can be of great help by sitting down, listening to their concerns, and helping them make a list of benefits and burdens specific to their relative's situation. The idea of withholding or withdrawing fluids is likely to arouse strong feelings. How, they may ask, can we take away water from our loved one? A helpful nursing response is to show them other ways they can show caring. For instance, consider the following response to Mrs. Conigliaro, who asks whether her dying husband, who has no signs of delirium and a long history of heart failure, should have an IV. She asks the nurse "Won't he die if he doesn't drink?" The nurse replies as follows:

> Mrs. Conigliaro, your husband's cancer is taking his life, not lack of water. I'm not sure that fluids would make him more comfortable. They might make his lungs wet and swell up his legs. There's no evidence that dehydration causes dying patients much discomfort. In my opinion, your husband doesn't need fluids anymore. We can offer him little sips and small pieces of ice. And we can continue caring for his mouth and lips to keep them moist. Can I show you and your daughters how to do that? (Zerwekh, 1997, p. 29).

Hypercalcemia

Artificial hydration is clearly indicated with elevated levels of serum calcium. Hypercalcemia is commonly seen with squamous cell carcinoma of the lung and breast, and with multiple myeloma (Berger, Portenoy, and Weissman, 2002). The patient commonly becomes anorexic, nauseated, and cognitively impaired. The best immediate intervention is rehydration with saline. Intravenous infusions of bisphosphonates such as pamidronate (Aredia) given over 4 to 6 hours will control hypercalcemia for as long as a month. Gallium nitrate and plicamycin (mithramycin) will also reduce serum calcium levels that do not respond to other therapies.

Some contemporary hospices have utilitarian policies that limit interventions and medication to those that are standardized, least expensive, and likely to comfort most patients. Unfortunately, such policies do not allow for investigation of individual circumstances or achieve maximum quality of life. The author recently watched a 61-year-old gentleman with newly diagnosed multiple myeloma admitted to one hospice unit within a large hospice corporation. The company had a standing policy against hydrating patients, and their formulary did not include bisphosphonates or zoledronic acid. The patient received morphine and lorazepam. He died without pain and with minimal nausea, but he never rose out of his hypercalcemia-induced confusion to say the words he needed to say and make the decisions he had a right to make. Nurses need to advocate for individualized care and individualized decision-making.

ᨀᨋ Planting the Seeds

Hospices that limit medications and interventions to those that are cost efficient and likely to benefit most patients should have policies that allow for careful consideration of exceptions. When the nurse believes there is compelling evidence for a treatment or medication outside standard protocols, such a policy creates an avenue for considering alternative approaches.

Impaired Skin Integrity

At the end of life, multiple risk factors for skin breakdown develop and worsen. The patient grows inactive and increasingly immobile, placing more and more pressure on bony prominences. Nervous system deterioration diminishes awareness of the need for position change. Malnutrition and weight loss predispose the skin over bony prominences to breakdown. Urinary and fecal incontinence results in excess moisture, tissue maceration, and erosion. Any patient who dies a lingering death with intact skin does so because of good nursing care by family, friends, or professional caregivers.

> *Any patient who dies a lingering death with intact skin does so because of good nursing care by family, friends, or professional caregivers.*

Prevention of pressure sores requires frequent repositioning, pillows, cushions, special mattresses, and maintenance of clean, dry skin. Skin breakdown becomes nearly inevitable with prolonged immobility, malnutrition, and emaciation. When the goal is comfort, and death is near, the preventive regimen and pressure sore treatment should be modified to avoid inflicting pain and to respect patient wishes. For instance, Louise has been bedridden for several months with metastatic disease. Despite careful nursing by her adult daughters, she now has a 5-mm-wide infected crater over her coccyx. It is summertime and Louise loves her garden. Every afternoon she asks to be lifted into a wheelchair to go out and be surrounded by flowers. The nurse, in collaboration with her daughters, has developed a plan of care that includes placing Louise directly on her coccyx for 1 hour every day. They choose to respect her final wishes rather than follow the usual requirements of pressure sore management. Louise's dressings are complex, using expensive wound-care products, purchased by the family. After examining the goals of care, the nurse and daughters jointly decide to switch to using Betadine-soaked gauze dressings, which completely control the odor, to be changed only when they are soaked with discharge. Betadine discourages granulation and wound healing, but Louise's wound will never heal. It is more important to Louise to completely eliminate the odor than to try to heal her wound; the goals of pressure sore management in the terminally ill should be assessed continually, with patient comfort and choice in mind.

Consult nurses who specialize in enterostomal and wound therapies for difficult wound management.

> 66 | *When the goal is comfort, and death is near, the preventive regimen and pressure sore treatment should be modified to avoid inflicting pain and to respect patient wishes.*

Malignant Wounds

A small number of dying patients suffer from cancerous skin lesions. Patients who seek initial medical care for malignancies very late in the disease process will sometimes present with malignant wounds, which may look like craterous ulcers or assume a cauliflower or fungus appearance. Such wounds are called "fungating" lesions. In patients receiving regular medical care, these lesions can usually be controlled with excision or radiation. They sometimes grow out of control at the end of life when radiation or chemotherapy no longer works. Such ugly tumors are terribly distressing; they are disfiguring and can be accompanied by offensive odors and discharge that repel loved ones and even professionals.

When excision or radiation is not possible, these wounds are managed with irrigation and moist dressing changes. Wound-care products are chosen to absorb odoriferous drainage; sometimes this may require pouching. Metronidazole gel or solution is an antiinfective that kills odor-causing anaerobic bacteria. Charcoal dressings may also be helpful to reduce odor. Nurses certified as wound and enterostomal specialists may need to become involved in treatment. A hospice nurse describes managing a difficult wound:

> He had a fungating malignant wound with secretions all over the place. I literally needed to spend half of my time on my knees in order to dress his wounds. Gradually, we got the secretions under control. The dressings were simplified to make them manageable. I got rid of all the excess bags of supplies and equipment so that his room didn't look like a hospital anymore.

The families of these patients need exceptional support in the hospital or nursing home, and to persist in providing physical care at home. Feelings of repulsion should be addressed compassionately, and the nurse should make every effort to control drainage and odor so that the patient is not shunned in his or her last days.

Impaired Thought Processes and Risk for Seizures

Terminal processes affecting the brain commonly impair thinking and occasionally cause seizures. Cognitive impairment is inevitable with progressive end-stage processes like hypoxia, azotemia, hepatic encephalopathy, cerebral lesions, drug side effects, depression, and fever. Impairments range from diminishing attention and problem-solving ability, to delirium and diminishing level of consciousness before death.

Delirium is an acute cognitive impairment that includes disorientation, attention and memory deficits, lethargy or agitation, and perceptual disturbances like illusions or hallucinations. Delirium may also involve labile emotions including fear and anxiety. Delirium is the main reason for cognitive failure at the end of life. Not only is impaired thought disturbing for loved ones to witness, but it is often unpredictable as death approaches. One moment a patient may be nonresponsive, and the next moment he or she may rouse to recognize loved ones visiting. The nurse should explain this cognitive roller coaster to friends and family members. For example, you might say, "Have you noticed how Lee sometimes seems completely alert and knows everything that is going on, and at other times, he gets confused and upset? That up-and-down pattern is normal. There are so many chemicals having bad effects on his brain, and things are constantly changing inside his body."

> ❝ *Not only is impaired thought disturbing for loved ones to witness, but it is often unpredictable as death approaches. One moment a patient may be nonresponsive, and the next moment he or she may rouse to recognize loved ones visiting.*

Assessment of cognitive changes should emphasize careful listening and observation of mental and behavioral changes, taking particular note of aggravating and relieving factors, such as pain or isolation. Palliative management of confusion and agitation includes reversing any processes that can be reversed (such as hypoxia or hypercalcemia), readjusting drug regimens, providing oxygen for hypoxia, and offering human presence. Antipsychotics, such as haloperidol (Haldol), and benzodiazepines, such as lorazepam (Ativan), are usually effective for terminal restlessness. Agitation at the end of life should be soothed by a familiar environment and familiar caregivers with reassuring voice and touch. Soothing music, individualized to the patient, and aromatherapy, especially essential oil of lavender, are often useful to calm frightened, restless patients. A hospice nurse describes how one of her patients was calmed:

> I find that patients really enjoy music. One of my patients was agitated and restless. We tried to figure out what would work with her. The moment her daughter turned on the Walkman, she mellowed out and was quiet. One day I walked in and they were playing Handel's Messiah for her. She died with the Messiah playing.

WWW. Internet Resource Box

The Mini-Mental State Examination (MMSE) and the Memorial Delirium Assessment Scale (MDAS) are well-known tools for assessing mental status. The MMSE can be accessed through an Alzheimer's Web site: *www.medafile.com*. The MDAS can be accessed through an AIDS information Web site: *www.hivguidelines.org/public*.

Cognitive Impairment due to Cerebral Lesions

Palliative management of primary and metastatic brain lesions, which occur frequently in terminal cancer, emphasizes reducing intracranial pressure and treating complications. Corticosteroids reduce the edema surrounding malignant masses and thus reduce the intracranial pressure and temporarily reverse neurological deficits. Long-term therapy inevitably runs into the many complications of steroid use. See Box 15-6. Pressure on the brain causes convulsions. Anticonvulsants are commonly needed, including phenytoin (Dilantin), carbamazepine (Tegretol), valproic acid (Depakote), or gabapentin (Neurontin). All have side effects that may manifest if survival is prolonged. Another problem with cancer of the brain is deep vein thromboses, which occur in about a quarter to nearly half of patients with cerebral metastases (Nguyen & DeAngelis, 2004). Some physicians will order prophylactic anticoagulation. Radiotherapy can prolong survival, as can resection of single brain lesions. Consider the following summary of nursing interventions after a home visit to a patient with an expanding terminal glioblastoma of the brain, whose condition had just taken a turn for the worse:

> Yesterday she walked to the bathroom and conversed slowly. Today she is mute, incontinent, and doesn't know how to stand. I called the doctor's office and suggested increasing the Decadron that she takes daily to reduce the fluid layer around the brain tumor. Maybe it will briefly stop this downhill skid. He agreed. Her husband and I discussed protecting her stomach from the steroid effects with the cimetidine she now cannot swallow. I taught him how to crush it between spoons and put it in pudding. Yesterday she ate dinner with the family. Today it's ice cream bars only. We discussed making high-fiber high-protein concoctions in their blender. To manage her sluggish bowels, I proposed 3 days of blenderized fruit, then Senekot if that hasn't worked. I showed him how to care for an incontinent bedridden person and ordered wheelchair, hospital bed, and adult size medium diapers from a medical equipment company. We talked about her husband's need for rest and the necessity to take advantage of his daughters' offer to relieve him. We also went over the signs that death might be close.

Risk for Seizures

Seizures are uncommon at the end of life, but do occur with brain tumors, advanced AIDS, medication side effects, and preexisting seizure disorders. Palliative care must emphasize seizure prevention in these patients. Seizures terrify family members, exhaust patients, and put them at risk of physical injury. Because of the risk of side effects, anticonvulsants usually are not prescribed until a seizure has occurred. Nevertheless, whenever the patient has expanding brain lesions, anticonvulsants should be available with an order to use as needed. When the patient cannot swallow, the benzodiazepines (diazepam, lorazepam) are the anticonvulsants of choice and can be administered by injection. For home care, the rectal route using diazepam gel or the sublingual route with lorazepam oral solution (2 mg/mL) is preferred. When seizures do occur, family members need to be taught to turn the patient on his side, and prevent trauma by attending to the surrounding environment and avoiding putting anything in the patient's mouth. Caretakers should expect incontinence during the seizure and diminished level of consciousness in the period immediately afterward.

𝓮𝕒 Planting the Seeds

Families caring at home for a seizure-prone patient need emotional support and systematic teaching. Witnessing a grand mal seizure in someone you dearly love is very frightening. Include the following teaching points:

- Put nothing in the mouth. This contradicts old first-aid advice.
- Turn the person on his side, if possible.
- Place pillows between the person and hard objects, such as along siderails of a hospital bed.
- Do not offer fluids or food until the person is completely awake and can swallow.
- Expect incontinence.
- Create a quiet reassuring environment afterward. The patient may sleep for several hours.

Risk for Hemorrhage

When tumors erode large blood vessels, some patients experience a final terminal hemorrhage from the stomach, bowel, urinary tract, or vagina. Head and neck tumors sometimes cause massive bleeding. Anticipate such a frightening event at home and in inpatient facilities by having anxiolytics, such as midazolam (2.5–5 mg SC prn), on hand to sedate the patient. Dark towels (black, red) should be available to absorb the blood and reduce the visually shocking effect. If there is great likelihood of this event, some families may ask that the patient be moved to an inpatient setting. It is an unusual family caregiver who can remain calm in such circumstances, even with careful anticipatory teaching.

Imbalanced Nutrition

Dying patients may be unable or disinterested in eating and drinking. Food and fluids are vital to living but not to dying. The provision of food and fluid has come to symbolize nurturance, but it is not nurturing to force them on the dying. See Chapter 9 for an ethical discussion on artificial nutrition for the dying patient. This section examines caring for patients experiencing end-of-life loss of appetite and weight, painful mouths and difficulty swallowing, and nausea and vomiting.

> 66 *Food and fluids are vital to living but not to dying. The provision of food and fluid has come to symbolize nurturance, but it is not nurturing to force them on the dying.*

Anorexia and Weight Loss

Anorexia is a common symptom in advanced disease. When the dying have a poor appetite, comfort, not better nutrition, is the goal. Although meals and food should be made as appealing as possible, there is no benefit to forcing calories, vitamins, or protein. If patients have an interest in maintaining their appetite, refer them to an experienced dietician. Diet should not be restricted unless it causes discomfort. One 21-year-old man, living with terminal leukemia, spent his last days eating small bites of pizza and drinking small swallows of beer with friends.

When patients want to eat but have no appetite, medications commonly used to enhance appetite include the antiemetics such as metoclopramide (Reglan); corticosteroids such as dexamethasone (Decadron); the progestational hormone megestrol acetate (Megace); medical marijuana (cannabinoids); and the newer antipsychotics. Marijuana has been demonstrated to increase appetite, but the evidence is inconsistent (Martin & Wiley, 2004). Tetrahydrocannabinol (THC) is responsible for the pharmacological effects of marijuana and is available legally in dronabinol (Marinol) or nabilone (Cesamet). The second generation antipsychotic agents, such as risperidone (Risperdal) and olanzapine (Zyprexa), are proving helpful to manage anorexia, weight loss, and nausea (Fisch & Kim, 2004). The most common second generation side effects are sedation and extrapyramidal side effects, but with a much lower incidence than in the first generation antipsychotics like haloperidol. The sedative and anxiolytic effects of an antipsychotic may actually be of great benefit to the dying patient. Nurses are often in a position to suggest these medications to the physician. When they are prescribed, we monitor appetite and weight gain.

Artificial nutrition can be delivered through both the parenteral and enteral routes. When the patient is still functioning cognitively with reasonable quality of life, most can benefit from artificial nutrition when oral nutritional intake becomes severely compromised. In contrast, when the patient is near death, artificial feeding offers no health benefit and does not prolong life (Abrahm, 2000; Ersek, 2003; Murphy & Lipman, 2003). Some sources actually note higher mortality rates in patients receiving tube feeding (Ersek, 2003). Actively dying patients do not experience hunger, so there is no need to use artificial means to relieve it.

The burdens of both total parenteral nutrition (hyperalimentation) and tube feeding outweigh any presumed benefits. In advanced disease, total parenteral nutrition (hyperalimentation) is associated with multiple complications, such as pneumothorax or hemorrhage related to insertion, infection, hyperglycemia, and occlusion of catheters. Likewise, there are many problems related to tube feeding, including the need to restrain the patient, skin excoriations around the tube, gastrointestinal erosions, peritonitis, aspiration, and diarrhea (Abrahm, 2000; Ersek, 2003).

It is troubling that the insertion of percutaneous endoscopic gastrostomy (PEG) tubes has dramatically increased in the United States (Shega, Hougham, Stocking, Cox-Hayley, and Sachs, 2003). They are particularly common in nursing home residents with advanced dementia. Physicians believe they will improve nutritional status, reduce aspiration pneumonia, improve healing of pressure ulcers, and extend survival. Nursing homes often request PEG insertion in response to regulatory guidelines that mandate maintaining nutritional intake and prevention of weight loss. In contrast, when demented bedbound patients with end-stage disease can no longer swallow on their own, they should receive active palliative caregiving, not a useless invasive procedure.

66 | *When the patient is near death, artificial feeding offers no health benefit and does not prolong life (Abrahm, 2000; Ersek, 2003; Murphy & Lipman, 2003).*

The feelings around providing food as nurturing should be separated from the compulsion to provide that food artificially when there is no evidence that the patient benefits at the end of life. The nursing role with family and nursing home staff is persistent listening to their concerns and explaining that food is necessary for life, but that artificially providing it can be burdensome and serve no good. Sometimes the feelings around providing food are so strong that a family will insist on artificial feeding. Their choice should be respected, and the patient continually monitored for complicating burdens.

66 | *The feelings around providing food as nurturing need to be separated from the compulsion to artificially provide food when there is no evidence that the patient benefits.*

Dysphagia and Stomatitis

Problems with swallowing and inflammation of the oral mucosa are common at the end of life. Swallowing difficulties are caused by neurological diseases, cancerous lesions, and chemotherapy or radiotherapy. The patient needs to be observed carefully for changes in oropharyngeal function and swallowing, such as avoiding eating, taking a long time for meals, chewing at length and swallowing several times, coughing or choking during meals, regurgitating, frequently clearing the throat, drooling, complaining of food getting caught in the throat, and/or complaining of pain with swallowing (Dahlin, 2004). Dysphagia can be relieved with corticosteroids to reduce swollen tissues, a diet modified to include soft food requiring little or no chewing, upright posture, speech-language consultation regarding other modifications during chewing and swallowing, and environmental modification to reduce distractions during eating.

Inflammation of the oropharyngeal mucosa is caused by radiation or chemotherapy, compromised immunity, and poor oral hygiene. Physical assessment reveals cracked lips, dry mouth, oral erythema, bleeding, pain, and abnormal tongue surfaces (Dahlin, 2004). Ulcers, vesicles of herpes simplex, or white patches of *Candida* may be present. Oral infection with *Candida* is characterized by burning pain when eating and a bright red tongue or white plaques on the tongue or elsewhere in the mouth. An oral antifungal, such as ketoconazole (Nizoral), or an antifungal troche, such as clotrimazole (Mycelex), is effective. Interventions include antiinfectives; topical steroids; oral rinses with sodium chloride or bicarbonate; oral anesthetics before meals; a bland, low-acid, high-protein diet; ice chips; opioids for severe pain; a water spray or saliva substitute; and lip balm. Mouthwashes should not contain alcohol.

Nausea and Vomiting

Much has been learned from managing the side effects of cancer chemotherapy that can now be applied to control of nausea and vomiting at the end of life. Like pain, nausea is a subjective experience that can be determined only by the patient's report. Although vomiting can be observed and measured, the degree of distress that it causes can likewise only be determined by patient's report. The following assessment questions are useful (Gates & Fink, 2001):

- How severe is your nausea? Try a 1 to 5 rating scale with 1 as mild and 5 as severe.
- How often are you nauseated during a 24-hour period?
- Are you also throwing up? How often in 24 hours?
- What triggered the nausea and/or vomiting?
- What relieved the nausea and/or vomiting?
- Are the anti-nausea drugs helping? Are they causing any side effects you don't like?

Nausea and vomiting are caused by transmission of impulses to the vomiting center in the medulla. Impulses are transmitted by the cerebral cortex and limbic system when stimulated by the senses and learned associations, by the chemoreceptor trigger zone in the medulla that responds to chemical stimuli in the spinal fluid, by the middle ear vestibular apparatus, and by peripheral pathways involving the gastrointestinal tract and the vagus nerve. The vagus responds to toxins in the blood and gastrointestinal tract, as well as to gastrointestinal compression. Serotonin receptors are located along the vagus nerve (Gates & Fink, 2001). When serotonin is released in response to toxins in the GI tract or bloodstream, it binds to the vagal serotonin receptors and a message to vomit is transmitted to the vomiting center. The vagus also has stretch receptors that respond to stretch of the gut or liver capsule.

End-of-life nausea and vomiting can be caused by increased intracranial pressure, by medication, by metabolic abnormalities, by constipation, and by bowel obstruction (Haughney, 2004). Increasing intracranial pressure triggers pressure receptors that carry impulses to the vomiting center. Patients who continue to receive emetogenic chemotherapy at the end of their life may have continuing difficulties with nausea and vomiting. Ironically, palliative medications can also stimulate vomiting; this includes steroids, nonsteroidal anti-inflammatory drugs (NSAIDs), and opioids. Steroids and NSAIDS irritate the lining of the stomach; they may need to be discontinued or taken in conjunction with a drug that suppresses gastric acid secretion, such as omeprazole (Prilosec). Opioids in the blood can stimulate the chemoreceptor trigger zone, especially when initially prescribed or when there are toxic accumulations due to kidney and liver failure. Metabolic abnormalities that cause accumulation of toxins that stimulate the chemoreceptor trigger zone include hypercalcemia, hyponatremia, and uremia.

Unfortunately, constipation is an all-too-common cause of nausea and vomiting at the end of life. Abdominal pressure and bowel distention cause vagal nerve response with transmission of impulses to the vomiting center. Bowel obstruction, due to expanding abdominal or pelvic masses, also causes nausea and vomiting as the bowel is stretched and compressed. Palliative management of constipation and bowel obstruction is discussed in the section, Impaired Elimination.

Nausea and vomiting can be relieved by using both pharmacological and nonpharmacological interventions. Antiemetics include the phenothiazines, haloperidol, metoclopramide, corticosteroids, serotonin antagonists, cannabinoids, anticholinergics, and antihistamines. See Table 16-1, Medications for Nausea and Vomiting. For persistent vomiting, medications should be scheduled around-the-clock. Several agents, chosen because they have different pharmacological actions, may need to be combined when single agents fail. For instance, an antihistamine and a corticosteroid might be added to Compazine. Olanzepine (Zyprexa) can be useful alone or in combination for nausea that does not respond to other interventions (Jackson & Tavernier, 2003). Be aware that high doses of the dopamine antagonists (phenothiazines, haloperidol, and metoclopramide) alone or in combination can cause extrapyramidal symptoms like akathisia and dystonia (Gates & Fink, 2001). Akathisia is manifested as restlessness progressing to inability to sit or lie still. Dystonia involves involuntary contraction of muscle groups in the head and neck. These reactions can be prevented or treated with lorazepam (Ativan) or diphenhydramine (Benadryl).

Table 16-1

MEDICATIONS FOR NAUSEA AND VOMITING

Class	Generic Name	Trade Name	Action	Comments
Phenothiazine	prochlorperazine chlorpromazine	Compazine Thorazine	Blocks dopamine receptors at CTZ	Inexpensive but sedative, extrapyramidal and anticholinergic effects
Butyrophenone Dopamine receptor antagonist	haloperidol metoclopramide	Haldol Reglan	As above Inhibits dopamine receptors in CTZ; increases GI motility	As above Lower expense Sedative, extrapyramidal effects, restlessness
Corticosteroid	dexamethasone	Decadron	Reduces cerebral edema	Risk of steroid side effects, especially GI
Serotonin (5HT3 receptor) antagonist	granisetron ondansetron	Kytril Zofran	Blocks serotonin receptors on vagus and in CTZ	Expensive Headache Few adverse effects
2nd generation antipsychotic	olanzapine	Zyprexa	Blocks serotonin	Sedation
Cannabinoid	dronabinol	Marinol	Peripheral and central nervous system	Dizziness and sedation Uneven effectiveness Use when other drugs ineffective
Anticholinergic	scopolamine	Transderm-Scop	Targets movement related N & V	Anticholinergic side effects
Antihistamine	hydroxyzine diphenhydramine	Vistaril Benadryl	Blocks histamine	Sedating

Source: Adapted from Haughney (2004).

It is important to maintain a continuous blood level of antiemetic in patients who are continuously nauseated. This often can be achieved by the use of sustained-release compazine spansules, administered every 12 hours. When the patient can no longer swallow, antiemetics can be formulated into suppositories. One example is BDR suppositories containing Benadryl 25 mg, Decadron 4 mg, and Reglan 20 mg (Gates & Fink, 2001). Likewise, metoclopramide (Reglan) and haloperidol (Haldol) can be given by subcutaneous infusion without local tissue irritation associated with the other antiemetics. One expert home hospice nurse describes taking the initiative to recommend a palliative approach for a patient with intractable vomiting:

> He was nauseated and vomiting and the doctor wanted to insert an NG tube and hook it up to suction. I recommended a suppository that our pharmacy makes up with Benadryl and Decadron and Reglan. The patient just didn't want that tube down. I said to the physician, "Can't we try this less invasive measure first?" I said that in my experience we rarely needed tubes. The patient stopped vomiting and died in 48 hours without unnecessary paraphernalia.

Special care needs to be taken in managing foods for people who are nauseated. Odors need to be minimized because they can trigger nausea. Bland foods close to room temperature are often preferred. Patients should be encouraged to eat small amounts slowly and should sip small amounts of fluid at frequent intervals. There is some evidence that fresh or dried ginger can reduce nausea and vomiting (Gates & Fink, 2001). Herbal remedies including chamomile, peppermint, and slippery elm relieve nausea for some patients. Clinical studies support the use of acupuncture, hypnosis, relaxation, and distraction as useful adjuncts to reduce nausea and vomiting (Deng, Cassileth, and Yeung, 2004).

Ineffective Breathing Pattern and Airway Clearance

Dyspnea (shortness of breath, breathlessness, or air hunger) is characterized by subjective awareness of uncomfortable breathing that many patients describe as terrifying. Dyspnea is caused by impaired gas exchange resulting in hypoxia due to cardiac, pulmonary, or neurological disease. Terminal dyspnea occurs in up to 75% of those close to death and should be anticipated in all dying patients (LaDuke, 2001). Objective signs include tachypnea, tachycardia, gasping, restlessness, agitation, use of accessory muscles, and grimacing. The experience of dyspnea must be understood as having psychosocial and spiritual dimensions, just like pain. Assessment involves comprehending the patient experience. Some patients live for months or years with repeated experience of dyspnea. Others experience it only during the final end-of-life events. Numeric, verbal, or visual analogue scales can be used for the patient to rate intensity of dyspnea. Other dimensions of symptom assessment include quality (words describing it), pattern, aggravating factors, relieving factors, and effects on life. Dyspnea affects ability to eat, sleep, converse, and move about.

With severe dyspnea, the patient is calmed by a caregiver staying at the bedside until the problem is brought under control. Basic nursing interventions that reduce apprehension and slow the respiratory rate include:

- Calm presence
- Positioning with head and chest elevated; may need to be positioned upright and leaning forward on pillows
- Guided pursed lip breathing and breathing exercises
- Open window or air conditioning to cool the air
- Bedside fan blowing air on face
- Cool compresses
- Relaxation, imagery, visualization, music, prayer

Oxygen by cannula may relieve distress but cannot be expected to relieve underlying pathophysiology that is impairing gas exchange. Medical therapies may be tried to control reversible causes of dyspnea. These include bronchodilators, diuretics, antibiotics, and radiation for obstructive lesions. Corticosteroids, particularly prednisolone (prednisone) and dexamethasone (Decadron) will often temporarily reduce pulmonary inflammation.

Because dyspnea is so distressing, aggressive measures to reverse the underlying processes may be indicated when the patient has months to live. These might include radiation therapy to relieve obstructions, blood transfusions when hypoxia is due to anemia, and pericardiocentesis for pericardial effusion (Abrahm, 2000). Recurrent pleural effusions can pose a particular problem since some people require repeated thoracenteses. For these, sclerosing agents to stop the fluid from leaking into the pleural cavity may be infused through a chest tube. For some with repeat pleural fluid accumulations, a pleuroperitoneal shunt is inserted to drain the fluid into the peritoneum.

Opioids are the mainstay of efforts to relieve terminal dyspnea. They work in two ways (LaDuke, 2001):

1. Alter perception of air hunger, thus reducing anxiety and associated oxygen consumption.
2. Improve oxygen supply and reduce pulmonary congestion by dilating pulmonary blood vessels.

Morphine works rapidly when given intravenously or absorbed as a concentrated liquid through the mucosa of the mouth (sublingual or buccal). Evidence of the effectiveness of nebulized morphine is inconclusive, but it is often used. As with pain, careful morphine titration is essential to manage dyspnea safely. A person who has not received opioids for pain should be given starting doses of 2 to 5 mg IV every 5 minutes until relief (Gates & Fink, 2001) or 5 to 6 mg immediate-release morphine p.o. every 4 hours. Patients receiving opioids for pain should have their dosage carefully titrated until air hunger is relieved. Opioids relieve symptoms before causing sedation and cause sedation before depressing respirations (LaDuke, 2001). A growing body of evidence reveals that oxygen saturations are maintained and carbon dioxide levels do not rise when opioids are carefully titrated (Opioid titration, 2004).

Anxiolytics, including benzodiazepines such as lorazepam (Ativan) and buspirone (BuSpar), and phenothiazines such as chlorpromazine (Thorazine) are also effective to manage dyspnea and should be titrated until relief is obtained. In some patients, midazolam (Versed) may be more effective than morphine (Midazolam beats, 2004). Severe dyspnea can be managed with a combination of anxiolytics and opioids titrated to comfort.

Ineffective Airway Clearance

Ineffective airway clearance, with or without an associated cough, is a common problem at the end of life. Secretions may accumulate due to malignant airway obstruction, infection, pulmonary edema, or impaired swallowing. The volume of secretions is often reduced by reduced fluid intake. Respiratory secretions can be diminished by administration of anticholinergics such as scopolamine IM, SC, or patch (Transderm-Scop); atropine drops; or hyoscyamine sulfate (Levsin). Tenacious mucus can be expectorated with the aid of nebulized saline with bronchodilators such as albuterol or terbutaline (Abrahm, 2000). To suppress cough itself, an elixir containing dextromethorphan or codeine is indicated. More potent opioids or nebulized anesthetics, such as lidocaine, can be used for stubborn coughs.

Impaired Bowel Elimination

The most common problems that impair intestinal function are constipation, diarrhea, bowel obstruction, and ascites.

Constipation

As mobility and intake of fiber and fluids diminish and opioids slow peristalsis, constipation is inevitable without a preventive regimen. Constipation is prevented by regular administration of a stool softener (docusate sodium) and bowel stimulant (senna or bisacodyl). A preventive bowel regimen is essential to avoid inflicting needless discomfort associated with constipation. When constipation has developed, bisacodyl suppositories or saline cathartics (Milk of Magnesia) may be effective. Removal of impacted stool may require multiple oil retention enemas followed by soapsuds. Before any manual disimpaction, administer an opioid and topical anesthetic.

Diarrhea

Diarrhea can be defined as increased volume and liquidity of stools, resulting in three or more loose or unformed stools per day (Kuebler, Berry, and Heidrich, 2002). Rectal cramping and rectal urgency are often associated with it. Uncontrolled diarrhea causes fluid and electrolyte imbalances, orthostatic hypotension, weakness, and eventual malnutrition and skin breakdown. As many as 10% of patients with advanced cancer complain of diarrhea, while as many as 50% of people with advanced AIDS suffer loose stools. Most diarrhea in AIDS patients is due to infection, particularly cryptosporidiosis (Heidrich, 2002). There are many causes of diarrhea in a person with advanced cancer. Tumors, impactions, and partial or complete bowel obstruction can cause excessive mucus production. Disease processes that cause fat malabsorption can yield large volume loose stools. Many therapies may result in diarrhea, including radiation, chemotherapy, stomach and bowel resections, enteral feedings, and excessive laxatives. Assessment includes determining character of the stools themselves as well as frequency, timing, and factors that precipitate and relieve diarrhea and associated discomfort. Abdominal and perineal physical examination is essential.

Diarrhea is managed by treating underlying causes to the extent possible, assuring hydration, and maintaining perineal skin integrity. Anticholinergics including hyoscyamine (Levsin) and dicyclomine (Bentyl) will reduce colicky pain (Kuebler, Berry, and Heidrich, 2002). Nonsteroidal anti-inflammatory drugs like ibuprofen may be prescribed because they inhibit mucosal prostaglandin. Opioids are prescribed to reduce intestinal motility. Loperamide (Imodium) is the drug of choice; it is three times more potent than diphenoxylate (Lomotil). Tincture of opium (paregoric) is a second line option, but it causes systemic opioid effects. When the diarrhea is refractory to these remedies, octreotide (Sandostatin) suppresses intestinal secretion and motility; it is quite expensive and is given subcutaneously by continuous infusions or in twice daily injections.

Bowel Obstruction

Bowel obstruction occurs when the intestinal lumen is occluded, a common complication of ovarian and colorectal cancers. The bowel is blocked by external pressure of the tumor, extension of the tumor into the bowel wall, or kinking of the bowel as a result of tumor adhering to it (Jatoi, Podratz, Gill, and Hartman, 2004). When the bowel is blocked, the intestinal contents above the blockage accumulate and distend the bowel. The patient is racked with cramping waves of peristalsis that are unable to overcome the blockage. Gastrointestinal secretions increase with nowhere to go. The abdomen becomes distended, the patient is nauseated and vomits, and the pain is often constant. When major surgery has been ruled out, palliative surgical interventions include placement of a stent to open up the lumen and PEG tube insertion to drain secretions (gastric venting).

Total bowel obstructions are treated palliatively with opioids to control pain and reduce peristaltic waves that cause cramping. Anticholinergics, including scopolamine (Transderm Scop), atropine, and hyoscyamine (Levsin), decrease smooth muscle tone, reduce peristalsis, and reduce bowel secretions. Another antisecretory agent, octreotide (Sandostatin), is highly effective in relieving the distention, nausea, vomiting, and pain in patients with bowel obstruction (Jatoi et al., 2004). It is available only by injection, but can be administered by continuous subcutaneous infusion if persistent vomiting is a problem. The whole range of antiemetics is appropriate, except for metoclopramide (Reglan), which increases gut motility and therefore would exacerbate cramping in total bowel obstruction.

Ascites

Ascites is the accumulation of fluid within the peritoneal cavity, caused by increased hydrostatic pressure when there is blockage of portal venous or lymphatic circulation. Tumors, heart failure, and reduced serum protein lead to movement of fluid out of the blood and into the peritoneal cavity. As fluid accumulates in the peritoneal cavity, the abdomen distends and intra-abdominal pressure causes anorexia, nausea, heartburn, and interference with bowel motility. Eventually, large fluid accumulations cause upward movement of the diaphragm, which interferes with chest expansion to cause dyspnea. Ascites requires palliation when it interferes with breathing or digestion, is painful, or is causing progressive fatigue and immobility (Berber, Portenoy, and Weissman, 2002). Management includes sodium restriction, diuretics (spironolactone to block aldosterone causing sodium retention), and paracentesis. At the end of life, repeated fluid accumulations may necessitate surgical intervention to implant a shunt that drains peritoneal fluid externally or into a thoracic vein (peritoneovenous shunt).

Impaired Urinary Elimination

As a person slows down on drinking, urinary output diminishes. Weakness makes it increasingly difficult to void using toilet, commode, or bedpan. Every effort should be made to adapt the patient's environment so that normal voiding is possible and requires minimal patient exertion. When close to death, a dehydrated patient may void only small amounts into diapers or incontinence pads. In contrast, an artificially hydrated patient is likely to need an indwelling catheter. Sometimes disease processes cause bladder retention, also necessitating a catheter.

WHEN SYMPTOMS ARE NOT CONTROLLED: PALLIATIVE SEDATION

Palliative sedation is also known as "sedation therapy," "terminal sedation" or "total sedation." It can be defined as sedation intended to induce and maintain deep sleep, but not cause death. The purpose of the deep sleep is to relieve physical symptoms when symptom management has failed. Some clinicians also use palliative sedation when a patient is experiencing profound emotional or spiritual anguish (Rousseau, 2004). A symptom is considered to be intractable or refractory when it cannot be adequately controlled despite intense efforts to find a tolerable therapy that does not seriously reduce consciousness (Braun, Hagen, and Clark, 2003). The most common reasons for palliative sedation include pain, dyspnea, uncontrolled vomiting, and agitated delirium; often more than one refractory symptom is present. Medications used for palliative sedation include benzodiazepines (lorazepam/Ativan), barbiturates (phenobarbital), neuroleptics (haloperidol), and anesthetics (propofol/Diprivan).

Proposing the use of palliative sedation elicits strong emotional and ethical reactions. The doctrine of double effect justifies an action with the good intention to relieve suffering, even if death is the unintended but predictable consequence. Nevertheless, some clinicians counter that palliative sedation is another name for active euthanasia. Family and staff decisions to use palliative sedation are difficult. Nurses have the right to conscientiously object to assisting with palliative sedation after they have transferred care to a competent colleague (HPNA, 2003). Rousseau (2004) proposes the following guidelines for choosing to induce sleep from which the person will not awaken:

- Terminal illness with a refractory symptom
- Exhaustion of palliative treatments
- Ethical, psychiatric, and spiritual consultation
- DNR in place
- Clarity about continuing nutrition or hydrating infusions
- Informed consent by patient/family
- Consideration of a trial of respite sedation for 24 to 48 hours to break cycle of anxiety and insomnia

When a patient's symptoms are not controlled, the distress of everyone involved escalates: patient, family, physician, nurse, and all other health-team members. In the midst of the turmoil, the nurse has an opportunity to assume a calming thoughtful role, helping everyone listen to each other and weigh the benefits and burdens of palliative sedation.

WHEN SYMPTOMS ARE NOT CONTROLLED: PATIENT ADVOCACY

End-of-life caregiving to relieve physical symptoms requires a high level of patient advocacy and close collaboration with physicians. The nurse needs to assume a courageous role and take the initiative to relieve ever-changing symptoms. We are the witnesses to the suffering and we cannot turn away. This requires a strong backbone, as one hospice nurse explained during an interview:

> You have to be tenacious even when a physician may feel that you're being a pain. You know that there are things that can be tried. You have to be knowledgeable and try to present information to physicians in a way that is acceptable to them. You recommend Plan A or Plan B (Zerwekh, 1995, p. 36).

When physicians resist ordering effective palliative medication to control symptoms, don't let the patient suffer alone and don't assume you are powerless. There is strength in numbers. Turn to knowledgeable colleagues, supervisors, or the hospice or palliative medical director. Develop a strategy together. Sometimes ethics consultation is available. Patient advocacy requires affirming the unique experience of the sufferer, clarifying the person's values about relief, and vividly documenting in oral and written report that the person is suffering. Nurses must articulate the experience of the patient so that it is never disregarded. Remember the proclamation of Elie Wiesel, Jewish Nobel Laureate and survivor of the Nazi death camps, "I swore to never be silent whenever and wherever human beings endure suffering and humiliation" (Wiesel's Speech, 1986). Consider making the same resolution.

CONCEPTS IN ACTION

You are making your first home visit to Fred, a 42-year-old physical therapist with bowel cancer. He has metastases to liver and lung. Fred is receiving an IV with 3 L of total parenteral nutrition managed by a home infusion company. Your physical assessment finds Fred lying flat in a rented hospital bed; he is breathless and apprehensive. He has reduced breath sounds bilaterally, massive ascites, 4+ edema toe to groin. He is incontinent of urine with a Stage 2 pressure sore over his right hip. His rectal temperature is 103.2°F. He made the decision to switch to hospice care at his last home-health visit. His new complaint today is persistent vomiting of fecal material. He is taking only sips of fluid. Despite receiving oxygen by cannula, he complains of feeling suffocated. His mother is sitting by his bed; she reveals no emotions. She tells you that "hospice is Fred's idea not mine. Don't even talk to me about taking away this IV." His wife and teen daughters are at work and school, respectively.

1. What additional assessment would be helpful?
2. What would you ask Fred? His mother?
3. How would you determine a priority list of problems?
4. What nursing strategies can be used to relieve Fred's physical complaints?
5. What would you report to the physician?
6. What pharmacological interventions would you recommend?

References

Abrahm, J. (2000). *A physician's guide to pain and symptom management in cancer patients.* Baltimore: Johns Hopkins University.

Berger, A., Portenoy, R., & Weissman, D. (2002). *Principles and practice of palliative care and supportive oncology.* Philadelphia: Lippincott.

Braun, T., Hagen, N., & Clark, T. (2003). Development of a clinical practice guideline for palliative sedation. *Journal of Palliative Medicine, 6*(3), 345–350.

Coyne, P. (2003). When the World Health Organization analgesic therapies ladder fails: The role of invasive analgesic therapies. *Oncology Nursing Forum, 30*(5), 777–783.

Dahlin, C. (2004). Oral complications at the end of life. *American Journal of Nursing, 104*(7), 40–47.

Dalal, S., & Bruera, E. (2004). Dehydration in cancer patients: To treat or not to treat. *Journal of Supportive Oncology, 2*(6), 467–483.

Deng, G., Cassileth, B., & Yeung, D. (2004). Complementary therapies for cancer-related symptoms. *Journal of Supportive Oncology, 2*(5), 419–426.

Ellershaw, J. (1995). Dehydration and the dying patient. *Journal of Pain and Symptom Management, 10,* 192–197.

Ersek, M. (2003). Artificial nutrition and hydration. *Journal of Hospice and Palliative Nursing, 5*(4), 221–230.

Fisch, M., & Kim, H. (2004). Use of atypical antipsychotic agents for symptom control in patients with advanced cancer. *Journal of Supportive Oncology, 2*(5), 447–452.

Gates, R., & Fink, R. (2001). *Oncology nursing secrets.* Philadelphia: Hanley & Belfus.

Haughney, A. (2004). Nausea and vomiting in end-stage cancer. *American Journal of Nursing, 104*(11), 40–48.

Jackson, W., & Tavernier, L. (2003). Olanzapine for intractable nausea in palliative care patients. *Journal of Palliative Medicine, 6*(2), 251–255.

Jatoi, A., Podratz, K., Gill, P., & Hartmann, L. (2004). Pathophysiology and palliation of inoperable bowel obstruction in patients with ovarian cancer. *Journal of Supportive Oncology, 2*(4), 323–334.

Kuebler, K., Berry, P., & Heidrich, D. (2002). *End-of-life-care: Clinical practice guidelines.* Philadelphia: WB Saunders.

LaDuke, S. (2001). Terminal dyspnea and palliative care. *American Journal of Nursing, 101*(11), 26–31.

Lanuke, K., Fainsinger, R., & DeMoissac, D. (2004). Hydration management at the end of life. *Journal of Palliative Medicine, 7*(2), 257–263.

Martin, B., & Wiley, J. (2004). Mechanism of action of cannabinoids: How it may lead to treatment of cachexia, emesis, and pain. *Journal of Supportive Oncology, 2*(4), 305–314.

Midazolam beats morphine in relieving dyspnea (2004, Fall). *The Oncology Report, 133*–134.

Murphy, L., & Lipman, T. (2003). Percutaneous endoscopic gastrostomy does not prolong survival in patients with dementia. *Archives of Internal Medicine, 163,* 1351–1353.

Nguyen, T., & DeAngelis, L. (2004). Treatment of brain metastases. *Journal of Supportive Oncology, 2*(5), 407–410.

Hospice and Palliative Nurses Association (HPNA). (2003) Palliative sedation at the end of life. *Journal of Hospice and Palliative Nursing, 5*(4), 235–237.

Opioid titration not tied to respiratory dysfunction (2004, Fall). *The Oncology Report, 133.*

Rousseau, P. (2004). Palliative sedation in the management of refractory symptoms. *Journal of Supportive Oncology, 2*(2), 181–186.

Shega, J., Hougham, G., Stocking, C., Cox-Hayley, D., & Sachs, G. (2003). Barriers to limiting the practice of feeding tube placement in advanced dementia. *Journal of Palliative Medicine, 6*(6), 885–893.

Wiesel, E. (1986, December 11) Speech: This honor belongs to all the survivors. *New York Times.*

Zerwekh, J. (1997). Do dying patients really need IV fluids? *American Journal of Nursing, 97*(3), 26–30.

Zerwekh, J. (2003). End-of-life hydration—benefit or burden? *Nursing 2003, 33*(2), 32hn1–32hn3.

Zerwekh, J. (1995). A family caregiving model for hospice nursing. *The Hospice Journal, 10*(1), 27–44.

CHAPTER 17

Caring in Different Settings When Death Is Imminent

Philosophical Reflections

"Death is the condition that makes it possible for us to live life in an authentic fashion."

YALOM, 1980, P. 31

Learning Objectives

1. Summarize the predictable underlying pathophysiology of signs and symptoms commonly seen at the end of life.
2. Explain the management of common end-of-life symptoms.
3. List the signs that are indicators of imminent death.
4. Explain how to humanize the final days.
5. Explain the process of letting go and the nursing role to support it.
6. Explore the spiritual implications of the last days.
7. Identify the challenges and possibilities for creating a caring palliative environment in the intensive care unit, nursing home, and home.
8. Explain how death is diagnosed and summarize responsibilities immediately afterward.

The End-of-Life Caregiving Tree has been illustrated with the foliage representing all of the different ways to manage symptoms. This final chapter examines the nursing role during the final days and hours of life. This period is a transitional time and is the final stage of growth. The chapter begins by examining the signs and symptoms of imminent dying, and presents the essentials of providing comfort in these last days. The chapter discusses the nurse's responsibility for humanizing the final period of waiting and supporting letting go by patient and family. The last hours of life are described from a spiritual perspective. The chapter explores the various challenges of providing care for those close to death in the ICU, nursing home, and home. Finally, this chapter addresses the diagnosis of death and responsibilities immediately thereafter.

THE LAST FEW DAYS: SYMPTOMS AND THEIR MANAGEMENT

The pathophysiology of dying organs was described in Chapter 13, which outlines the basic processes, signs and symptoms, and nursing diagnoses with failing cardiac, respiratory, renal, and hepatic functions. Death draws closer when irreversible failure of normal integrated bodily functions occurs. Whatever the underlying disease process, cardiopulmonary failure is always the final cause of death. The lungs or heart must fail for death to occur.

Pulmonary failure has multiple causes, including pneumonia, thromboembolism, pulmonary edema, pleural effusion, obstruction in the respiratory tract, obstructive lung disease, and depression of the medullary respiratory centers as the central nervous system fails. Ventilation fails to the point of being unable to sustain life. The consequence is hypoxemia and hypercapnia, and the heart works harder to circulate diminishing amounts of oxygen. Signs and symptoms of end-of-life pulmonary failure include apprehension, disturbed thought processes, and deteriorating level of consciousness coupled with orthopnea, use of accessory muscles, dyspnea, rapid or irregular breathing, and tachycardia. Excessive secretions from infection or pulmonary edema can cause frequent ineffective cough and fears of choking or drowning.

Circulatory failure can be sudden, due to myocardial infarction, arrhythmias, or loss of blood. Without prior myocardial damage, the heart will eventually fail because of the overwhelming workload imposed at the end of life. The diminished cardiac output causes reduced perfusion of the brain, kidneys, and periphery. Left ventricular failure causes the blood to back up into the pulmonary circulation, resulting in pulmonary edema. Right ventricular failure causes blood to back up into the vena cava, jugular vein, hepatic vein, and general circulation. If the patient is not dehydrated, this can cause pitting peripheral edema and ascites.

As a consequence of failing lungs and heart, the most common symptom management concerns at the end of life are shortness of breath, ineffective airway clearance, disturbed thought processes, and anxiety. Preexisting pain usually persists into the final days, even when consciousness diminishes and the patient is immobilized.

> *As a consequence of failing lungs and heart, the most common symptom management concerns at the end of life are shortness of breath, ineffective airway clearance, disturbed thought processes, and anxiety.*

Shortness of Breath and Ineffective Airway Clearance

In the final days of life, the patient may experience an intense hunger for air, frequent cough, and audible chest congestion with each breath.

Shortness of Breath

Dyspnea or shortness of breath is often the most common troubling symptom in the final days of life (Rousseau, 2002). The patient's desperation mounts, as he is unable to bring in enough air. Sometimes patients feel like they are drowning. Families despair as they witness the breathless struggle of those they love. The first nursing response is to position the patient in an upright position to allow full chest expansion. A chair with a high back and arm rests works well. A hospital bed should be adjusted to a High Fowler's position. Mountains of pillows will not work over time, as they collapse when a patient tosses and turns. Airflow against the face, using a fan or air conditioning, comforts some patients. Oxygen by nasal cannula may make more oxygen available, but remember that little gas exchange is possible in lungs filled with tumor or fluid, or when the blood flow to the lungs is failing.

Opioids, benzodiazepines, phenothiazines, and corticosteroids are the primary medications used to relieve dyspnea in the actively dying patient (Rousseau, 2002). Opioids reduce the perception of air hunger. When the patient can no longer swallow, sublingual, rectal, subcutaneous, and intravenous routes should be used. For acute severe dyspnea in the opioid naïve patient, 2 to 5 mg is administered every 15 or 20 minutes subcutaneously or intravenously until the patient is comfortable. Patients already receiving opioids may need their dose increased by 25% to 50% until the dyspnea is relieved. When the parenteral route is not available at home, use sublingual or buccal administration. Benzodiazepines (lorazepam, midazolam, diazepam) are also effective and can be given sublingually and rectally, as well as by injection. For acute severe dyspnea, midazolam can be administered intravenously and subcutaneously in doses ranging from 0.5 mg to 2.5 mg every 15 minutes until the patient is comfortable. Corticosteroids (dexamethasone, prednisone) will relieve bronchospasm associated with inflammation and can be useful for dyspnea associated with airway obstruction.

Ineffective Airway Clearance

In the last hours of life, when the patient can no longer swallow saliva or expectorate sputum, pharyngeal secretions accumulate to cause wet bubbling sounds referred to as a "death rattle." The sound is heard when the breath passes through the accumulated pharyngeal and pulmonary secretions in the back of the throat. Usually, the patient's reduced level of consciousness prevents distress from this problem, but the family and caregivers suffer as they must listen to the telling rattle.

> *In the last hours of life, when the patient can no longer swallow saliva or expectorate sputum, pharyngeal secretions accumulate to cause wet bubbling sounds referred to as a "death rattle."*

If possible, the patient with a death rattle should be placed in a comfortable position on his side so that the secretions drain out of the mouth. Anticholinergic drugs (scopolamine, atropine, hyoscyamine, and glycopyrrolate) are used to dry up oral, pharyngeal, and bronchial secretions. Scopolamine is administered subcutaneously every 2 to 4 hours by injection or continuously by infusion or transdermal patch. Atropine is administered subcutaneously, or atropine drops can be administered sublingually. Hyoscyamine sulfate (Levsin) and glycopyrrolate (Robinul) can be administered sublingually and subcutaneously. Be cautious about initiating oropharyngeal suctioning for a dying person. It traumatizes the mucosa and causes coughing and gagging, which increase patient suffering rather than relieve it. Just the sound of suctioning can be disturbing to everyone in the room. The exception to this general rule is patients who already have endotracheal tubes or tracheotomies and need occasional suctioning to maintain their airway.

Disturbed Thought Processes and Anxiety

When the dying trajectory is moving downhill, activity and consciousness slowly go downhill also. Sometimes anxiety dominates thinking. Likewise, restlessness and delirium can become problems.

Diminished Level of Consciousness

As death draws near, a person's energy is drained by even the simplest tasks of daily living. Naps become more and more frequent. Morning may not bring any sustained times of wakefulness. Most people come to a time when they are no longer able to rise out of bed; they speak very little. As consciousness drops, the person may respond only to shaking or pain.

> *Most people come to a time when they are no longer able to rise out of bed; they speak very little. As consciousness drops, the person may respond only to shaking or pain.*

Many become more and more difficult to arouse, until they are completely comatose. Normal level of consciousness is determined by a delicate balance of blood chemicals and gases interacting with the nervous system. Heart, lung, liver, kidneys, and nervous system are unable to maintain this balance, so the brain is no longer able to maintain alertness.

The dying individual sometimes will arouse when a situation feels compelling. For example, consider an expert nurse's experience with Sara:

> She was a 36-year-old woman, who lay for days in a deep coma. Her eyes needed to be protected with artificial tears, because her eyelids would not stay closed. On the evening before Sara died, her family gathered with the parish priest to celebrate a family mass at her bedside. During the communion, she began to weep out loud. Tears covered her cheeks. She died within the hour. Her family never stopped talking to her. They were convinced that she heard them.

Planting the Seeds

Level of consciousness can change from hour to hour. Just when you decide that your patient has become completely unresponsive, he or she may rouse to smile, squeeze a hand, or say a few words. If a beloved friend or relative comes to the bedside, comatose patients sometimes mobilize energy to respond briefly. Teach friends, family, and caregivers to speak to the dying person, and to choose words with care. Even when the person is in a deep coma, hospice professionals recommend assuming that the person may be able to hear our parting words.

Anxiety

Anxiety commonly besieges patients close to death, precipitated both by end-stage pathologies and fears related to death itself. Human presence and attentive listening are essential to comfort. We are companions to the dying, assuring them that they are not abandoned. The major medications providing relief of anxiety include the benzodiazepines (lorazepam, diazepam, midazolam), neuroleptics (haldoperidol, chlorpromazine), and antihistamines (hydroxyzine) (Rousseau, 2002). In the absence of an intravenous or subcutaneous route, lorazepam (Ativan) can be administered sublingually and diazepam (Valium) can be administered rectally.

Restlessness and Agitation

It is not uncommon for the dying person to begin to toss and turn, perhaps to pick at bed linens. Sometimes there may be muscle spasms or twitching. The brain is bathed in toxic metabolic byproducts; cerebral perfusion and oxygenation have both diminished. Restlessness may also be due to a reversible cause such as constipation, urinary retention, or pain. Sometimes palliative medications can be causing neuroexcitability. Drugs with anticholinergic or extrapyramidal side effects may need to be changed. Patients receiving high doses of opioids and whose kidneys are failing may benefit from opioid rotation to avoid neuroexcitability caused by opioid accumulation.

Nursing responsibilities for the restless patient include protecting him from injury. An agitated patient needs someone at the bedside until calming medication is effective. The bed should be arranged to prevent falls. It can be lowered to the floor, or the patient may need to be restrained to prevent injuries. Every effort should be made to avoid a person dying while tied down. Severe restlessness is exhausting to family and patient. Benzodiazepines (lorazepam, diazepam, midazolam) or neuroleptics (haloperidol, chlorpromazine) are the usual choices to control terminal restlessness. However, they occasionally cause paradoxical agitation.

Disorientation

Dying people gradually lose touch with reality. They may become disoriented to time and place. They may lose track of time, perhaps believing it to be some time in the past. They may mistake the current place for a place in the past or for whatever is familiar. Visitors may be misidentified and confused with each other. The person may have conversations with people from the past or hear voices or see something not apparent to observers at the bedside. Many people believe that the dying are making a transition to another reality that they will experience after they die, that they are reorienting to another time and place.

Acute delirium with reduced awareness of the environment, disorientation, and perceptual disturbances, such as hallucinations and delusions, is uncommon but troubling at the end of life. When extreme disorientation is distressing, it may be helpful to remind the dying person of the present moment: time, place, nearby loved ones. However, as attention to the present moment fails, do not deny the person's visions. Respond honestly by offering your own observations.

Sometimes disorientation leads to outbursts that are frightening and angry. Remember that multiple physiological variables are at the root of delirium; the pathophysiology is the same as that causing reduced level of consciousness and restlessness. The family needs to understand that disturbed behavior has a physiological cause. Otherwise, they can be profoundly troubled by the loved one's outbursts.

66 | *The family needs to understand that disturbed behavior has a physiological cause. Otherwise, they can be profoundly troubled by the loved one's outbursts.*

Create a comforting environment with familiar people, good lighting, and perhaps calming music. Haloperidol is the drug of choice; it is administered by mouth or injection. Continuous intravenous or subcutaneous infusion may be indicated with agitated delirium (Rousseau, 2002). Benzodiazepines may be added, but remember to watch for the occasional paradoxical side effect of exacerbating delirium. Agitated delirium is sometimes an indication for continuous palliative sedation, discussed in Chapter 16.

Pain

Pain from preexisting pathologies will persist in the last hours of life. Management of pain in the final hours of life can be challenging because the patient can no longer report pain and it is difficult to distinguish pain from other causes of distress (Panhke, 2003). Expect pain when the patient has a disease process known to cause it. Around-the-clock analgesia should not be discontinued as the patient's level of consciousness drops. In the final hours, comforting requires frequent reassessment. Watch and listen for patient distress. Medicate for breakthrough pain and titrate around-the-clock dosing as needed. When the patient grows agitated and restless, suspect pain and medicate based on that assumption. If the patient becomes calm, pain was probably the cause of agitation (Panhke, 2003). If agitation persists, delirium may be developing.

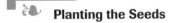

Planting the Seeds

When performing a procedure that would hurt anyone who can verbalize distress, be sure the patient is appropriately medicated. Pay attention to nonverbal cues, including restlessness, crying, moaning, and grimacing. Ask family and friends at the bedside whether they detect behavior that they believe indicates pain in their loved one. When pain appears not to be controlled, analgesics should be carefully titrated upward while noting whether they diminish the nonverbal indicators of distress.

In the final days of life, expert management of pain and other symptoms will control distress in most patients. During this time, the nurse should be continually watchful for signs that death is imminent.

SIGNS OF DEATH DRAWING CLOSE

Recognizing the signs of imminent death is essential practice wisdom for those working in hospice and palliative care. In fact, most hospices provide families and friends with literature describing the cardinal signs of dying. See Box 17-1, Cardinal Signs of Imminent Death. The nurse who is familiar with these indicators can be extremely helpful in guiding the plans of patient, family, and professional team. For patient and family, the nurse's

Box 17-1 ■	CARDINAL SIGNS OF IMMINENT DEATH

Reduced level of consciousness
Taking no fluids or only sips of fluids
Decreased urine output
Progressing coldness and mottling in legs and arms
Irregular labored breathing; periods of no breath
Death rattle

anticipatory guidance helps them to know that this is the time for final religious practices, family gathering, final decisions, and last words. The professional team readies itself to control any exacerbation of symptoms and to support the bereaved.

Sometimes the patient has been ill for a long time, but with pathology that does not predispose her to cardiopulmonary failure. When these signs of cardiopulmonary deterioration finally do appear, it is realistic to begin plans for the last hours and days.

66 *Sometimes the patient has been ill for a long time, but with pathology that does not predispose her to cardiopulmonary failure. When these signs of cardiopulmonary deterioration finally do appear, it is realistic to begin plans for the last hours and days.*

Friends and family need frequent explanation to understand and anticipate the dramatic physical changes affecting the person they love. They should be encouraged to come to the bedside to touch and hold the patient, bathe the skin, clean the mouth, care for the lips, speak sincere words of comfort, and initiate final religious and cultural rituals.

Irreversible deterioration of consciousness is one of the prominent cardinal signs of imminent death. The person can no longer drink and swallow. Decreased intake means decreased urine output. Because the person no longer controls urination, incontinence is inevitable. This is easily managed with adult diapers and bed protectors. If he is artificially hydrated, the volume of urine usually requires catheterization when he becomes incontinent. Diminishing circulation is seen first in the periphery, with cold and mottled extremities. If blood pressure is being monitored, it will gradually descend. Even if he is given vasopressors, they will eventually fail. Respiratory rate will either increase or decrease, eventually becoming irregular with lengthening periods of apnea. When he can no longer swallow or effectively cough, secretions will pool in the pharynx to cause a death rattle.

Consider how the nurse intervened with Mr. Lopez, a married 73-year-old gentleman with metastatic cancer of the bowel that had metastasized to the inguinal nodes. He had developed massive lower extremity edema refractory to diuretics. He also had a fungating-ulcerated lesion over the left iliac crest. These conditions had been worsening for months, severely impairing Mr. Lopez's mobility and quality of life. He lingered over those months, however, with no evident cardiac or pulmonary involvement emerging to take his life. One evening his breathing became wet and labored; cyanosis was present in his feet and legs. His wife was unable to wake him up. The nurse made a home visit and went over all the cardinal signs of imminent death with the wife and daughter. They agreed that he had suffered enough; they did not want to bring him to the hospital for diagnosis or treatment that would only prolong his suffering. The nurse applied a scopolamine transdermal patch, which had been ordered in the hospice protocol, and taught the family how to use lorazepam sublingually if Mr. Lopez showed any signs of respiratory distress. She switched his MS Contin to rectal administration and taught his wife how to insert it. Alerted by the nurse who recognized by these cardinal signs that death was imminent, they called the immediate family and parish priest to his bedside. He died 2 days later.

During the last hours of life, in addition to watching the signs and controlling the symptoms of the dying person, the nurse cares for the family and loved ones as they wait at the bedside.

THE DEATH VIGIL

A vigil is a time of deliberate watchfulness; it often involves staying awake through the nighttime hours. Family and close friends frequently maintain a vigil in the final hours of dying. They may be at the bedside, or they may be waiting by the telephone.

As death hovers, the dying person usually withdraws from active involvement in everyday living. The last days of life are not a time to expect many words to be spoken, even from the fully conscious. It is not the time for loved ones to have any expectations of the dying. It can be helpful for those who surround the dying person to say whatever has not been said, to express appreciation as well as forgiveness. They can be encouraged to heal old hostilities. Loved ones who arrive after the person has lost consciousness should be encouraged to make their peace verbally. Nurses should intervene whenever anyone at the bedside switches to speech that refers to the person near death as a body and no longer a person. When observers make dehumanizing comments, and converse over him about their own lives, remind them of the patient as person:

> "This is Mr. _____ and he is still here. Treat him like you want your father/mother/sister/brother to be treated."

As possible, try to create a peaceful environment at the bedside. Surround the person with those things she finds beautiful and satisfying. For example, one social worker spent her last evening in her own living room while her friends sipped wine, discussed oil paintings, and listened to

Beethoven playing in the background. In contrast, a 25-year-old police officer died in a hospice bed with his friends smoking and playing poker beside him. The patient should be surrounded by the environment he would choose, not the one we might like.

As everyone sees clearly that death is very close—release may be welcomed after a long struggle—the last few days often seem to take forever. Friends and family may grow weary. The longer the lingering, the greater the strain on everyone.

> 66 | *The patient should be surrounded by the environment he would choose, not the one we might like.*

When loved ones have been very involved in the vigil awaiting death, they may become preoccupied with the hope that they can be present at the moment of death. In reality, hospice nurses report that it is common for people to die just in the moments after a spouse, child, or friend has left the room. Help families understand this and realize that it is their persistent help and everyday sharing that count, the harvest of a lifetime. Affirm all that they did do with the person.

Letting Go as Death Nears

Experienced hospice nurses describe helping patients "let go of attachments to life as they have known it and life itself. This competency also involves anticipating the dying process and providing guidance at the time of death" (Zerwekh, 1993, p. 29). Letting go of life, as they have known it, is a challenge. People nearing death have faced successive losses in the process of detaching from relationships, roles, independence, control over body functions, material things, the past, and the future they had hoped to live. Nurses can be helpful simply by courageously listening to the fears and pain that need to be expressed. Refer to Chapter 5 to understand the experience of the dying person and Chapter 7 to understand the grief process. Remember that American society encourages us to remain positive. Therefore, it is a great relief for a dying person to be able to express grief over losses without being blocked by encouraging words that deny reality of imminent dying. Nurses can coach families to listen to and acknowledge difficult words like, "This is the last time we'll be together," without contradicting.

Letting go of medical interventions is also extremely challenging. It means giving up and stopping a process that may have been perceived as a heroic battle. Some physicians and some patients never let go of medical possibilities. For example, Barbara had metastatic lung cancer with metastases to bone and brain; she chose the most aggressive chemotherapy and radiation, which her physician encouraged. He always spoke of remission, and Barbara hoped targeted radiation to the 14 tiny lesions in her brain would significantly extend her life. After that procedure, her physician predicted she would be home in 2 days. Unfortunately, the complicating cerebral edema led to an extremely low level of consciousness from which she never recovered to say good-bye. In contrast, many patients nearing death want to talk about stopping chemotherapy or hemodialysis or forgoing more surgery. We need to listen and quiet our instinctual, "Oh no, you shouldn't give up."

Guidance to let go of life itself involves support for those who rage and fight against death, as well as those who calmly accept it. When dying is a struggle and the patient lingers, nurses look for underlying issues or unfinished business that may be keeping the person from letting go. When death has been accepted, the nurse should respect the person's intuition that it is close. One nurse shared a memorable example from her own experience:

> One day she called me out of the blue and said, "This is the day I am going to die." I was skeptical and she seemed fine at first. We were talking about the things that were important to her and needed to be done before she died. Then she just started becoming less and less responsive and her vital signs were changing. She wanted to say good-bye to her son, whom we were able to reach. She died 10 minutes after he came (Zerwekh, 1993, p. 30).

The experience of letting go for family and friends involves learning to say good-bye. Loved ones need the feeling of having done everything possible as a necessary preliminary to letting go (Kruse, 2004). For them, letting go involves witnessing a downward decline and finally being able to move forward in their view of life after the loved one has died.

In the last hours, guidance to let go may involve the nurse's presence at the death itself. Emergency availability at the death bed is a standard hospice practice, albeit somewhat limited by resources and geography when the person is at home. The nurse at the deathbed assists by:

- Recognizing and interpreting indicators of imminent death
- Encouraging family gathering
- Urging the family to share words of reconciliation
- Encouraging touching and grieving as culturally appropriate
- Supporting deathbed rituals as culturally and religiously indicated
- Staying in the background, with family in the foreground
- Managing emerging symptoms

A nurse describes encouraging touch as a fragile infant with severe congenital defects died in his grandmother's arms:

> He had been on life support since birth. One day the grandmother called and said he was having a real difficult time breathing. They didn't want CPR or antibiotics. He was getting dusky despite suctioning. She asked what to do. I said to unhook all the tubes (the oxygen, trach, and feeding tube), pick him up, sit in the rocking chair, and hold him until I get there. He died in her arms. That was the first time since he was a tiny baby that she could hold him in her lap.

Box 17-2 ■

Fear not for I have redeemed you; I have called you by name, you are mine. When you pass through the waters I will be with you; and through the rivers, they shall not overwhelm you; when you walk through the fire you shall not be burned; and the flame shall not consume you (Isaiah 43:1–2).

THE SPIRITUAL JOURNEY

Mystical teachings of the major religions emphasize fostering a special quality of awareness at the time of death. Hindu scripture describes a person's dying thoughts as influencing his or her spiritual journey after death. In great detail, the Buddhist Tibetan Book of the Dead instructs the dying person in the recognition and union with the Clear Light. Many Eastern traditions require chants and meditations before, during, and after death to assist the person to avoid the suffering of reincarnation and instead experience union with God. Orthodox Jewish law requires the gathering of 10 men (a minyan) to be present to read the Psalms, to pray, to light candles, and to pronounce a blessing and rend their garments at the time of death. "Afterlife is said to be a reunion and all of life a preparation for it" (Heschel, 1974, p. 64). For centuries, the 23rd Psalm has provided comfort at the bedsides of the dying, as have verses from Isaiah 43. See Box 17-2.

Medieval Christianity stressed conscious decisions at the time of death, with much use of imagery depicting the emissaries of heaven and hell struggling around the bedside. Family and clergy gathered for final good-byes, to vigil, and to pray. Theological debate continues to this day as to whether conscious deathbed repentance and conversion, or the moral and spiritual choices of a lifetime, determine the journey of the soul after death. Regardless, faithful Christians of all creeds continue to find strength and blessing by gathering, praying, and reading scriptures that comfort the dying and surviving:

> Let not your hearts be troubled; believe in God, believe also in me. In my Father's house are many rooms; if it were not so, would I have told you that I go to prepare a place for you? And when I go and prepare a place for you, I will come again and will take you to myself, that where I am you may be also. (John 14:1–3)

Many people who have no particular religious conviction will find reminders in the eternal rhythms of all that lives, the endless circles and seasons of birth and death, decay, and life rising up again from soil and water. Ohiyesa, a Dakota Indian physician, in 1911, described his peoples' celebration of the unity and mystery of life:

In the life of the Indian there was only one inevitable duty . . . the daily recognition of the Unseen and Eternal. His daily devotions were more necessary to him than daily food. He wakes at daybreak, puts on his moccasins and steps down to the water's edge. Here he throws handfuls of clear, cold water into his face, or plunges in bodily. After the bath, he stands erect before the advancing dawn, facing the sun as it dances upon the horizon, and offers his unspoken orison. . . . Each soul must meet the morning sun, the new sweet earth, and the Great Silence alone (Blues & Zerwekh, 1984).

Nurses working at the end of life develop unique spiritual practice wisdom through keeping company with people who are transcending beyond this mortal life. In the days and hours immediately before death, we are physically present and have the opportunity to be spiritually present in a kind of nonverbal connection, as explained by an expert hospice nurse:

The essence of me is sharing with the essence of them beyond the words. . . . (Zerwekh, 1993, p. 27)

In these final moments, listen and leave silent spaces for patient and families to speak if they choose. Foster reconciliation as families choose and recognize that the final moments of life are ultimately spiritual events and not medical events. Spirituality has been described as the essence of personhood and meaning, as well as the experience of God and the transcendent. Ultimately, this means connection with reality more enduring than oneself as an individual. Be still. The passing of another human being is a sacred moment.

> 66 | *In these final moments, listen and leave silent spaces for patient and families to speak if they choose. Foster reconciliation as families choose and recognize that the final moments of life are ultimately spiritual events and not medical events.*

WHERE WILL DEATH OCCUR?

A comfortable and dignified environment can be created in either a hospital, nursing home, or home. However, the challenges of institutional dying are greater. This section addresses issues related to dying in the ICU, nursing home, and home, and the nurse's role in each setting.

Death in the ICU

ICUs combine the latest technology with intensive medical and nursing staff in order to save lives of the sickest patients. These patients would die without aggressive efforts to rescue them. "Critical-care settings symbolize a cultural commitment to heroically prevent death, even at great costs. In this context of fighting to save lives, death appears as the enemy, and its naturalness is over-looked" (Benner, Hooper-Kyriakidis, and Stannard, 1999, p. 364). Contemporary ICUs usually treat patients aggressively until death is acknowledged as inevitable, and then goals are redirected toward palliation (Prendergast, 2002). Because of prognostic uncertainty, many ICU patients die without ever being identified as dying. Whatever the prognosis, palliative care should be integrated into aggressive critical care. Individual personhood and the mandate to comfort should not be lost in the technological regimen.

> 66 | *Because of prognostic uncertainty, many ICU patients die without ever being identified as dying. Whatever the prognosis, palliative care should be integrated into aggressive critical care. Individual personhood and the mandate to comfort should not be lost in the technological regimen.*

Acknowledging suffering and providing palliative care for ICU patients with life-threatening illnesses encompasses three goals (Prendergast, 2002):

1. Control pain and other symptoms.
2. Communicate effectively with patient and family.
3. Acknowledge uncertainty and face the real likelihood of impending death.

Caring for those dying in intensive care requires aggressive symptom control and a developing rapport with families. Systematic pain and nonpain symptom assessment must be incorporated into critical-care nursing practice. Research evidence reveals that moderate to severe pain is frequently ignored in the ICU (Prendergast, 2002). Because pain is subjective and critically ill patients are often unable to report their experience, assessment for potential sources of pain is particularly important. Agitation is a common indicator that pain is present in the nonverbal critically ill. It is important to recognize that sedation without analgesia reduces agitation without relieving the underlying pain.

Ironically, critical care itself often causes pain and suffering. The nurse in ICU risks moral distress when she feels that her actions conflict with her commitment to compassionate practice (Volbrecht, 2002). Her patients are dying and not being cared for as dying. Often, the nurse at the bedside is compelled to perform invasive and painful procedures that she fears may be futile: dressing changes, wound irrigation, debridement, venipunctures, gastric tube insertions, catheterizations, turning, positioning, and restraining patients. Accommodating the demand for ongoing monitoring and bedside interventions, nurses are compelled to deny privacy, modesty, and visitors. "The nurse wants to be true to her responsibility to the patient and neither create unnecessary suffering nor omit possible lifesaving treatment" (Benner, Hooper-Kyriakidis, and Stannard, 1999). Nurses cause suffering because we believe we are accomplishing a long-term good. Therefore, the expert ICU nurse must continually evaluate the effectiveness of interventions to achieve realistic goals of care.

> *The nurse in ICU risks moral distress when she feels her actions conflict with her commitment to compassionate practice (Volbrecht, 2002).*

> *Remember that these are the last hours of a fellow human being.*

Remember that these are the last hours of a fellow human being. To remain true to our own convictions, we must break out of silence to become patient advocates in the ICU. Clinical leaders must support staff nurses to speak out on behalf of each patient:

"Is it possible to meaningfully prolong his life?"
"What can we realistically accomplish?"
"He's hurting. How can we keep him comfortable?"
"What good can we accomplish with this procedure?"
"He needs to be premedicated before we do this procedure."
"How about transferring him to the palliative-care unit?"
"We need to call the palliative-care/hospice/pain team."
"He may die soon. The family should be at his side."
"Let's take these tubes out."

Critical-care nurses are at the bedside bearing witness to the patient and families deciding whether they should focus on death or seek more aggressive curative interventions. Families desperately need to understand the implications of ever-changing prognoses and interventions. They seek to uncover the human implications of biomedical events and decisions. Families do not know whether to keep fighting or say good-bye. The nurse's role is to work with them and support them in making these decisions.

In order to help, the nurse should act as an interpreter, explaining the human implications of medical matters to patient and family. Likewise, we need to interpret the patient's suffering experience to physicians. We can coach each to understand the other's thinking.

> *The nursing role is to be an interpreter, explaining the human implications of medical matters to patient and family. Likewise, we need to interpret the patient's suffering experience to physicians. We can coach each to understand the other's thinking.*

Nurses bridge the gap between the discussion of medical possibilities and the significance of death as a human passage for the person and his network of loved ones (Benner et al., 1999). Thus, we must listen and understand the family's tumultuous emotional reactions as they face the unfolding tragedy and struggle to make decisions. Box 17-3 summarizes key features of promoting family-centered communication in the ICU.

The culture of the intensive care unit often does not support nurse or family participation in decision-making (Miller, Forbes, and Boyle, 2001). Nurses frequently withdraw from these issues and do not inquire about

Box 17-3 ■ NURSES' ROLE IN PROMOTING FAMILY-CENTERED COMMUNICATION IN THE ICU

- Question the goals of care
- Continually seek truth, recognizing that possibility of survival is delicately balanced with possibility of imminent death
- Listen to patient and family
- Explain the patient and family truth to the physician
- Explain medical truths to the patient and family in understandable language
- Encourage critical reasoning that merges medical and human truths
- Support ongoing family participation in decisions
- Encourage family at the bedside to touch, hold, talk, and participate in physical care as they wish
- Make the family comfortable. Bring chairs and cots to the bedside

patients' preferences or initiate discussions about prognoses and preferences. When we have no voice, we cannot speak for those who no longer have a voice. Without the essential nursing role of bridging the gap, families may be abandoned to misunderstanding and fear. Shifting the culture toward active participation of physicians, nurses, and families requires a strong multidisciplinary effort. From admission forward, policies should require regular family conferences that clarify ever-changing goals.

Withdrawing Therapies

Therapies are withdrawn when they are considered medically futile, having no reasonable chance of therapeutic benefit. Weighing benefit and burden, the following therapies are most frequently withheld or withdrawn: blood products, kidney dialysis, vasopressors, ventilator, parenteral nutrition, antibiotics, intravenous fluids, and tube feeding (Prendergast & Puntillo, 2002). Other life support should be stopped before the ventilator. An anticholinergic, such as atropine or glycopyrrolate (Robinul), should be ordered to control secretions. It is now established practice to use opioids and benzodiazepines (midazolam, lorazepam) to prevent agonal dyspnea and anxiety when ventilatory support is removed. Some participants may perceive that these drugs are being used to kill the patient (active euthanasia); they need to understand that they are not being given to hasten death, but to relieve symptoms.

The endotracheal tube must be left in place to foster comfort for those with excessive secretions or those who are completely incapable of breathing on their own. Removing the endotracheal tube, for those who can briefly breathe on their own, may encourage closer physical contact and communication with loved ones. When the patient is awake, has few secretions, and the airway

---

Box 17-4 ■   **STEPS TO REMOVING THE VENTILATOR FROM A DYING PATIENT**

1. Goals of care and final decision discussed with family. Physician, nurse, social worker, and chaplain work collaboratively to promote communication as needed.
2. Do-not-resuscitate order and decision to remove ventilator documented.
3. Date and time for removal of ventilator established.
4. Cultural and religious rituals encouraged as family wishes.
5. Tests and medications that are not palliative discontinued.
6. Artificial feeding and fluids discontinued.
7. Family counseled and decision made to be present when tube is removed, come to bedside immediately afterward, or be called.
8. Organ donation discussed if appropriate.
9. Senior physician and respiratory therapist scheduled to be present.
10. Method of removal determined and order written.
11. Suction and towels for secretions made available.
12. Patient premedicated.
13. All medical devices and restraints removed.
14. Ventilator alarms silenced.
15. Ventilator removed and patient continuously monitored for discomfort; opioids and benzodiazepines administered for comfort.
16. Family supported, whether they are at bedside or waiting elsewhere.
17. Family given time to say good-bye after death. Bereavement support plan in place.
18. Staff debriefed to evaluate process.

Source: Adapted from Marr & Weissman (2004), p. 284.

---

can be maintained, immediate extubation and removal of the ventilator creates the possibility of communication (Marr & Weissman, 2004). Patients often are weaned slowly from the ventilator (terminal weaning) as medications are adjusted to maintain comfort. All alarms are silenced and all tubes and lines removed except for an IV route. Encourage the family to be present, but remember that it is their choice. Box 17-4 outlines steps to use in removing ventilatory support.

Death in the Nursing Home

For many in contemporary society, the question of death at home or in the hospital has become a moot point. Lengthy terminal courses and family inability to provide care have necessitated nursing home placement, where dying is often prolonged. Family may be faithful visitors, occasionally present, or estranged and conspicuously absent. The challenge of the nursing home nurse is to maintain a personalized approach in the last days of life, both in direct attention to the individual and through teaching, supervising, and supporting nonprofessional caregivers to work constructively with their own grief and give special attention to patients very close to death.

Contemporary nursing homes are compelled by regulations to focus on a medical task-oriented model of care, instead of the nursing model of care that creates a home-like environment. Dying is often not acknowledged and nutrition, fluids, activity, and complex drug regimens are enforced in an attempt to improve function. Extreme under-staffing often leads to patients dying alone and in pain. This situation causes chronic sorrow among many nurses and nursing assistants in nursing homes, who truly desire the time and ability to care for the residents entrusted to their care.

More than 20% of U.S. deaths occur in skilled nursing facilities (SNFs) and 25% of nursing home residents die every year (Reynolds, Henderson, Schulman, and Hanson, 2002). Frequently, pain, personal cleanliness, and emotional symptoms are poorly managed. In the United States, only 5.6% of nursing home residents receive hospice care under the Medicare benefit, in which a hospice agency contracts with the SNF to offer hospice nursing, social work, pastoral care, and medical consultation by the hospice medical director. This low percentage may be attributed to three disincentives for a nursing home to work with a community hospice (Evans, 2002):

1. Cash flow is slowed since Medicare pays the hospice agency, which then pays the nursing home.
2. If the patient's SNF can be covered under Medicare skilled care reimbursement, that provides more money than under the lower Medicare hospice reimbursement.
3. Hospice recommendations often go against nursing home routines and culture; a serious conflict of authority can result.

Box 17-5 identifies requirements for effective end-of-life care in a nursing home setting. Improving end-of-life care in the nursing home setting requires a systematic collaborative plan by nurse leaders, nurse practitioners, and physicians. Everyone needs training in end-of-life care. End-stage disease should be identified early and appropriate palliative plans developed with the family. Advance directives must be discussed to avoid futile resuscitation attempts. Protocols should be adapted to focus on comfort when restorative care is no longer possible. Certified nursing assistants (CNAs), who provide most of the bedside care, must be valued for their contributions, trained in care focusing on comfort, and regularly included in care planning. A volunteer program can educate volunteers to offer human presence at the bedside so that patients do not die alone. For instance, the Jewish Home and Care Center in Milwaukee, Wisconsin, has organized community volunteers called "Caring Partners" who sit with dying residents who have no loved ones to vigil at the bedside (Evans, 2002).

Box 17-5 ■	REQUIREMENTS FOR EFFECTIVE END-OF-LIFE CARE IN THE NURSING HOME SETTING

- Physicians, nurse practitioners, and nurse leaders identify individuals with end-stage disease and are able to acknowledge treatment futility.
- Physicians, nurse practitioners, nurse leaders, social workers, and spiritual counselors communicate effectively with family members to agree on end-of-life plans.
- Advance directives are discussed with patient and family, specifically explaining why resuscitation does not work in patients with advanced chronic diseases.
- Certified nursing assistants (CNAs), who provide most of the bedside care, are valued for their contributions and trained in care focusing on comfort. They are respected members of the caregiving team.
- The minimum data set (MDS) and resident assessment protocols (RAPs), which drive the care provided in nursing homes, are adapted to focus on comfort and symptom relief instead of current emphasis on restoring function.
- The supervisory staff of licensed practical and registered nurses are systematically educated in palliative assessment and intervention.
- Palliative care is rewarded throughout the facility.

Source: From Evans (2002); and Travis et al. (2002).

WWW.   Internet Resource Box

See the Hospice and Palliative Nurses Association Web site to learn about their certification program for nursing assistants: *www.hpna.org*.

Death at Home

Managing a death at home is possible with:

- A capable primary caregiver who knows what to expect and how to manage.
- A support network for the caregiver/s.
- Necessary equipment, medicines, and supplies.

In the absence of family or friends as caregivers, capable paid caregivers can also manage a comfortable home death. All must be supported by professionals educated in palliative care.

Teaching the family caregiver to manage during the final days is an extraordinary challenge. Fear and uncertainty impair learning. An expert nurse explained the teaching process:

> They are teachable, but you have to be calm and take it slowly. Their energies are being used so intensely in dealing with their emotions that the learning process is severely limited. You have to teach over and over again, teaching only limited amounts at a time. People usually understand only about half at one time.

Teaching should include role-modeling and demonstration by the nurse, followed by return demonstration by caregivers. For instance, show them how to turn the patient. Show them how to crush the pills. Show them how to talk to a person who no longer can respond verbally. Written instructions should be clear, simple, and left in the home. Some patients have symptoms that are ever-changing at the end of life; in these situations, caregivers need active nursing oversight to modify medication regimens continuously. Even families and individual caregivers who communicate well and have a history of problem-solving will tend to decompensate. When death is imminent, the burden on caregivers accelerates. Caregiver health should be an ongoing priority. They will need relief from the 24-hour-a-day, 7-day-a-week caregiving demands. Chapter 11 describes family caregiver burden and the process of strengthening the family. A nurse describes the process of encouraging a weary family caregiver:

> The caregiver said she couldn't do it. I suggested we take it one day at a time. I give a lot of encouragement and feedback. I reinforce that they are giving excellent care and write in their log at home. I think it's reassuring when a registered nurse tells someone that they're doing everything possible.

If there is any family money saved, it may be the time to recommend tapping into the financial reserve to buy private-duty nursing. A night shift is especially helpful to enable family members to sleep. Home hospice programs offer short periods of continuous care in the home during times of crisis when death is imminent.

Decisions about desired place of death and whether to initiate cardiopulmonary resuscitation or call 911 should be made before the final stretch so that caregivers have clear goals. Family decision-makers must understand that if they call 911, trained paramedics will initiate aggressive resuscitative efforts.

Planning for a death at home includes anticipatory guidance to have needed medications ready in the home for expected symptoms. However, unexpected symptoms that require aggressive management can precipitate crises requiring the nurse to first make a home visit, get an order, and then obtain needed medication. This can take hours while the patient suffers. To eliminate that kind of ordeal, hospices are developing standardized emergency or crisis kits. One example is the inexpensive emergency kit assembled by the Cleveland Clinic to manage pain, dyspnea, nausea, and seizures that may present acutely (LeGrand, Tropiano, Marx, Davis, and Walsh, 2001). See Box 17-6, Emergency Kit

Box 17-6 ■	**EMERGENCY KIT CONTENTS**			
DRUG	FORMULATION	ROUTE	QUANTITY	FOR CONTROL OF
Morphine solution	20 mg/mL	PO, SL	30 cc	Emergent pain and dyspnea
Chlorpromazine (Thorazine)	25 mg suppos	PR	2	Restlessness, nausea, dyspnea (with MS)
Diazepam (Valium)	10 mg suppos	PR	2	Anxiety and siezures
Hyoscyamine (Levsin)	0.125 tab	SL	4	Excessive secretions

Source: From LeGrand, Tropiano, Marx, Davis, and Walsh (2002).

Contents. This kit includes 30 cc of morphine solution 20 mg/mL that can be swallowed or absorbed through the oral mucosa to manage pain or dyspnea; 2 chlorpromazine 25 mg suppositories that can be used for restlessness, nausea, and dyspnea; 2 diazepam 10 mg suppositories used to manage seizures and anxiety; and 4 hyoscyamine 0.125 mg tablets used sublingually or orally to control secretions. The contents are bagged, labeled as Emergency Kit, and refrigerated to be used only as instructed by the nurse. The nurse discards remaining medication after the death. Crisis kits are cost effective, eliminate emergency hospital visits, and prevent the suffering of a long wait to obtain new medication.

When death at home is planned, the nurse or another team member helps the family develop an after-death checklist that identifies action plans for the first few hours. The plan might include calling key family and friends, clergy, and funeral home. It is vital that the nurse know the law regarding home death in the local community. Sometimes the police or medical examiner needs to be called. Hospices may need to make prior arrangements regarding an anticipated death under medical management. A local service-oriented funeral director is an excellent source of information for planning. Before the death, the family should be encouraged to begin coordinating with the funeral home chosen.

DIAGNOSIS OF DEATH

Traditionally, death has been defined by the cessation of breath or heart beat. In the absence of life support technology, cardiopulmonary assessment reveals the best indication of imminent death. Death can be expected within the hour if extremities are cold and cyanotic, if breath is extremely irregular with long periods of apnea, if the pulse is very weak or cannot be felt, and if the blood pressure is very low or cannot be heard. Some people will gradually deteriorate in all these areas. Others will have only some of these signs before breath stops. Loss of bowel and bladder control often occurs immediately before or after death.

🐚 Planting the Seeds

Immediately after death, the eyelids may remain slightly open; the jaw will relax and keep the mouth open. It may be easier for loved ones to look upon the person's body if the eyes are gently closed and the head propped up by a towel or small pillow so that the mouth closes.

For contemporary professionals, the cessation of cardiac or respiratory function has become an automatic herald to start cardiopulmonary resuscitation. The more technological the environment, the more likely resuscitation attempts will proceed. Clarify the patient/family choices with regard to resuscitation by reviewing advance directives and requesting physician documentation in the patient record.

WWW.   Internet Resource Box

Learn about the State of Oregon's one-page Physician Orders for Life-Sustaining Treatment (POLST), a one-page physician order form that follows patients back and forth from home to nursing home to hospital, wherever they receive care. It has been highly successful in preventing unwanted intensive medical interventions for patients who do not want them. See *www.ohsu.edu/polst/background.*

When death occurs at home, with symptoms controlled and families prepared, many will choose not to call for help until after the death has occurred. When symptoms and emotional distress are a problem in the hours preceding death, it is best if the family has a lifeline to a nurse who can advise them or come over. This is one of the essential services of a hospice program. Without such service or because of stress and a need to feel that everything is being done, some families may respond by calling an ambulance or dialing 911 for emergency help from trained paramedics. Remember that they will try to restore life to the dying unless nurse or family or clear advance directives inform them of other wishes.

IMMEDIATELY AFTER DEATH

Family members should do what they feel is comfortable and appropriate at the time of death. The nurse encourages staying at the bedside. Many will want to gather around the bed to pray, meditate, cry, be silent, or reminisce. Some will want to leave the bedside to regain their own balance. Some nurses with extensive experience at the moment of death tell us that they continue to feel strongly the presence of the person, sometimes outside of the body but lingering in the room. Final words and good-byes can be spoken.

Some people will choose to hug, caress, or bathe the body. Others will find this fearful and strange. It is a normal way of working through the finality of death and should not be discouraged. Traditional cultures and religions have rules about respectful care of the body; these rules must be strictly observed. The funeral home need not pick up the body right away if there are still family members who have not come or need more time at the bedside to grieve. In the home, an electric blanket can be used for a few hours to keep the body from getting cold to touch. Often, the hospital or nursing home settings exert pressure to remove the person's body as quickly as possible; when possible, nurses should advocate for family needs.

CONCEPTS IN ACTION

Imagine you are making a home visit to Sophie, a 66-year-old mother of three adult children. Her youngest daughter, Heather, age 41, has been caring for her. Sophie suffers from end-stage chronic obstructive lung disease and heart failure. During her last difficult hospitalization, her heart stopped twice, she was intubated, and she had difficulty being weaned from the ventilator. She developed a small pressure sore over her right coccyx and required several antibiotics to control complicating sepsis. Sophie now has an advance directive requesting no hospitalization, antibiotics, intubation, or resuscitation. When you examine Sophie, you find that she has stopped eating and is taking only sips of fluid. She is difficult to arouse. The family reports that she has not voided since the previous day.

- What other physical assessment data do you need to conclude that death is imminent? What lay language could you use to teach Heather the signs to expect?

Sophie's breathing is labored with disturbing gurgling sounds coming from the back of her throat. Her temperature is 103.4°F. She is restless, picking at the bedclothes, and keeps trying to get out of bed.

- What nursing measures should you implement?
- What medications do you need?

Heather tells you that her mother is hallucinating. "She keeps talking about setting sail and yelling, 'Papa, papa, come here and help me untie the boat.'"

- How should you respond?
- What advice would you give the children and grandchildren as they gather at Sophie's bedside?
- How should you prepare this family for Sophie's imminent death?
- What might Heather need during this period?

References

Benner, P., Hooper-Kyriakidis, P., & Stannard, D. (1999). *Clinical wisdom and interventions in critical care.* Philadelphia: WB Saunders.

Blues, A., & Zerwekh, J. (1984). *Hospice and palliative nursing care.* Orlando, FL: Grune & Stratton.

Evans, B. (2002). Improving palliative care in the nursing home: From a dementia perspective. *Journal of Hospice and Palliative Nursing, 4*(2), 91–99.

Heschel, A. (1974). Death as homecoming. In J. Riemer (Ed.), *Jewish reflections on death.* New York: Schocken.

Kruse, B. (2004). The meaning of letting go. *Journal of Hospice and Palliative Nursing, 6*(4), 215–222.

LeGrand, S., Tropiano., Marx, J., Davis, M., & Walsh, D. (2001). Dying at home: Emergency medications for terminal symptoms. *American Journal of Hospice and Palliative Care, 18*(6), 421–423.

Marr, L., & Weissman, D. E. (2004). Withdrawal of ventilatory support from the dying adult patient. *Journal of Supportive Oncology, 2*(3), 283–288.

Miller, P., Forbes, S. & Boyle, D. (2001). End of life care in the intensive care unit: A challenge for nurses. *American Journal of Critical Care,* 10(4), 230–237.

Panke, J. (2003). Difficulties in managing pain at the end of life. *Journal of Hospice and Palliative Nursing,* 5(2), 83–90.

Prendergast, T. (2002). Palliative care in the intensive care unit setting. In A. Berger, R. Portenoy & D. Weissman (Eds.), *Principles and practice of palliative care and supportive oncology* (pp. 1087–1102). Philadelphia: Lippincott Williams & Wilkins.

Prendergast, T., & Puntillo, K. (2002). Withdrawal of life support: Intensive caring at the end of life. *Journal of the American Medical Association,* 288(21), 2732–2740.

Reynolds, K., Henderson, M., Schulman, A., & Hanson, L. (2002). Needs of the dying in nursing homes. *Journal of Palliative Medicine, 5*(6), 895–901.

Rousseau, P. (2002). Management of symptoms in the actively dying patient. In A. Berger, R. Portenoy & D. Weissman (Eds.), *Principles and practice of palliative care and supportive oncology* (pp. 789–796). Philadelphia: Lippincott Williams & Wilkins.

Travis, S., Bernard, M., Dixon, S., McAuley, W., Loving, G., & McClanahan, L. (2002). Obstacles to palliation and end-of-life care in a long-term care facility. *The Gerontologist, 42*(3), 342–349.

Volbrecht, M. R. (2002). *Nursing ethics: Communities in dialogue.* Upper Saddle River, NJ: Prentice-Hall.

Yalom, I. (1980). *Existential psychotherapy.* New York: Basic Books.

Zerwekh, J. (1993). Transcending life: The practice of nursing hospice experts. *The American Journal of Hospice and Palliative Care, 10*(5), 26–31.

Index

Note: Page numbers followed by *b* indicate boxed material; page numbers followed by f refer to figures; and page numbers followed by t refer to tables.

A

Acceptance, of terminal prognosis, 133*b*
Acquired immunodeficiency syndrome (AIDS), 303–305
  late–stage symptoms of, 304*b*
Active euthanasia, 201, 202, 202*b*
Addiction, 354*b*
  to opioids, 355
    fear of inducing, as reason for undertreatment of pain, 354–356
Adjuvant medications, in pain relief, 370–373
Adolescent(s). *See also* Child(ren).
  conceptualization of death by, 267*b*
  grief felt by, 272–273
    aids to expression of, 274, 275
    myths about, 268*b*
Advance directives, 190, 191
  internet sources of, 191
Advance planning
  in end–of–life care, 187*b,* 190
  of funerals, 146
African–American patient(s)
  conceptualization of death by, 145*b*
  end–of–life care for, 167, 170
    barriers to, 164*b*
    cultural aspects of, 168*b*
  perceptions of pain by, 166, 323*b*
Age–related differences, in perception of pain, 321, 322
Agitation, at end of life, 423–424
AIDS (acquired immunodeficiency syndrome), 303–305
  late–stage symptoms of, 304*b*
Airway clearance, ineffective, 413, 421–422
  management of, 413
Alzheimer's disease, 301
Analgesics, for terminal patient, 348–370. *See also* Pain management, opioids in.
Anesthetics, for pain, 373
Anger, terminal patient's, 107–109, 133*b,* 137
  nursing responses to, 108*b*
Anorexia, 406
Antianxiety agents, for terminal patient, 102–103, 372, 413, 423
Anticipatory grief, 142–143, 144*b*
Anticipatory guidance, in end–of–life care, 310–311, 339, 392
Anticonvulsants, indications for, 372, 405
Antidepressants, for terminal patient, 104–105
  in management of pain, 371–372

Anxiety, terminal patient's, 100–103, 423
  interpersonal interventions for, 101–102
  pharmacotherapy for, 102–103, 372, 423
Anxiolytics, for terminal patient, 102–103, 372, 413, 423
Appetite, loss of, 406
Arab–American cultural perceptions, of pain, 323*b*
Art therapy, for grieving child, 274
Artificial hydration, for impaired fluid balance, 396*b*
Ascites, 415
Assisted death, 201–206
  arguments for and against, 203*b*
Assisted suicide, 201, 202*b*
  in Oregon, 106, 204–206, 205*b*
    internet information on, 206
Attachment theory, of healthy vs. unhealthy grief, 135
Autonomy issues, at end of life, 183, 186
Awareness, of dying, 88–89

B

Bargaining, by terminal patient, 133*b*
Behavioral symptoms, of grief, 136*b*
  in children, 267–268
Beneficence, 182
Benzodiazepines
  for anxiety, 102, 413
  for dyspnea, 421
  for muscle spasms, 373
Bereavement, 132. *See also* Grief.
  myths about, 149*b*
  support groups dealing with, referrals to, 150
Biphosphonates, for pain, 373
Blaming–style family communication, as unhealthy, 247
Bleeding, from vessels eroded by tumors, 405
Body–vs.–personhood issues, 207
Bone, metastasis of cancer to, and pain, 374
Bowel cancer, 299
Bowel elimination, impaired, 413–415
  management of, 361*b,* 413, 414, 415
  nausea and vomiting due to, 409
Brain lesions
  cognitive impairment due to, 404
  vascular, 300
Breakthrough pain, 369
  opioids for, 369–370, 370*b*
Breast cancer, 299